The Cerebral Palsies
Causes, Consequences, and Management

Geoffrey Miller, M.D., FRCP, FRACP
Professor of Pediatrics and Neurology, Department of Pediatrics, Baylor College of Medicine, Houston; Child Neurology Section, Texas Children's Hospital, Houston

Gary D. Clark, M.D.
Assistant Professor of Pediatrics, Neurology, and Neuroscience, Department of Pediatrics, Baylor College of Medicine, Houston; Child Neurology Section, Texas Children's Hospital, Houston

Butterworth–Heinemann

Boston   Oxford   Johannesburg   Melbourne   New Delhi   Singapore

Every effort has been made to ensure that the drug dosage schedules within this text are accurate and conform to standards accepted at time of publication. However, as treatment recommendations vary in the light of continuing research and clinical experience, the reader is advised to verify drug dosage schedules herein with information found on product information sheets. This is especially true in cases of new or infrequently used drugs.

Library of Congress Cataloging-in-Publication Data
The cerebral palsies : causes, consequences, and management / [edited by] Geoffrey Miller, Gary D. Clark.
     p.   cm.
     Includes bibliographical references and index.
     ISBN 0-7506-9964-7
     1. Cerebral palsy. I. Miller, Geoffrey, 1947– . II. Clark, Gary D.
     [DNLM: 1. Cerebral Palsy—diagnosis. 2. Cerebral Palsy—etiology.
     3. Cerebral Palsy—rehabilitation.   WS 342 C411 1998]
RC388.C47   1998
616.8'36--dc21
DNLM/DLC
for Library of Congress   97-52631
     CIP

British Library Cataloguing-in-Publication Data
A catalogue record for this book is available from the British Library.

The publisher offers special discounts on bulk orders of this book.
For information, please contact:
Manager of Special Sales
Butterworth–Heinemann
225 Wildwood Avenue
Woburn, MA 01801-2041
Tel: 781-960-2500
Fax: 781-960-2620

For information on all Butterworth–Heinemann publications available, contact our World Wide Web home page at: http://www.bh.com/

10 9 8 7 6 5 4 3 2 1

Printed in the United States of America

Contents

Contributing Authors

James F. Bale, Jr., M.D.
Professor of Pediatrics and Neurology, Division of Pediatric Neurology, University of Utah School of Medicine and Primary Children's Medical Center, Salt Lake City

Patrick D. Barnes, M.D.
Associate Professor of Radiology, Harvard Medical School, Boston; Chief, Division of Neuroradiology, Director of Magnetic Resonance Imaging, Children's Hospital, Boston

William E. Bell, M.D.
Professor of Pediatrics and Neurology, University of Iowa Hospitals, Iowa City

Timothy B. Boone, M.D., Ph.D.
Assistant Professor, Scott Department of Urology, Baylor College of Medicine, Houston; Medical Director, Urodynamic Laboratory, Methodist Urology Institute, Houston

Kerrie K. Browning, M.S., CCC-SLP
Clinical Instructor of Otorhinolaryngology and Communicative Sciences, Baylor College of Medicine, Houston; Speech Pathologist, Department of Speech, Language, and Learning Disorders, Texas Children's Hospital, Houston

Gary D. Clark, M.D.
Assistant Professor of Pediatrics, Neurology, and Neuroscience, Department of Pediatrics, Baylor College of Medicine, Houston; Child Neurology Section, Texas Children's Hospital, Houston

Linda S. de Vries
Consultant in Neonatology, Wilhelmina Children's Hospital, Utrecht, The Netherlands

Jan Goddard-Finegold, M.D.
Associate Professor of Pediatrics and Pathology, Division of Pediatric
Neurology, Baylor College of Medicine, Houston; Associate Professor of
Pediatrics and Pathology, Division of Pediatric Neurology, Texas
Children's Hospital and Harris County Hospital District, Houston

Sharon M. Greis, M.A., CCC-SLP
Director of Pediatric Feeding Program, Therapy Coordinator, United
Cerebral Palsy Association, Children's Services, Philadelphia

Carlos H. Lifschitz, M.D.
Associate Professor of Pediatrics, Baylor College of Medicine, Houston;
Chief, Feeding Disorders Clinic, Section of Gastroenterology and
Nutrition, Texas Children's Hospital, Houston

Ingrid Linge, O.T.R., B.C.P.
Occuaptional Therapist, Department of Physical Medicine and
Rehabilitation, Texas Children's Hospital, Houston

Linda Pax Lowes, Ph.D., P.T., P.C.S.
Assistant Professor, School of Physical Therapy, Texas Women's University,
Houston

Ann R. McMeans, M.S., R.D., L.D.
Pediatric Clinical Dietitian, Food and Nutrition Services, Texas Children's
Hospital, Houston

Geoffrey Miller, M.D., FRCP, FRACP
Professor of Pediatrics and Neurology, Department of Pediatrics, Baylor
College of Medicine, Houston; Child Neurology Section, Texas Children's
Hospital, Houston

Van S. Miller, Ph.D., M.D.
Associate Professor of Neurology, University of Texas Southwestern
Medical Center, Dallas

Michael J. Noetzel, M.D.
Associate Professor of Neurology, Neurological Surgery, and Pediatrics,
Washington University School of Medicine, St. Louis; Medical Director,
Clinical and Diagnostic Neuroscience Services, St. Louis Children's
Hospital

Richard L. Robertson, M.D.
Instructor in Radiology, Harvard Medical School, Boston;
Neuroradiologist, Department of Radiology, Children's Hospital, Boston

Mark Romness, M.D.
Newington Department of Orthopaedic Surgery at Connecticut Children's
Medical Center, Hartford; Assistant Professor of Orthopaedics, University
of Connecticut School of Medicine, Farmington

Barry S. Russman, M.D.
Professor of Pediatrics and Neurology, University of Connecticut School of
Medicine, Farmington; Director, Muscle Disease Program, Connecticut
Children's Medical Center, Hartford

Stuart K. Shapira, M.D., Ph.D.
Associate Professor of Molecular and Human Genetics and of Pediatrics,
Baylor College of Medicine, Houston

John W. Swann, Ph.D.
Professor of Pediatrics, Baylor College of Medicine, Houston; Director,
Cain Foundation Laboratories, Texas Children's Hospital, Houston

Barry R. Tharp, M.D.
Professor of Pediatrics and Neurology, Baylor College of Medicine,
Houston; Medical Director, Blue Bird Clinic for Pediatric Neurology, The
Methodist Hospital, Houston

Catherine Loren Turk, Ph.D.
Speech-Language Pathologist, Department of Speech, Language, and
Learning Disorders, Texas Children's Hospital, Houston

Preface

"I don't know what you mean by *glory*," Alice said.

Humpty Dumpty smiled contemptuously. "Of course you don't—till I tell you. I meant 'there's a nice knock-down argument for you!' "

"But *glory* doesn't mean 'a nice knock-down argument,' " Alice objected.

"When I use a word," Humpty Dumpty said in a rather scornful tone, "it means just what I choose it to mean—neither more nor less."

"The question is," said Alice, "whether you can make words mean so many different things!"

—Lewis Carroll, *Alice Through the Looking Glass*

This book deals with the causes, consequences, and management of cerebral palsy, a condition that may arise at any time during the development of the brain. Cerebral palsy is thus a relatively common disorder and an important topic. In one way or another, many disciplines are involved in the diagnosis, management, and care of children with cerebral palsy. Although it is beyond the scope of this book to provide a fully comprehensive overview of every discipline related to the diagnosis and treatment of cerebral palsy, this book is pertinent to pediatricians, child neurologists, developmentalists, physiatrists, and allied health professionals. It has been written so that individual chapters of interest may be read without the need to refer to other parts of the book. That is, each chapter stands on its own by providing appropriate background material, some of which may also be dealt with in greater detail in another chapter.

We hope that when you have read the book you will know more about cerebral palsy, and unlike Alice in her conversation with Humpty Dumpty, you will understand what is meant by the term and its causes, consequences, and management.

Geoffrey Miller
Gary D. Clark

The Cerebral Palsies

1

Cerebral Palsies: An Overview

Geoffrey Miller

Cerebral palsy is neither a disease nor a pathologic or etiologic entity, and the use of the term does not imply causation or severity. Rather it denotes a heterogeneous collection of clinical syndromes that are characterized by abnormal motor actions and postural mechanisms. These syndromes are due to nonprogressive abnormalities of the developing brain. Though the appearance of neuropathologic lesions and their clinical expression may change with time as the brain matures, no active disease is present. Clearly, a 3-month-old infant differs from a 3-year-old child, but more important for the understanding and management of children with cerebral palsy is the fact that poor or aberrant environmental interactions further impair appropriate developmental expression of such children's nervous systems. Although the cerebral palsy syndromes usually coexist with other manifestations of static brain dysfunction, the diagnosis of these syndromes is important as it implies specific treatment programs and prognosis and triggers a search for associated disabilities.[1]

CLINICAL MANIFESTATIONS

The cerebral palsy syndromes are classified according to the type and distribution of motor abnormality. The various forms can be divided into spastic, dyskinetic, ataxic, atonic, and mixed (Table 1.1). This phenomenologic approach has changed little since Freud's treatise in 1897.[2] However, it should be appreciated that often the clinical picture is not pure. Involuntary abnormal movements may be seen in the spastic syndromes, and pyramidal signs may be seen in dyskinetic and ataxic syndromes. Furthermore, all the cerebral palsy syndromes are characterized, to some extent, by disordered motor action and posture such that a voluntary movement that normally is complex, coordinated, and varied becomes uncoordinated, stereotypic, and limited. In the more severely affected individual, an attempt at voluntary movement may evoke a primitive reflex, cocontraction of agonist and antagonist muscles, and mass movements. Discrete movements may be impossible.[3] For example, individual finger movements cannot be performed, wrist extension may be associated with extension of all the fingers, and attempts at flexion may involve all segments of a limb. The simplest of actions performed unconsciously by the able-bodied requires marked effort

Table 1.1 Cerebral Palsy Syndromes

Spastic
    Diplegia
        Good hand function
        Poor hand function
        Asymmetric
    Hemiplegia
        Arm involved more than leg
        Leg involved as much as or more than arm
    Quadriplegia
Dyskinetic
    Mainly dystonic
    Mainly athetoid
Ataxic
    Simple ataxia
    Ataxic diplegia
Atonic

Source: Adapted with permission from G Miller. Cerebral Palsies. In G Miller, JC Ramer (eds), Static Encephalopathies of Infancy and Childhood. New York: Raven, 1992;11–26.

and concentration and meets with frequent failures in those with cerebral palsy.[3] All the syndromes are best recognized after age 5 years.

Spastic Syndromes

The spastic syndromes are either symmetric or asymmetric and may predominantly involve the legs, as in diplegia, or only three limbs or one limb on either side of the body. Recognition of these variations is important in terms of etiology, associated findings, and prognosis.[4] Patients with spastic cerebral palsy exhibit features of an upper motor neuron syndrome, which are composed of positive and negative signs. Positive signs include spastic hypertonia, hyperreflexia resulting from hyperexcitability of the stretch reflex, extensor plantar responses, and clonus. Negative signs include slow effortful voluntary movements, impaired fine-motor function, difficulty in isolating individual movements, and fatigability.[5,6] Spastic hypertonia is a velocity-dependent increase in resistance to passive muscle stretch. It decreases during sleep and is increased by stress and during voluntary movement when cocontraction of agonist and antagonist muscles may occur. In its classic form, spastic hypertonia is described as *clasp-knife*. That is, when a joint is moved passively, maximum resistance is felt after a few degrees. This resistance gives way after some effort by the examiner. The degree of resistance is increased, and its time of onset decreased, by more rapid movement. In its most severe form, however, spastic hypertonia causes the affected part to be rigid in flexion or extension. The character and distribution of signs in the adult-onset upper motor neuron syndrome may differ from those seen in cerebral palsy, which is a reflection of the differing responses to insult of the maturing nervous system.[7]

The spastic cerebral palsy syndromes are classified according to the distribution of abnormal upper motor neuron signs. *Spastic diplegia* is defined as greater involvement of the lower limbs than the upper limbs, *quadriplegia* as an equal or greater involvement of the upper limbs, and *hemiplegia* as involvement of one side of the body. In all the spastic syndromes, some mild dyskinetic signs may be present. The term *paresis* may be used instead of *plegia*. Although by strict definition the former means less paralysis, in common usage it does not imply any difference in severity.

In many cases of spastic diplegia in full-term infants, a specific cause may be uncertain, although neuroimaging may show evidence of prenatal insult. In preterm infants, the risks of spastic diplegia increase with increasing prematurity. Preterm infants with mild periventricular leukomalacia have relatively good hand function and fewer associated disabilities. In others, upper limb function varies and depends on the degree of spasticity, presence of contractures, sensory loss, associated involuntary movements, and intelligence. Frequently, dwarfing is present below the waist, and vasomotor and sensory disturbances of central nervous system origin, such as astereognosis and poor two-point discrimination, are common.[8] These sensory findings are frequent in all the spastic syndromes, in which there are also varying degrees of flexion, adduction, and internal rotation of the hips and flexion at the elbows and knees. An equinovalgus or calcaneovarus deformity of the foot may be present, and extension of the fingers, abduction of the thumb, extension of the wrist, and supination of the forearm may be limited. These features may be accompanied by poor grasp release and involuntary or associated movements. A diplegic group exists that exhibits asymmetric findings and usually more severe associated disabilities than are seen in the patient with symmetric spastic diplegia and relatively good hand function. Some patients in this group are preterm infants with periventricular leukomalacia plus unilateral hemorrhagic infarction.

The majority of spastic hemiplegia in full-term infants is related to prenatal circulatory disturbances, neonatal stroke, or maldevelopment.[9-12] As the problem usually is a cortical lesion, the arm is involved more than the leg. Congenital hemiplegias may be missed during the newborn period and become evident during examination for another reason. Alternatively, a caregiver might notice hand dominance, reduced movement, or abnormal posturing on one side in an infant. Occasionally, the disorder is found after a seizure occurs. Initially, movement and tone on the affected side decrease before tone and, sometimes, tendon reflexes become abnormally increased. The hand is held closed, and the typical posture appears as the child ages.[3] The arm is adducted at the shoulder and flexed at the elbow, the forearm is pronated, and the wrist and fingers exhibit flexion. In the leg, the hip is partially flexed and adducted, and the knee and ankle are flexed because of increased tone in the hamstring and plantar flexor muscles. The foot may be in the equinovarus or calcaneovalgus position. In the mildly affected child, these postures are more easily seen on walking or running. More than a slight delay in independent walking is unusual unless severe mental retardation is present. In postnatally acquired cases, in addition to spasticity, athetotic posturing is sometimes seen, an observation made by Freud and others in the last century.[13,14] In general, handicap is usually only mild or moderate, and those patients with normal computed tomographic (CT) findings are more likely to be less impaired. In those term infants with a postnatal cause for hemiplegia, such associated disabilities as intellectual impairment, hemianopia, and seizures may be greater. In those infants who experience seizures, cognitive deficits tend to be worse.[15] Undergrowth of the affected side is found, and its degree correlates with the severity of sensory deficit. However, the degree of sensory loss does not mirror the severity of the motor deficit.[16] In general, language development is related to cognitive ability. Language is preserved after early damage to either hemisphere, although some impairment of visuospatial skills may occur,[17,18] and the side of the lesion in congenital hemiplegia does not appear to affect the individual's IQ or any verbal-performance discrepancy.[15,18] However, insults acquired in a child younger than 5 years are more likely to have a deleterious effect on IQ,[18] probably because this period coincides with peak synaptic production and elimination.[19,20]

The spastic quadriplegias usually affect term infants who are often small, although extremely low-birth-weight infants are contributing to this group in increasing numbers.[21,22] These are the most severe of the syndromes, and the use of the term *spastic quadriplegia* implies a seriously multiply handicapped infant. Marked spastic paresis affects all four limbs, and dystonia may also be present. Common associated abnormalities include marked mental retardation, little or no speech, pseudobulbar palsy with feeding and respiratory difficulties, microcephaly, hip subluxation, contracture, and scoliosis. Visual impairment may be present, and many patients have seizures.

Dyskinetic Syndromes

The dyskinetic syndromes are characterized by the involuntary movements of athetosis, chorea, and dystonia. An infant with this type of cerebral palsy syndrome usually presents with hypotonia, retention of primitive reflexes, a tendency to drool, involuntary grimacing, and delayed psychomotor development. Contractures, unless positional, are not a particular feature, as they are in the spastic syndromes. Typical features appear as the child ages. In athetosis, slow, smooth, writhing movements are seen that involve distal muscles, with dyssynergia of opposing muscle groups, such as flexion and extension or pronation and supination. The abnormal movements are accentuated or induced by emotion, change in posture, or intended movement. They are best seen during reaching, when the fingers extend and abduct. Retention of primitive reflexes and facial grimacing with oropharyngeal difficulties are present. Choreiform movements are rapid, irregular, unpredictable contractions of individual muscles or small muscle groups, involving the face, bulbar muscles, proximal parts of the extremities, and fingers and toes. Chorea is worsened by stress, excitement, and fever, and this exacerbation may include ballismus.[23] In dystonia, twisting of the body results in the persistence of trunk and limb distortions. Tone is variable in the dyskinetic syndromes. Initially,

hypotonia may be present during infancy; if hypertonus develops later, it is of the "tension" type, which may be reduced with relaxation or changes in posture. This is true also of spastic hypertonus, though to a lesser extent. *Tension* is sudden involuntary hypertonus affecting both flexor and extensor muscles, the limbs becoming stiff during attempted movement or with emotion. Tendon reflexes are normal or difficult to elicit, and clonus and extensor plantar responses are absent, although athetoid movements of the toes may be misleading.

More than one form of involuntary movement is commonly found in the dyskinetic syndromes. However, these syndromes can generally be divided into two types[24]: *mainly athetoid*, in which movements are choreiform, athetoid, or a combination of both, and the muscle tone is normal or hypotonic, particularly in the early years; and *mainly dystonic*, which is dominated by dystonic traits, tension, and persistent neonatal reflex patterns. Patients with the mainly dystonic type of dyskinesia are usually severely disabled in all four limbs and in the trunk and pharyngeal muscles. Transitional cases exist between the two types. Varying degrees of dysarthria and motor and intellectual disability exist. These disabilities are usually much more marked in those with the dystonic type, who may also exhibit some pyramidal signs and who frequently have anarthria.

Ataxic Syndromes

Those with ataxic syndromes are usually term infants with an early prenatal etiology. They are a clinically and etiologically heterogeneous group.[25] Some cases are due to simple genetic inheritance. Autosomal recessive conditions include cerebellar hypoplasia, granule cell deficiency,[26] and Joubert syndrome.[27] An autosomal dominant form of nonprogressive ataxia has also been described.[28] A small number of patients have congenital hypoplasia of the cerebellum and what might be termed a *pure ataxia*.[3] However, although the term *ataxia* implies an incoordination of cerebellar or sensory origin, in cerebral palsy it more likely reflects a widespread disorder of motor function. Neuroimaging may be normal or might show biparietal or infratentorial lesions.[25] In practice, the diagnosis is made by exclusion, as all patients with cerebral palsy have some incoordination and disturbance of posture. The clinician needs to be confident that these signs are not primarily due to weakness, spasticity, dystonia, or choreoathetosis. Furthermore, progressive neurodegenerative disorders may initially look like an ataxic cerebral palsy. Most patients with ataxic cerebral palsy are hypotonic from birth and display delayed motor and language skills. The ataxia improves in most patients over time. In general, but not always, the more severe is the motor impairment, the worse are the associated disabilities. Speech acquisition is related to intellectual ability and may be characteristically slow, jerky, and explosive.

Atonic Syndromes

There is a heterogeneous group of infants who are usually full term and remain hypotonic for many months. These infants develop extremely slowly and never stand or walk. They often have cerebral dysgenesis and microcephaly and are profoundly mentally retarded. Neurologic examination reveals an absence of the findings that characterize the other cerebral palsy syndromes. Tone is variable and may feel increased, but the character of this increase is not that which is found in spasticity; rather, it is described as *paratonic*: That is, when a joint is moved passively, an increasing resistance occurs that is proportional to the amount of pressure applied. At times, this resistance may falsely feel as if it is volitional. This atonic group has been recognized for many years but is rarely mentioned in modern classifications.[29,30]

ASSOCIATED DISORDERS

The cerebral palsies, although characterized by their motor dysfunction, are almost always accompanied by other disorders of cerebral function. Among these are abnormalities of cognition, vision, hearing, language, cortical sensation, attention, vigilance, and behavior. Epilepsy often is present, as are defects in gastrointestinal function and growth. Dyspraxias and agnosias can interfere with skilled tasks, regardless of the extent of motor deficit. For example, an affected child may be unable to voluntarily close his or her eyes or mouth or to protrude the tongue, although these actions can be easily performed in an involuntary fashion. These disorders of higher cortical function may have an important impact on activities of daily living and affect such tasks as dressing or managing buttons in a child who appears to be only relatively mildly affected.

Approximately 65% of the total cerebral palsy population have mental retardation.[31,32] Although the severity of mental retardation often correlates with the degree of motor handicap, individual variation occurs and mental development is often uneven. In those without frank mental retardation, specific learning disabilities may affect educational potential.[33] While it might be specious to compare the results of psychometric assessments of multiply handicapped children with those that are derived from a population of able-bodied children, such comparison is important because strategies for devising communication techniques, activities of daily living, and education are based on what a disabled child will understand. Assessments require time, repetition, and experience and the use of a multidimensional approach that combines results from norm-, criterion-, and observation-referenced tests.[34] Those patients with dyskinetic cerebral palsy of the mainly athetoid type are more likely to have better cognitive function than those with bilateral spastic syndromes, and children with spastic quadriplegia are generally the most severely affected. In children with hemiplegia, language development is related to cognitive ability and, as a group, those with a postnatally acquired hemiplegia do less well than do those born at term with congenital hemiplegia.[3]

Children with cerebral palsy are more likely to exhibit behavioral and emotional disorders, and the presence of physical and intellectual handicaps does not exclude psychiatric disorder. The causes are complex and attributable to both primary neurologic symptomatology, which includes emotional lability,

poor attention and vigilance, and obsessive-compulsive traits, and to the secondary effects of dependency, frustration, and low self-esteem.[35]

Approximately one-third of patients develop epilepsy,[36] which most often has its onset during the first 2 years of life. The incidence is greatest in patients with spastic quadriplegias and acquired hemiplegias and is lowest in patients with mild symmetric spastic diplegia and mainly athetoid cerebral palsy. The most common seizures are partial with secondary generalization. Infantile spasms may occur, particularly in infants with microcephaly and spastic quadriplegic or atonic cerebral palsy.[37] Mental retardation is more likely to be associated with the presence of seizures, and those patients with multiple seizure types are more likely to be more severely retarded. Epilepsy can cause additional handicap as its control may be difficult or it might require the use of sedative doses of anticonvulsant, which further impair learning and socialization.

Ocular and visual abnormalities are common in cerebral palsy and include strabismus, abnormalities of saccadic and pursuit movements, refractive errors, congenital structural defects, nystagmus, field defects, amblyopia, and cortical visual impairment.[38–43]

All types of speech and language abnormalities, from aphasias to dysarthria, may be encountered. The disorders may be complex. Causes include hearing loss; poor intelligence, experience, and language development; and abnormal integration of motor mechanisms of the oropharynx and coordination of breathing patterns.

Many patients, especially those with dyskinetic and spastic quadriplegic cerebral palsy, fail to thrive and, in general, growth is stunted. This is related to poor nutritional status caused by inadequate intake, recurrent vomiting with aspiration secondary to gastroesophageal reflux, and pseudobulbar palsy.[44–46] Poorly understood central nervous system factors also play a role,[47] and these factors seem to be associated with hirsutism (unrelated to phenytoin), acne, and precocious puberty. Dental disease, including malocclusion and caries, is common. In the more severely affected patient, chronic respiratory disease is usually present.[48] This is due to reflux, palatopharyngeal incoordination, chest deformity, and poor coordination of respiratory muscles. In those children with cerebral palsy who are immobile, the risk of spontaneous fractures due to osteopenia and osteoporosis is increased.[49,50]

Enuresis, frequency, urgency, and stress incontinence occur in many children with cerebral palsy. These disorders are related to reduced mobility and communication, poor cognition, low expectations of caregivers, and neurogenic dysfunction.[51] Urodynamic assessment has demonstrated bladder hyperreflexia, detrusor sphincter dyssynergia, bladder hypertonia with leakage, and periodic relaxation of the distal sphincter during filling.[52]

Deterioration or change in neurologic signs may occur in older children. In some, such signs are due to an acquired cervical spondylotic myelopathy secondary to exaggerated neck flexion or extension.[53,54] Patients with cerebral palsy also may later develop disabling dystonia in the absence of any myelopathy.[55] This may rarely be due to an undiagnosed dopa-responsive dystonia, and

Table 1.2 Aids to Early Diagnosis

Increased suspicion from obstetric and perinatal history
Abnormal behavior
Psychomotor delay
Retention or asymmetry of primitive reflexes
Hypotonia disproportionate to muscle power
Hyperreflexia and clonus
Deviant oromotor patterns
Oculomotor abnormalities
Delayed postural reactions

Source: Reprinted with permission from G Miller. Cerebral Palsies. In G Miller, JC Ramer (eds), Static Encephalopathies of Infancy and Childhood. New York: Raven, 1992;11–26.

an inborn error of metabolism or a neurodegenerative disorder should be considered,[56] although the more common cause is continuing aberrant development of the nervous system.[57] Dystonic reactions have also been reported after ingestion of carbamazepine or phenytoin in children with preexisting brain damage.[58,59] In the adult with cerebral palsy, for whom fewer services are available than are in place for children, additional common complaints include increasing musculoskeletal problems that cause back, neck, and joint pain.[60]

EARLY AND DIFFERENTIAL DIAGNOSIS

Although the lesion in cerebral palsy is nonprogressive, the clinical signs are not unchanging. Abnormal patterns emerge as the damaged nervous system matures. A definite diagnosis of cerebral palsy may be delayed during early infancy, particularly in preterm infants, and serial examinations are required.[61] Evidence of spasticity may not be noted until age 6 months, and dyskinetic patterns generally are not obvious until approximately age 18 months. Ataxia, as opposed to the incoordination and motor delay associated with mental retardation, may not be apparent until even later. Nonspecific aids to early diagnosis are listed in Table 1.2.

Neurobehavioral signs that should raise suspicion are excessive docility and irritability. A common history is one in which the baby is a poor feeder during the neonatal period. This may be followed by a baby who is irritable, sleeps poorly, vomits frequently, is difficult to handle and cuddle, and has poor visual attention. Deviant oromotor patterns include tongue retraction and thrust, tonic bite, oral hypersensitivity, and grimacing. Early motor signs include poor head control with normal or increased tone in the limbs. Persistent or asymmetric fisting is abnormal. Gross- and fine-motor development are not only delayed[62] but usually are qualitatively abnormal. In addition to the formal neurologic examination, infant assessment includes observation in prone and supine positions. Posture and tone are observed on pulling to sit, in supported sitting, and in vertical and ventral suspension. Skill in propping on arms and hands and the ability to rotate within the body axis are noted, as are the emergence and quality of protective postural reactions. Particular signs that at 4 months are associated with an increased risk of cerebral palsy are failure to support weight on the forearms in a prone position, failure to sit supported with head erect, or failure to show interest in surroundings or social responsiveness.[63] Increased neck extensor and axial tone may give a false impression of good head control.

The development of normal posture and movement in a child requires the integration and inhibition of primitive brain stem reflexes. Those reflexes principally concerned with posture are the tonic labyrinthine, tonic neck, and neck- and body-righting reflexes.[64] An early indication of the presence of motor disability may be delay in the disappearance of a primitive reflex or the presence of one to an abnormal degree.[63,65] Most primitive reflexes disappear between 3 and 6 months of age. An obligatory primitive reflex is abnormal at any age. For example, a tonic labyrinthine response occurs when the neck is extended and, when in supine, leads to shoulder retraction, leg extension, and either elbow flexion or extension and pronation of the arms. Flexion of the neck causes flexion of the extremities. An excessive tonic labyrinthine response may manifest as opisthotonic posturing or apparent early rolling over. Other signs that can easily be elicited occur when the infant is held in vertical suspension. During the early months, the baby should "sit in the air." An abnormal response is persistent leg extension, which may be followed by or associated with an abnormal positive support reaction. When the anteromedial areas of the soles are placed on a firm surface, plantar flexion should occur. The feet should return to neutral within a few seconds. Continued plantar flexion, particularly with equinus posturing, is abnormal if obligate or maintained for more than 30 seconds. Absence may also indicate a central or peripheral nervous system lesion.

Early diagnosis of a particular type of cerebral palsy may be difficult.[66] In hemiplegia, asymmetry of movement appears early, often with some retraction of the shoulder on the affected side. The fingers tend to flex, and the thumb adducts. Initially, little spasticity may be present, but spasticity develops later with a decrease in abduction at the hip, plantar flexion at the ankle, clawing of the toes, and a flexion-pronation pattern affecting the upper limb. Other early signs are a lack of use of both hands in the midline and an inability to reach out on the affected side. In the prone position, support on the affected upper limb is decreased, and diminished movement of the affected leg is noted. When such a child is pulled to sitting, this leg will tend to extend. Later, the protective reactions are asymmetric. In spastic quadriplegia, moderate or severe psychomotor delay with poor head control is seen. Spasticity can begin as early as 2–3 months and can involve the antigravity muscles, particularly the biceps, forearm pronators, wrist flexors, thumb adductors, and finger flexors. In the lower limbs, hip flexion, thigh adduction, and knee flexion occur with equinus of the feet and adduction of the forefoot. Marked adduction of the thighs produces the typical scissoring of the lower limbs. In spastic diplegia, infants often have hypotonia of the lower limbs with delayed functional maturation for several months. Usually at approximately 6 months, spasticity involving ankle plantar flexors and hip adductors is noted and usually is followed by contractures of the hip flexors and hamstring muscles. The young infant with dyskinetic cerebral palsy may experience reduced spontaneous movement, oromotor incoordination, hypotonia at rest, but varying tone on movement and with emotion. Retention of primitive reflexes occurs and includes extension patterns in the supine position, and flexion when prone with shoulder retraction, and persistent head turning to one side.[67]

In the older infant, diagnosis is easier. For example, in the spastic syndromes at approximately 9–10 months, in addition to the classic signs, the infant who is pulled to sitting exhibits an inability to flex the legs and poor truncal balance. Instead of developing a pincer grasp, the hand splays when attempting to reach for an object and, if this is achieved, an ulnar grasp is used.

Although microcephaly occurs after severe hypoxic-ischemic encephalopathy in full-term infants, it may be delayed for more than 12 months. However, a decreased rate of head growth in the first 4 months of life correlates closely with the development of secondary microcephaly and an adverse neurologic outcome.[68]

Early diagnosis does not rely on the presence of isolated abnormal signs but on a combination of findings that include motor delay, positive neurologic signs, primitive reflex activity, and abnormal postural reactions. A degree of hypertonia or hyperreflexia in an infant whose functional development and behavior are normal is an indication for observation. If these observations remain isolated on future examination, the findings most likely will be transitory and will disappear progressively after 9 months. They may, however, be harbingers of later abnormalities of language and attention.[69]

The diagnosis of cerebral palsy implies that no active disease is present and that the responsible pathology is in the brain. It is a diagnosis of exclusion and should not be made on the basis of a single examination. The differential diagnosis includes neurodegenerative disorder, inborn errors of metabolism, developmental or traumatic lesions of the spinal cord, neuromuscular disorder, movement disorder, neoplasm, progressive hydrocephalus, and subdural hematoma. Repeated examination is necessary to detect any changes that might be consistent with a progressive disorder. Some inborn errors of metabolism may be misdiagnosed as cerebral palsy. Glutaric aciduria type 1 may present during early infancy, particularly after an infectious illness, and may appear similar to a dystonic cerebral palsy.[70] Similarly, conditions such as arginase deficiency or 3-methyl glutaconic aciduria may present with ataxia and spasticity, sometimes in a diplegic pattern, or with extrapyramidal features.[71,72] Quantitative amino and organic acid analysis should be considered when unexplained cerebral palsy is seen. Among other disorders that should be considered are progressive spastic paraparesis, dopa-responsive dystonia,[73] congenital stiffness (hyperekplexia) in infants, and Lesch-Nyhan disease. Clinical deterioration may not be due to a progressive disorder. As previously mentioned, new signs might be due to continuing aberrant development of the nervous system or to an acquired cervical myelopathy. Other causes of clinical deterioration include an increase in contracture formation, anticonvulsant toxicity, and undiagnosed or intractable epilepsy. Hypotonia in association with weakness suggests a neuromuscular disorder. Rapidly evolving signs suggest a neurodegenerative disorder.

Extrapyramidal signs in early infancy or marked worsening during periods of catabolism also make the diagnosis of cerebral palsy suspect. Practically every infant with a severe intellectual handicap has some motor disorder that is expressed as motor development inappropriate to his or her chronologic age. If a cerebral palsy syndrome is not present, the presence or absence of primitive reflexes usually is appropriate. Cerebral palsy is present when, in addition to the intellectual handicap, a motor disorder is noted that deviates completely from normality at any age.[74]

No specific tests exist for the diagnosis of cerebral palsy. In addition to a complete history, differential diagnosis is aided by an examination for dysmorphic and neurocutaneous features; for organomegaly associated with storage disorders or infection; and for abnormal fundi associated with infection, cerebral dysgenesis, or an inborn error of metabolism. In those with unexplained cerebral palsy, quantitative assessments of amino and organic acids should be performed, in addition to acid-base status and ammonia and lactic acid values. Endocrine abnormalities should also be considered, and thyroid function tests and calcium and phosphate levels should be obtained. Other tests such as renal and liver functions should be ordered where appropriate. Magnetic resonance imaging (MRI) of the brain may provide useful diagnostic information and, in one study, was reported to detect an abnormality in 93% of patients with cerebral palsy.[75]

At present, prediction or prevention of most cases of cerebral palsy in full-term infants is difficult.[76,77] Individual events at birth, such as meconium-stained liquor, delayed onset of respirations, and acidosis in the absence of persisting neurologic abnormalities, do not reliably predict later cerebral palsy.[77] An Apgar score of 3 or less at 10 minutes is associated with a more than 50% risk of cerebral palsy but, even in these infants, more than 40% do not develop cerebral palsy.[78] A low Apgar score may be produced by many factors including asphyxia, prematurity, neuromuscular disorder, cerebral dysgenesis, maternal drugs, and severe illness due to organ failure. In addition, persisting neurologic signs after a low Apgar score may be due to conditions other than severe perinatal asphyxia, such as cerebral dysgenesis and seizures, or metabolic disorder.

Despite sophisticated fetal monitoring and increased cesarean section rates during the last two decades, the frequency of cerebral palsy in full-term infants has changed little, although perinatal mortality rates have fallen.[79–82] Fetal heart rate monitoring has a very high false-positive rate for predicting long-term neurologic disability,[83] and pH at birth is a poor indicator of later disability as it does not indicate reliably the onset or duration of any damaging hypoxia-ischemia that may have occurred many hours or days before delivery.[84,85] If a serious persistent neonatal encephalopathy is not present, cerebral depression at birth preceded by abnormal heart rate patterns in labor or acid-base derangement is *not* predictive of later impairment.[86] Furthermore, in some cases of cerebral palsy, a history of fetal distress may be an indication of previous brain damage, before the fetal distress, rather than a cause of cerebral palsy.[87]

EPIDEMIOLOGY, ETIOLOGY, AND BIOLOGICAL BASIS

Epidemiology

The prevalence of cerebral palsy is approximately 2.5 per 1,000 live births.[32] The cerebral palsy rate in infants with a birth weight of less than 1,500 g is between 5% and 15%, and an additional 25–50% show other developmental disabilities.[88–90] After the mid-1970s, a rise in cerebral palsy occurred due to the increased survival of very preterm babies, many of whom were severely disabled.[91,92] This epidemiologic change was found in a regional study from England, in which investigators reported that because the prevalence of cerebral palsy had increased among low-birth-weight infants but the number of cases among normal-birth-weight infants remained unchanged, the relative proportion that each birth-weight group contributed to the whole sum had altered.[93] This study found that during the late 1980s, more than 50% of all cerebral palsy cases were in low-birth-weight infants, and those infants weighing less than 1,000 g at birth were making an important contribution to the total. The study also noted that the severity of disability in the lower-birth-weight groups had increased, whereas little change was noted in the disability level of affected normal-birth-weight infants.

Etiology

The cause of cerebral palsy in full-term infants is usually of prenatal origin.[94,95] Intrapartum events play only a limited role and may be influenced by a preexisting abnormality.[78,96] The proportion of cerebral palsy cases associated with intrapartum asphyxia has been estimated to be approximately 10–20%.[77,97] A small number of such cases are due to prepartum hypoxic-ischemic events, such as a large placental abruption, fetomaternal hemorrhage, placental infarction, and maternal shock.[98] However, careful examination of these children may reveal evidence of a possible earlier adverse prenatal event.[98,99] Such evidence includes an excess of minor congenital anomalies, a short umbilical cord, or neuroimaging that demonstrates cerebral dysgenesis or a cerebrovascular accident.[100,101] Examination of the placenta may support a prenatal cause or contribution to the cause,[102] and neuroimaging and neuropathologic studies have demonstrated that antepartum adverse events may play a role in later neonatal neurologic morbidity.[75,103–105] Some 10–18% of cerebral palsy cases, usually of the spastic type, are acquired after the neonatal period.[106] Causes include central nervous system infection, trauma, cerebrovascular accidents, and severe hypoxic events such as near-drowning.

The risk of developing cerebral palsy increases with decreasing gestational age. This risk increases 20-fold in those neonates weighing less than 1,500 g.[107] Nonetheless, even in the preterm population, a contributing causative role may have been played by prenatal factors.[108,109] The principal lesions that are associated with the later development of cerebral palsy in the preterm baby are periventricular leukomalacia, intracranial hemorrhage, posthemorrhagic hydrocephalus, and pontosubicular necrosis. Posthemorrhagic hydrocephalus is a serious complication of intraventricular hemorrhage and frequently leads to cerebral palsy.[110] Bronchopulmonary dysplasia affects many preterm infants who require mechanical ventilation, and many of these infants are subjected to prolonged periods of hypoxemia. In those who suffer from severe disease, 15–25% develop cerebral palsy, and 17–35% develop severe neurodevelopmental impairment.[111] Some babies with bronchopulmonary dysplasia develop a dyskinetic disorder characterized by choreiform and akathitic movements, most prominent distally, and extensor posturing of the neck with an oro-buccolingual dyskinesia.[112] However, bronchopulmonary dysplasia probably is not independently associated with adverse neurodevelopmental outcome.[113] A similar disorder is seen after cardiopulmonary bypass and profound hypothermia in infants who undergo correction of complex congenital heart defects.[114] In this post–cardiac surgery choreic syndrome, if the patient does not survive, examination of the brain shows neuronal loss, reactive astrocytosis, and degeneration of myelinated fibers, primarily in the outer segment of the globus pallidus.[115]

Severe asphyxia in the full-term infant causes parasagittal cortical injury and infarction in the brain stem and basal ganglia and is associated with the development of spastic quadriparesis. Concurrent ischemic necrosis may also occur in the spinal cord gray matter and can contribute to the flaccidity, hypokinesia, and absent reflexes found in the asphyxiated infant.[116] The degree of intrapartum asphyxia sufficient to lead to cerebral palsy is also associated with a marked neonatal encephalopathy (which includes stupor, flaccidity, poor suck, and a poor or absent Moro reflex), signs of damage to other organs apart from the brain,[117,118] persistent neurologic signs at 7 days of life, and the frequent occurrence of poorly controlled early-onset seizures.[78,119] Although a spectrum of clinical findings follows a hypoxic-ischemic insult in a full-term infant, dividing the severity into mild, moderate, and severe has prognostic value.[118,120,121] In those findings classified as mild, the baby displays irritability, jitteriness, brisk Moro and tendon reflexes, and sympathetic overactivity that lasts fewer than 24 hours. Those babies with a moderate encephalopathy experience lethargy, hypotonia, reduced primitive reflexes and, sometimes, seizures. A severe encephalopathy is characterized by coma, hypotonia, brain stem and autonomic dysfunction, seizures, and sometimes, increased intracranial pressure. The mild form of encephalopathy is associated with a good outcome, whereas a moderate encephalopathy is followed by later neurologic abnormality in 20–40%, and this is more likely if the condition persists for more than 1 week.[122] Outcome is usually poor after a severe encephalopathy.

The electroencephalogram (EEG) is another useful prognostic instrument for predicting outcome after a peripartum hypoxic-ischemic insult in a full-term newborn.[120,123] During the first few hours after a severe insult, amplitude decreases and electrical activity slows. This is followed within 24–48 hours by a burst-suppression pattern. The duration of suppression increases over the next 1–2 days, and the tracing may become isoelectric. Seizures indicate a poor outcome. Conversely, rapid resolution of EEG abnormalities or a normal interictal pattern implies a good prognosis. A CT scan of the brain can also aid in prognosis after a severe perinatal hypoxic-ischemic insult in a full-term infant. When the scan is performed between 48 and 96 hours after the insult, no differentiation between gray and white matter correlates strongly with later significant neurologic deficit.[118,124] Similarly, MRI scanning of the brain 2 weeks after a hypoxic-ischemic insult that shows blurring of the gray and white matter interface and lesions of the thalamus and basal ganglia is associated with a poor outcome. Conversely, a normal MRI scan is associated with a good outcome.[125] Magnetic resonance spectroscopy is another useful method for predicting a normal outcome.[126]

Some other prenatal and perinatal causes of cerebral palsy include mechanical injury; ischemic insult[127,128]; intracranial hemorrhage from coagulopathies; prenatal exposure to various environmental toxins such as methyl mercury and irradiation[129–131]; cerebral dysgenesis and neuronal migration defects; congenital infections with organisms such as cytomegalovirus, syphilis, varicella virus, and toxoplasmosis; and bacterial, viral, and fungal neonatal infections.

Kernicterus, which leads to choreoathetosis and sensorineural deafness, is now a rare cause of cerebral palsy in industrialized nations. Hyperbilirubinemia causes the pathologic correlate, which is yellow pigment deposition and loss of neurons in the basal ganglia, dentate nuclei, mammillary bodies, hippocampus, inferior olives, and some cranial nerve nuclei. The encephalopathy associated with kernicterus is characterized by a poor Moro response, hypertonus, arching, a high-pitched cry, and poor feeding. If the infant survives, kernicterus is followed by a later persistent neurologic deficit.[3,132] The encephalopathy usually occurs within the first week in full-term infants and sometimes later in premature infants. The increase in tone continues for a few months but, by 6 months, hypotonia and retention of primitive reflexes become apparent, as are seen in dyskinetic cerebral palsy from other causes. During the second and third years of life, athetosis develops. Sensorineural hearing loss is present, and paralysis of upward gaze is a characteristic feature. Almost total ophthalmoplegia has been described.[3] Although it may be reduced, intellect often is within the normal range. Premature infants now rarely develop kernicterus, but for many years it has been known that this can occur in the absence of hemolytic disease[133] and that it generally is confined to neonates whose serum bilirubin levels are greater than 20–24 mg/dl.[134] Though kernicterus can occur at lower levels in the sick, very low–birth-weight neonate, its incidence in this group has decreased, which may be due to the discontinuation of benzyl alcohol inclusion in intravenous solutions.[132]

Children who have major and minor malformations are at increased risk for developing cerebral palsy, presumably reflecting early prenatal abnormalities in development.[101,135] Many of these infants have a breech presentation, which is itself a risk factor for later cerebral palsy and which probably occurs as a result of a prior fetal abnormality.[94]

Intracranial hemorrhage in full-term neonates is an uncommon but important cause of later cerebral palsy.[136] A common site of hemorrhage in this group is thalamic and residual germinal matrix. Sometimes no definite source can be identified, and the hemorrhage is presumed to originate from the choroid plexus. This disorder may have a sudden and dramatic clinical onset marked by vomiting, seizures, apnea, lethargy, irritability, bulging fontanelle, and abnormal movements. Most infants who suffer thalamic hemorrhage have uneventful birth histories and present between 3 and 28 days of age. Roland and colleagues[136] found that predisposing factors for cerebral vein thrombosis (sepsis, congenital heart disease, coagulopathy, electrolyte disturbance) were identified in 50%. Follow-up at 18 months reveals that hydrocephalus, seizures, and cerebral palsy, especially hemiplegia, occur in the majority.

There is an association between brain damage and multiple gestations. The prevalence of cerebral palsy is reported to be much higher in twins than in singletons, particularly in the survivors of intrauterine deaths and in monochorionic twins,[137–139] and antenatal white matter necrosis is more common in monozygous than in dizygous twins.[140] The risk of cerebral palsy is also increased the higher the multiple gestation.[141,142] Causes include low birth weight, congenital anomalies, cord entanglement, vascular shunts between twins, and abnormal vascular connections.[140] If one twin dies in utero, a release of thromboplastin and emboli may occur and, if the death occurs during early pregnancy, cerebral dysgenesis has been reported in the surviving twin.[143] Furthermore, evidence for the existence of the dead twin may be gone by the time birth takes place.[144–147]

Biological Basis

Approximately 5–15% of surviving low-birth-weight infants develop cerebral palsy.[148] In many, the disorder is related to the presence of periventricular leukomalacia, which predicts cerebral palsy much better than do grades 1 and 2 intraventricular hemorrhage. Periventricular leukomalacia refers to necrosis of white matter dorsolateral to the external angle of the lateral ventricles, particularly in the area of the trigone and in the white matter near the foramen of Monro.[149,150] One mechanism that causes periventricular leukomalacia, which is sometimes hemorrhagic, is ischemic infarction in watershed regions. This infarction leads to varying degrees of cell damage and necrosis, followed by cystic change. The cysts resolve, leaving gliosis, a reduction in white matter, and ventriculomegaly. The motor deficit typical of periventricular leukomalacia is spastic diplegia. The legs are affected more than are the arms because the fibers subserving leg function lie medially and thus are more likely to be involved first by this form of ischemic infarction. More extensive insults, however, involve the more lateral fibers. Varying degrees of intellectual impairment occur in this form of spastic diplegia, visuomotor and perceptual abilities being more extensively involved than verbal abilities.[151,152] As many as 25–50% of small preterm infants later develop learning or attentional difficulties. Involvement of association fibers may play a role in the etiology of these learning difficulties. In addition, Volpe[153] hypothesizes that interference with or damage to subplate neurons affects cerebral cortical organization and neuronal connectivity and that this may be an important cause of intellectual impairment in the preterm infant.

The immature brain is more vulnerable to various insults in certain locations that lack this same degree of vulnerability when the brain is more mature. These developmental periods of selective vulnerability are based on both cellular and vascular factors.[154] As previously mentioned, in the premature infant, the periventricular region is a watershed area. In addition, it is the site for immature oligodendrocytes, which are particularly sensitive to the oxidative stress that occurs after metabolic insults such as hypoxia-ischemia.[155,156]

Two systems supply blood to the cerebral hemispheres in the preterm infant. Both course from the brain surface. The ventriculofugal system travels down to the ventricles and then back into the brain toward the cortex. The ventriculopetal system penetrates into the brain toward the ventricles. The systems form a boundary zone around the ventricles, which, in the right circumstances, can become a watershed region.[157] This vascular anatomy renders the periventricular region vulnerable to ischemia and failure of cerebrovascular autoregulation. Causes of this failure may include asphyxia, hypotension, handling, and hypocapnia.[148,158] Hypotension may be related to sepsis, a patent ductus arteriosus, apnea spells, and cardiac failure.[159,160] Furthermore, during the days following premature delivery, hypoxia plus hypotension is related to ultrasonographically detectable white matter lesions and to adverse neurodevelopmental outcome at 1 year.[161–164] The periventricular region is also intrinsically vulnerable to damage because of actively differentiating astrocytes and oligodendrocytes.[148] Most neonatal cortical neurons have been produced by 20 weeks of gestation.[165] However, the late germinative zone produces migrating glial precursors after major neuronal migration has ended.[166] Thus, in the preterm infant, projection and association fibers are damaged by germinal matrix–intraventricular hemorrhage, and ischemic or hemorrhagic infarction in the periventricular white matter impairs myelination by damaging or preventing migration of oligodendroglial precursors and adversely affects cortical neuronal development by similarly affecting astrocytic precursors bound for the upper layers of the cortex.[167]

Periventricular leukomalacia begins as a focal area of necrosis that shows coagulative change in the neuropil, followed by swollen axons, encrustation of axons, and increased numbers of microglial cells, macrophages, and reactive astrocytes. The lesions become cystic, and some demonstrate hemorrhage.[168] In some preterm infants, periventricular leukomalacia has a prenatal origin.[169–172] Furthermore, examination of fetuses that have died in utero after 20 weeks' gestation demonstrates that prenatal ischemic lesions are frequent and commonly are associated with placental lesions.[173] It is now clear that antenatal factors can increase the risk of preterm birth and thus are associated with periventricular leukomalacia.[174,175] In very low–birth-weight infants, this increased risk appears to be associated with a history of prolonged rupture of membranes, chorioamnionitis, and antepartum hemorrhage.[174,175] Leviton[176,177] proposed that placental infection leads to a release of endotoxin into amniotic fluid and an increase in cytokines such as tumor necrosis factor and interleukin-1, which may be associated with not only preterm birth but also direct white matter damage. Periventricular leukomalacia of prenatal origin also may be found in full-term infants. Results from total population studies in Sweden have shown that in mild diplegics and some hemiplegics born at term, with uneventful deliveries and neonatal periods, neuroimaging in many cases reveals lesions consistent with periventricular leukomalacia.[178,179] This is in contrast to lesions found in full-term children with spastic quadriplegia or diplegia who were severely asphyxiated at birth. In this group, parasagittal or multicystic encephalomalacia is found.[178]

Hypoxia-ischemia also causes selective neuronal necrosis which, in the preterm infant, occurs in the inferior olivary nuclei, ventral pons, and subiculum of the hippocampus.[150] In the full-term infant, neuronal necrosis is most evident in the depths of sulci and parasagittal areas of the cerebral cortex, in the basal ganglia, and in the CA1 region of the hippocampus. These patterns are believed to be related to the synaptic distribution of excitatory amino acids such as glutamate. These amino acids accumulate after the insult and trigger a calcium influx, which leads to destructive intracellular events including the generation of toxic free radicals,[155] the release of proteolytic enzymes, lipase activation, release of free fatty acids, and protein kinase C activation.[180] The changing distribution and character of excitatory amino acid receptors during brain development influences selective neuronal vulnerability.[181] As the brain matures, areas of increased vulnerability change and, as with periventricular leukomalacia, this is related to cellular and vascular factors. By term, different areas, such as the basal ganglia, have now become more prone to damage. In addition, agents of hypoxic-ischemic damage such as glutamate or nitric oxide can induce apoptosis, and cells may be triggered to undergo this process hours after the initial insult and thereby contribute to delayed cerebral injury. Thus, excitotoxicity leads to a cascade of events that cause neuronal death by both necrosis and the triggering of apoptosis.[156,182–185]

Periventricular leukomalacia may be visualized during the neonatal period by ultrasonography, CT scan, or MRI. Of these three, ultrasonography is the cheapest and most convenient as it does not require transport of the infant. Echodensities are seen adjacent to the external angles of the lateral ventricles on coronal projection and are distributed throughout the periventricular region or at the level of the foramen of Monro and trigone of the lateral ventricles on parasagittal projection.[148] Echodensities around the ventricles are followed by the appearance of periventricular cysts between 10 days and 3 weeks after the insult.[186,187] The usual time given is 10–14 days.[188] The cysts disappear after approximately 6 weeks.[189] Thus, established cavitation seen at, or shortly after birth, indicates a prepartum insult. Some preterm infants who develop cerebral palsy have normal perinatal and neonatal ultrasound scans.[76] Although this might be due to lesions below the resolution of ultrasonography, it might also be because the causative insults occurred prenatally. However, premature infants who have undergone repeated ultrasound scans during the neonatal period and who show no evidence of cerebral abnormality and have normal neurologic examinations at term are at low risk for developing a major neurodevelopmental handicap.[190,191] Abnormal echoes confined to the regions of the germinal matrix have a strong pathologic correlation with hemorrhage in this area but carry no increased risk for major adverse outcome.[191] Persistent ventriculomegaly carries a significant risk of later cerebral palsy.[192] The most important ultrasound determinant of long-term outcome is the degree of parenchymal injury, identified as one or more intraparenchymal echodensities. Volpe[193] reported that among 37 infants who exhibited extensive intraparenchymal echodensities (which includes frontoparieto-occipital regions), 81% died, all the survivors had motor deficits, and only one of these had an IQ greater than 80. Of 38 infants with localized intraparenchymal echodensities (confined to frontal, parietal, or occipital regions), 37% died and only 10% with a known outcome had both normal motor and cognitive function subsequently.[193]

CT scanning of the preterm infant with periventricular leukomalacia reveals periventricular hypodensities that may be difficult to differentiate from hypodense areas that are normally present.

Although it reveals the early changes of periventricular leukomalacia, MRI is used rarely because of the difficulties of transporting and monitoring a neonate in the scanner. MRI is able to detect the extent of lesions, particularly in the basal ganglia and brain stem, and in this respect is superior to both CT and ultrasonography and may be a more sensitive indicator of later outcome.[194] The later MRI scans of periventricular leukomalacia show periventricular increased intensity in T_2-weighted scans and ventriculomegaly with a bumpy configuration of the lateral ventricles. These findings are due to glial scarring, inadequate myelination of periventricular axons, and white matter loss.[76,195] The images also show deep cortical sulci and high-intensity areas in the white matter adjacent to the trigone body of the lateral ventricles. A marked degree of white matter reduction in this area is related to a more severe motor impairment.[196] In addition, the severity of ventricular dilation, the degree and extent of white matter reduction, optic radiation involvement, and the thinning of the corpus callosum are reported to correlate with full-scale and performance IQ but not with verbal IQ.[152] In general, MRI is more sensitive than other neuroimaging modalities for determining abnormalities in children with cerebral palsy. Such abnormalities in full-term children include parasagittal cortical change, status marmoratus, brain stem infarcts, neuronal migration defects, cerebral white matter hypoplasia, and defects in the posterior fossa.[75]

In preterm infants, periventricular hemorrhagic infarction usually is unilateral or asymmetric and occurs in the periventricular white matter dorsal and lateral to the lateral ventricle.[197] An ipsilateral intraventricular hemorrhage usually is present and is believed to lead to venous infarction, which probably originates in the area where the medullary veins drain into the terminal vein in the subependymal region.[198] This venous infarction evolves to a single large cyst, unlike the multiple smaller cysts of periventricular leukomalacia. In addition, this large cyst usually does not disappear and may become confluent with the lateral ventricle.[148] The clinical correlate is a hemiparesis in which the leg is involved more than or as much as the arm. This is in contrast to a congenital hemiparesis, in which the arm usually is involved more than the leg. If periventricular leukomalacia coexists, the child may have an asymmetric diplegia. Severe intellectual deficits often accompany venous infarction.

Congenital spastic hemiparetic cerebral palsy is more likely to occur in full-term infants of normal birth weight. Lesions in the middle cerebral artery distribution are often found. Causes include abnormal development of blood vessels, hypercoagulable states, vasculopathies, and emboli secondary to disorders affecting the placenta or fetus.[199] Causes of postnatal strokes during early infancy include venous sinus thrombosis, disseminated intravascular coagulation, sepsis, and congenital heart disease and emboli.[200,201] Other findings in hemiparetic cerebral palsy include cerebral dysgenesis and periventricular atrophy. In some patients, neuroimaging is normal, suggesting maldevelopment at a microscopic level.[10,76]

Dyskinetic forms of cerebral palsy tend to occur in full-term infants.[202] This cerebral palsy syndrome often, but not always, is associated with severe, acute perinatal asphyxia that leads to lesions in the basal ganglia and thalamus that later show a marbled appearance known as *status marmoratus*. This condition may be seen as high-intensity areas on T_2-weighted MRI.[196,203] During the neonatal period, affected infants show evidence of damage to multiple organs and have an encephalopathy characterized by lethargy, decreased spontaneous movement, hypotonia, and suppressed primitive reflexes. They develop dyskinetic cerebral palsy secondary to selective neuronal necrosis in the hippocampus, thalamus, basal ganglia, reticular formation, and Purkinje cells of the cerebellum.[121,150] Status marmoratus of the basal ganglia and thalamus is a pathologic condition characterized by hypermyelination, neuronal injury, and gliosis. The basal ganglia and thalamus are vulnerable during the perinatal period because of active neuronal differentiation and a transient dense concentration of glutamate receptors.[148,180,204]

The spastic quadriplegias usually affect full-term infants who often are small. Extremely low–birth-weight infants are contributing to this group in increasing numbers. Spastic quadriplegia in most full-term infants has a prenatal origin such as cerebral dysgenesis or infection. A lesser number is due to perinatal or prenatal plus perinatal causes or postnatal events.[22] As discussed earlier, children with ataxic cerebral palsy are usually full-term infants in whom a prenatal etiology for the condition exists. They are a clinically and etiologically heterogenous group.[25]

The specific biological basis of most brain malformations is unknown and is discussed in detail in Chapter 2. During brain development, abnormalities may occur that affect cell proliferation, migration, differentiation, survival, or synaptogenesis. Brain cells that fail to make proper synaptic connections die by apoptosis. As many as 50% of cells in some parts of the brain may die in this way during normal cerebral development.[205] Some malformations are known to be genetic in origin and follow mendelian inheritance patterns.[206–210] A small number may result from radiation, toxins, or infectious agents acting during a critical period of gestation.[211] Other malformations may be associated with chromosomal abnormalities; one example is the relationship between holoprosencephaly and trisomy 13 and 18. Some neurocutaneous syndromes may be associated with brain malformations (e.g., hemimegalencephaly and hypomelanosis of Ito or the linear sebaceous nevus syndrome).[212] Studies of the nematode *Caenorhabditis elegans* and the *Drosophila* fruit fly have demonstrated that abnormal expression of several genes or groups of genes leads to aberrant nervous system development.[211] Some of these genes influence growth factors, cell adhesion molecules, and cell-surface receptors, which play an important role in brain development.[213]

PROGNOSIS

Early prognostication may be difficult, except at the extremes of involvement. Social and environmental factors play an important role and accentuate the importance of early support and guidance for the family with an affected child. In general, prognosis is related to clinical type of cerebral palsy, pace of motor development, evolution of infantile reflexes, intellectual deficit, sensory impairment, and emotional-social adjustment.[214] Those patients who walk by less than 2 years of age are more likely to have normal or borderline IQs. In general, the more severe the motor deficit, the more likely is a significant intellectual impairment, although this is not always the case. The prognosis for ambulation in children with cerebral palsy who do not achieve head balance by 20 months, who exhibit retention of primitive reflexes or absence of any postural reactions by 24 months, or who fail to crawl by approximately age 5 years usually is poor. Those children who sit by 2 years of age and crawl before 30 months usually become community walkers, as do many who sit by 4 years. However, most of those who sit between age 3 and 4 years walk only with aids or braces or have restricted functional ambulation. In general, those children who achieve independent ambulation do this by approximately age 3 years, but those who walk only with support may not achieve that goal for up to 9 years. After age 9 years, a child with cerebral palsy is unlikely to start to walk, even with support. Virtually all children with hemiplegic cerebral palsy will learn to walk, as will many with athetosis or ataxia.[3,214–217]

More than 90% of infants with cerebral palsy now survive into adulthood.[218,219] Individual achievement is related to many factors, such as intelligence, physical function, ability to communicate, and personality attributes. The availability of training, jobs, sheltered employment, and counseling also contribute to the adjustment of adults with cerebral palsy. The presence of a supportive family and the availability of specialist medical care are other important factors. Long-term planning and preparation are required, particularly when all indications point toward dependency.

Most patients with cerebral palsy have a long life expectancy; exceptions are those with severe multiple handicaps.[220] The mortality rate in this group is affected, to some extent, by the aggressiveness and quality of care. Studies on life

Table 1.3   Priorities of Management

Communication
Social and emotional development
Education
Maximal independence in activities of daily living
As near-normal appearance as possible
Nutrition
Mobility

Source: Reprinted with permission from G Miller. Cerebral Palsies. In G Miller, JC Ramer (eds), Static Encephalopathies of Infancy and Childhood. New York: Raven, 1992;11–26.

expectancy have reported that children with cerebral palsy who were immobile, had not mastered toilet skills, and were tube-fed usually died within 5 years. By 10 years, 80% had died and, even if survival lasted until age 15, life expectancy was still only 4 years more.[221] The most common cause of death is respiratory disease.

MANAGEMENT

No single professional can effectively carry out the multiple medical, social, psychological, educational, and therapeutic needs of the child with cerebral palsy.[222] Comprehensive management requires a multidisciplinary team made up of members who take a goal-oriented approach that is based on an adequate fund of knowledge and an understanding and appreciation of the contributions from other involved disciplines. If this does not occur, the team becomes a "multiprofessional tower of Babel."[223] The priorities of management are listed in Table 1.3. Further details on neurohabilitation and treatment are discussed in later chapters in this book.

Initial realistic functional goals for the child with cerebral palsy must be set and periodically re-evaluated. These goals should be based on expert assessment and knowledge of prognosis. The aim is to achieve maximal potential in all areas of development and to encourage independence in a child in whom experience has been curtailed and dependency encouraged. The interdependence of various aspects of development must be appreciated; management should not become a series of unrealistic treatment sessions in which the principal caregivers and teachers are not involved. Concentrating exclusively on a child's disability may also be detrimental: At times, the parents' emotional needs and child's recreational needs should come first.

Social and Psychological Services

Early social and psychological services are vital. Chronic grief exacts a high price on parents and, secondarily, on professionals. Parents may limit themselves socially, placing stress on marital relationships and the nurturing of other children. Parents may later deny having received certain information, or they may fail to assimilate information about their child's disorder.[223,224] Parents frequently express dissatisfaction with and, at times, resentment toward various health care professionals. They react with chronic sorrow, as well as denial, guilt, frustration, anger, resentment, and embarrassment.[225]

Information should be given honestly and sensitively to parents and should be delivered with skill and tact. Investigations should be described and a second opinion offered. Early review is important so that parents have an opportunity to ask questions and vent feelings. Much of what was originally said in conferences with parents may have been forgotten or misunderstood, and the physician must be prepared to repeat information with patience and compassion. The physician is wise to avoid being too dogmatic or offering uncertain long-range prognoses. An important aspect of parent counseling is to try to alleviate any guilt that parents may feel as a result of fantasies of causation. Parents may need to find some cause for the damage, as the unknown and the feeling of being victimized by fate are more distressing to some than a specific cause, no matter how inappropiate.[226] Health professionals should be aware that counseling is an ongoing process and should ensure that parents understand that counseling services are always readily available.

Practical Aims of Therapy

Little good evidence exists that various therapies improve final functional motor outcomes in children with, or who are at risk for developing, cerebral palsy.[227,228] The goals of therapy should be to aid parents and caregivers in interacting with and effectively handling a disabled child in a functional manner. The minimal aims should be to learn how best to seat, dress, feed, communicate with, transfer, transport, and toilet the child.[229] Such support should be provided in a consistent fashion from the earliest possible date.

The role of the orthopedic surgeon is to relieve and prevent deformity and to maximize function.[230–232] Gait analysis, using a combination of videotaping and electromyography, demonstrates patterns of abnormal gait and the phasic muscle contractions during the gait cycle. This analysis allows the surgeon to determine which muscles might require surgical lengthening and permits postoperative analysis of gait, and thus can be used to measure the success of surgical procedures.[233,234]

Care and management of the patient with cerebral palsy includes longitudinal social, language, and psychometric assessment, the aims of which are to provide a rational basis for training in communication and activities of daily living and to gain the maximum benefit from formal education.[34,235] As the child grows older, prevocational assessment and training, based on informed prognostication, become most important. Psychological development, communication, and education become the main priorities.

Approaches to Feeding and Nutritional Concerns

Severely disabled children with cerebral palsy are at considerable risk for poor growth and weight gain and require regular assessments of feeding skills and nutritional status.[236,237] Details are discussed in Chapter 12. Many children with cerebral palsy, particularly those with significant intellectual impairment, have feeding difficulties, which can become a major part of their management, requiring caregivers to devote many hours to nutritional concerns. Time constraints and the degree of feeding difficulties can contribute to undernutrition. This problem may be relieved, to some extent, by the provision of a gastrostomy, usually in addition to a fundoplication.[238,239] Such measures improve nutrition and weight gain, reduce aspiration, and provide a reliable route for medication. Before provision of, or in addition to, a gastrostomy, videofluoroscopy of feeding and swallowing can be used to train caregivers in more efficient feeding of a child.[240]

Oromotor dysfunction, such as incomplete lip closure during swallowing, low suction pressure, and prolonged delay between suction and propelling stages, leads to drooling.[241] Many procedures have been tried to alleviate drooling, including oromotor training and behavioral approaches and various surgical methods.[242,243] Pharmacologic approaches include the use of anticholinergic agents such as benztropine or benzhexol hydrochloride and transdermal scopolamine.[244,245] A combination of behavioral and pharmacologic approaches seems to be the best initial method before surgery is contemplated, as drooling may improve with age. Complications of surgery include ranula formation, complaints of a dry mouth, difficulty with swallowing, and changes in the consistency of oral secretions.[246]

Medications

Medications may help to reduce the disabling effects of the positive signs of the upper motoneuron syndrome (e.g., hyperreflexia, spasticity, and clonus) but have little effect on the negative signs (e.g., weakness and incoordination).[6,247] Dantrolene sodium inhibits release of calcium ions from sarcoplasmic reticulum, reducing muscle contraction. It may improve range of motion and decrease tone, tendon reflexes, and scissoring.[248] Side effects include weakness, drowsiness, lethargy, paresthesias, nausea, and diarrhea.[249] Liver damage also has been reported but usually is reversible with cessation of treatment.[250]

Diazepam is a frequently used benzodiazepine in cerebral palsy. It is thought to exert its antispasticity effect by increasing the presynaptic effect of the inhibitory neurotransmitter gamma-aminobutyric acid (GABA). Some of its efficacy is due to its tranquilizer effect, which also makes it useful in dyskinetic cerebral palsy.[251] All the benzodiazepines may produce sedation, weakness, ataxia, memory disturbances, and dependence after prolonged use.

Baclofen is an analog of GABA and binds to the GABA-B receptor. It inhibits the influx of calcium into presynaptic terminals and suppresses the release of excitatory neurotransmitters. Monosynaptic and polysynaptic reflexes are inhibited, and gamma efferent activity is reduced.[251] Side effects include confusion, sedation, nausea, paresthesias, hypotonia, and ataxia. Sudden withdrawal may lead to seizures and hallucinations.[252] Intrathecal baclofen instilled via a pump has been used to decrease spasticity. Although baclofen may improve activities of daily living and gait in ambulatory patients whose gait is impaired by spasticity and might aid in the management of those with severe spasticity, complications related to the catheter are common, and infection requiring pump removal is reported to occur in 5% of patients so treated.[253] Dose-related side effects include confusion and lethargy.[254]

Injections of phenol or alcohol into muscle motor points have a temporary effect on spasticity but have been replaced by botulinum toxin, which is very effective in reducing spasticity or dystonia.[255–257] Botulinum toxin blocks the presynaptic release of acetylcholine and, when injected into muscle, decreases tone by reducing muscle contraction. Its early use, in addition to reducing tone, may also modify the effects of spasticity on soft tissue and bone and reduce the extent of later surgery.[258,259] Injections usually must be repeated every 2–4 months, and approximately 4% of adults develop antibodies to the toxin after repeated injections.[260]

Neurosurgical Procedures

Posterior rootlet rhizotomy is sometimes performed to reduce spasticity. The procedure reduces tone, may aid in nursing management, and may improve function in a selected group of patients.[261,262] Other neurosurgical approaches include stereotactic operations on the basal ganglia, which will decrease dystonia or hyperkinesia, particularly where this is unilateral, but reportedly the procedure does not lead to significant improvement in function.[263]

Technological Devices

Sophisticated technological aids play an important role in the lives of those with cerebral palsy. These include motorized wheelchairs, various switching devices that can be used to activate communication systems, voice-activated computers, and various environmental control systems.

REFERENCES

1. Levine MS. Cerebral palsy in children over 1 year: standard criteria. Arch Phys Med Rehabil 1980;61:385–389.
2. Freud S. Infantile Cerebral Paralysis. Translated by LA Russin from the original, published 1897. Coral Gables, FL: University of Miami Press, 1968.
3. Crothers B, Paine S. The Natural History of Cerebral Palsy. Cambridge, MA: Harvard University Press, 1959.
4. Michaelis R, Edebol-Tysk K. Zerebralparesen. Paediatr Prax 1988;36:199–205.

5. Burke D. Spasticity as an adaptation to pyramidal tract injury. Adv Neurol 1988;47:401–423.
6. Landau WM. Parable of palsy pills and PT pedagogy. Neurology 1988;38:1496–1499.
7. Mykleburst BM. A review of myotatic reflexes and the development of motor control and gait in infants: a special communication. Phys Ther 1990;70:188–203.
8. Lesny I, Stencik A, Tomasek J, et al. Sensory disorders in cerebral palsy: two point discrimination. Dev Med Child Neurol 1993;35:402–405.
9. Uvebrant P. Hemiplegic cerebral palsy, aetiology and outcome. Acta Paediatr Scand 1988;345:S45–S47.
10. Wiklund LM, Uvebrant P. Hemiplegic cerebral palsy: correlation between CT morphology and clinical findings. Dev Med Child Neurol 1991;33:512–523.
11. Niemann G, Wakat JP, Krageloh-Mann I, et al. Congenital hemiparesis and periventricular leukomalacia: pathogenetic aspects on magnetic resonance imaging. Dev Med Child Neurol 1994;36:943–950.
12. Koelfen W, Freund M, Varnholt V. Neonatal stroke involving the middle cerebral artery in term infants: clinical presentation, EEG and imaging studies, and outcome. Dev Med Child Neurol 1995;37:204–212.
13. Freud S. Die Infantile Cerebrallähmung. In S Nothnagel (ed), Specielle Pathologie und Therapie. Vienna: Holder, 1897;1–327.
14. Cazauvieilh JB. Recherches sur l'agénésie cérébrale et le paralysie congénitale. Arch Gén Méd 1827;14:5–33.
15. Vargha-Khadem F, Isaacs E, van der Werf S, et al. Development of intelligence and memory in children with hemiplegic cerebral palsy: the deleterious consequences of early seizures. Brain 1992;115:315–329.
16. Cooper J, Majnemer A, Rosenblatt B, Birnbaum R. The determination of sensory deficits in children with hemiplegic cerebral palsy. J Child Neurol 1995;10:300–309.
17. Teuber HL. Recovery of Function After Brain Injury in Man. In R Porter, DW Fitzsimmons (eds), Outcome of Severe Damage to the Central Nervous System (Ciba Foundation Symposium 34). Amsterdam: Elsevier, 1975;159–190.
18. Goodman R, Yude C. IQ and its predictors in childhood hemiplegia. Dev Med Child Neurol 1996;38:881–890.
19. Huttenlocher PR, DeCourten C, Garey LJ, Vander Loos H. Synaptogenesis in human visual cortex—evidence for synapse elimination during normal development. Neurosci Lett 1982;33:247–252.
20. Huttenlocher PR. Synaptic density in human frontal cortex—developmental changes and effects of aging. Brain Res 1979;163:195–205.
21. Ferrara TB, Hoekstra RE, Graziano E, et al. Changing outcome of extremely premature infants (<26 weeks' gestation and <750 gm): survival and follow-up at tertiary center. Am J Obstet Gynecol 1989;161:1114–1118.
22. Edebol-Tysk K. Epidemiology of spastic tetraplegic cerebral palsy in Sweden: 1. Impairments and disabilities. Neuropediatrics 1989;20:41–45.
23. Harbord MG, Kobayashi JS. Fever producing ballismus in patients with choreoathetosis. J Child Neurol 1991;6:49–52.
24. Hagberg B, Hagberg G, Olow I. The changing panorama of cerebral palsy in Sweden, 1954–1970: I. Analysis of the general changes. Acta Paediatr Scand 1975;64:187–192.
25. Miller G, Cala LA. Ataxic cerebral palsy. Clinico-radiologic correlations. Neuropediatrics 1989;20:84–89.
26. Matthews KD, Afifi AK, Hanson JW. Autosomal recessive cerebellar hypoplasia. J Child Neurol 1989;4:189–193.
27. Joubert M, Eisenring JJ, Robb JP, et al. Familial agenesis of the cerebellar vermis: a syndrome of episodic hyperpnea, abnormal eye movements, ataxia, and retardation. Neurology 1969;19:813–825.

28. Kornberg AJ, Shield LK. An extended phenotype of an early onset inherited non-progressive cerebellar ataxia syndrome. J Child Neurol 1991;6:20–23.

29. Yannet H, Horton FH. Hypotonic cerebral palsy in mental defectives. Pediatrics 1952;9:204–211.

30. Foerster O. Der atonisch-astatische typus der infantilen cerebrallahmung. Eur J Clin Invest 1910;98:216–244.

31. Lipkin PH. Epidemiology of the Developmental Disabilities. In AJ Capute, PJ Accardo (eds), Developmental Disabilities in Infancy and Childhood. Baltimore: Brookes, 1991;43–47.

32. Murphy CC, Yeargin-Ausopp M, Decoufee P, Drews CD. Prevalence of cerebral palsy among ten year old children in metropolitan Atlanta, 1985 through 1987. J Pediatr 1993;123:513–519.

33. Dorman C, Hurley AD, Laatsch LK. Prediction of reading and spelling achievement in cerebral palsied adolescents using neuropsychological tests. Int J Clin Neuropsychol 1984;6:142–144.

34. Bagnato SJ, Campbell TF. Comprehensive Neurodevelopmental Evaluation of Children with Brain Insults. In G Miller, JC Ramer (eds), Static Encephalopathies of Infancy and Childhood. New York: Raven, 1992;27–46.

35. Hurley AD, Sorner R. Psychiatric aspects of cerebral palsy. Psychiatr Ment Retard Rev 1987;6:1–5.

36. Aksu F. Nature and prognosis of seizures in patients with cerebral palsy. Dev Med Child Neurol 1990;32:661–668.

37. Aicardi J. Epilepsy in brain injured children. Dev Med Child Neurol 1990; 32:191–202.

38. Black P. Visual disorders associated with cerebral palsy. Br J Ophthalmol 1982; 66:46–52.

39. Jan J, Groenveld M, Sykanda AM, Hoyt CS. Behavioral characteristics of children with permanent cortical visual impairment. Dev Med Child Neurol 1987;29: 571–576.

40. Thurston SE, Leign RJ, Crawford T, et al. Two distinct deficits of visual tracking caused by unilateral lesions of cerebral cortex in humans. Ann Neurol 1988; 23:266–273.

41. Schenk-Rootlieb AJ, van Nieuwenhuizen O, van der Graaf Y, et al. The prevalence of cerebral visual disturbance in children with cerebral palsy. Dev Med Child Neurol 1992;34:473–480.

42. Buckley E, Seaber JH. Dyskinetic strabismus as a sign of cerebral palsy. Am J Ophthalmol 1981;91:652–657.

43. Katayama M, Tamas LB. Saccadic eye movements of children with cerebral palsy. Dev Med Child Neurol 1987;29:36–39.

44. Sondheimer JM, Morris BM. Gastroesophageal reflux among severely retarded children. J Pediatr 1979;94:710–714.

45. Stallings VA, Charney EB, Davies JC, Cronk CE. Nutrition related growth failure of children with quadriplegic cerebral palsy. Dev Med Child Neurol 1993; 35:126–138.

46. Stevenson RD, Hayes RP, Cater LV, Blackman JA. Clinical correlates of linear growth in children with cerebral palsy. Dev Med Child Neurol 1994;36:135–142.

47. Stevenson RD, Roberts CD, Vogtle L. The effects of non-nutritional factors on growth in cerebral palsy. Dev Med Child Neurol 1995;37:124–130.

48. Ishida C, Fujiita M, Umemoto H, et al. Respiratory function in handicapped children. Brain Dev 1990;12:372–375.

49. Shaw NJ, White CP, Fraser WD, Rosenbloom L. Osteopenia in cerebral palsy. Arch Dis Child 1994;71:235–238.

50. Vilmshurst S, Ward K, Adams JE, et al. Mobility status and bone density in cerebral palsy. Arch Dis Child 1996;75:164–165.

51. Borzyskowski M. Cerebral palsy and the bladder. Dev Med Child Neurol 1989; 31:682–689.
52. Decter RM, Bauer SB, Khoshkin S, et al. Urodynamic assessment of children with cerebral palsy. J Urol 1987;138:1110–1112.
53. Reese M, Msall ME, Owen S, et al. Acquired cervical spine impairment in young adults with cerebral palsy. Dev Med Child Neurol 1991;33:153–158.
54. Fletcher NA, Marsden CD. Dyskinetic cerebral palsy: a clinical and genetic study. Dev Med Child Neurol 1996;38:873–880.
55. Scott BL, Jankovic J. Delayed-onset progressive movement disorders after static brain lesions. Neurology 1996;46:68–74.
56. Burke RE, Fahn S, Gold AP. Delayed onset dystonia in patients with "static encephalopathy." J Neurol Neurosurg Psychiatry 1980;43:789–797.
57. Saint Hilaire MH, Burke RE, Bressman SB, et al. Delayed-onset dystonia due to perinatal or early childhood asphyxia. Neurology 1991;41:216–222.
58. Chalhub EG, DeVivo DC, Volpe JJ. Phenytoin induced dystonia and choreoathetosis in two retarded epileptic children. Neurology 1976;26:494–498.
59. Crosley CJ, Swender PT. Dystonia associated with carbamazepine administration: experience in brain damaged children. Pediatrics 1979;63:612–614.
60. Murphy KP, Molnar GE, Lankasky K. Medical and functional status of adults with cerebral palsy. Dev Med Child Neurol 1995;37:1075–1084.
61. Burns YR, O'Callaghan M, Tudehope DI. Early identification of cerebral palsy in high risk infants. Aust Paediatr J 1989;25:215–219.
62. Allen MC, Alexander GR. Using motor milestones as a multistep process to screen preterm infants for cerebral palsy. Dev Med Child Neurol 1997;39:12–16.
63. Capute AJ. Identifying cerebral palsy in infancy through study of primitive-reflex profiles. Pediatr Ann 1979;8:589–595.
64. Foley J. Physical Aspects. In SM Blencowe (ed), Cerebral Palsy and the Young Child. London: E&S Livingstone, 1969;15–31.
65. Zafeiriou DI, Tsikoulas IG, Kremenopoulos GM. Prospective follow-up of primitive reflex profiles in high-risk infants: clues to an early diagnosis of cerebral palsy. Pediatr Neurol 1995;13:148–152.
66. Scherzer AL, Tsharnuter I. Early Diagnosis and Therapy in Cerebral Palsy. New York: Marcel Dekker, 1982.
67. Yokochi K, Shimabukuro S, Kodama M, et al. Motor function of infants with athetoid cerebral palsy. Dev Med Child Neurol 1993;35:909–916.
68. Cordes I, Roland EH, Lupton BA, Hill A. Early prediction of the development of microcephaly after hypoxic-ischemic encephalopathy in the full-term newborn. Pediatrics 1994;93:701–707.
69. Dargassies SS. Neurodevelopmental symptoms during the first year of life: I. Essential landmarks for each key-age. Dev Med Child Neurol 1972;14:235–246.
70. Haworth JC, Booth FA, Chudley AE, et al. Phenotypic variability in glutaric aciduria type 1: report of fourteen cases in five Canadian Indian kindreds. J Pediatr 1991;118:52–58.
71. Scheuerle AE, McVie R, Beaudet AL, Shapira SK. Arginase deficiency presenting as cerebral palsy. Pediatrics 1993;91:995–996.
72. Costeff H, Gadoth N, Apter N, et al. A familial syndrome of infantile optic atrophy, movement disorder, and spastic paraplegia. Neurology 1989;39:595–597.
73. Nygaard TG, Waran SP, Levine RA, et al. Dopa-responsive dystonia simulating cerebral palsy. Pediatr Neurol 1994;11:236–240.
74. Mackenzie ICK. The use of neurological terms in cerebral palsy studies. Cereb Palsy Bull 1959;5:47–51.
75. Truwit CL, Barkovich AJ, Kock TK, Ferriero DM. Cerebral palsy: MR findings in 40 patients. Am J Neuroradiol 1992;13:67–78.
76. Kuban KCK, Leviton A. Cerebral palsy. N Engl J Med 1994;330:188–195.

77. Perlman JM. Intrapartum hypoxic-ischemic cerebral injury and subsequent cerebral palsy: medicolegal issues. Pediatrics 1997;99:851–859.
78. Freeman JM, Nelson KB. Intrapartum asphyxia and cerebral palsy. Pediatrics 1988;82:240–249.
79. Carter BS, Haverkamp AD, Merenstein GB. The definition of acute perinatal asphyxia. Clin Perinatol 1993;20:287–304.
80. Paneth N, Bommarito M, Stricker J. Electronic fetal monitoring and later outcome. Clin Invest Med 1993;16:159–165.
81. Painter MJ. Fetal heart rate patterns, perinatal asphyxia, and brain injury. Pediatr Neurol 1989;5:137–144.
82. Colditz PB, Henderson-Smart DJ. Electronic fetal heart rate monitoring during labour. Does it prevent perinatal asphyxia and cerebral palsy? Med J Aust 1990; 153:88–90.
83. Nelson KB, Dambrosia JM, Ting TY, Grether JK. Uncertain value of electronic fetal monitoring in predicting cerebral palsy. N Engl J Med 1996;334:613–618.
84. Madsen H, Bjerrum P, Lose G, et al. The relationship between low pH in the umbilical cord artery in neonates and later development of cerebral paresis. Ugeskr Laeger 1991;153:2610–2612.
85. Naeye RL. Can meconium in the amniotic fluid injure the fetal brain? Obstet Gynecol 1995;86:720–724.
86. Yudkin PL, Johnson A, Clover LM, Murphy KW. Clustering of perinatal markers of birth asphyxia and outcome at age 5 years. Br J Obstet Gynaecol 1994; 101:774–781.
87. Richmond S, Niswander K, Snodgrass CA, Wagstaff I. The obstetric management of fetal distress and its association with cerebral palsy. Obstet Gynecol 1994; 83:643–646.
88. The Scottish Low Birthweight Study Group. The Scottish Low Birthweight Study: I. Survival, growth, neuromotor and sensory impairment. Arch Dis Child 1992; 67:675–681.
89. Volpe JJ. Brain injury in the premature infant—current concepts. Preventive Med 1994;3:638–645.
90. Aziz K, Vickar DB, Sauve RS, et al. Province-based study of neurologic disability of children weighing 500 through 1249 grams at birth in relation to neonatal cerebral ultrasound findings. Pediatrics 1995;95:837–844.
91. Bushan V, Paneth N, Kiely J. Impact of improved survival of very low birth weight infants on recent secular events in the prevalence of cerebral palsy. Pediatrics 1993;91:1094–1100.
92. Blaymore-Bier J, Pezzulo J, Kim E, et al. Outcome of extremely low birth weight infants: 1980–1990. Acta Paediatr 1994;83:1244–1248.
93. Pharaoh PD, Platt MJ, Cooke T. The changing epidemiology of cerebral palsy. Arch Dis Child 1996;75:169–173.
94. Nelson KB, Ellenberg JH. Antecedents of cerebral palsy: multivariate analysis of risk. N Engl J Med 1986;315:81–86.
95. Gaffney G, Sellars S, Flavell V, et al. Case-control study of intrapartum care, cerebral palsy, and perinatal death. Br Med J 1994;308:743–750.
96. Brann AW. Factors During Neonatal Life That Influence Brain Disorder. In JM Freeman (ed), Prenatal and Perinatal Factors Associated with Brain Disorders (NIH Pub. No. 85-1149). Washington, DC: U.S. Government Printing Office, 1998;263–358.
97. Nelson KB. What proportion of cerebral palsy is related to birth asphyxia? J Pediatr 1988;112:572–573.
98. Naeye RL, Peters EC. Origins of cerebral palsy. Am J Dis Child 1989;143:1154–1161.
99. Torfs CP, van den Berg BJ, Oechsli FW, Cummins S. Prenatal and perinatal factors in the etiology of cerebral palsy. J Pediatr 1990;116:615–619.

100. Naeye RL. Umbilical cord length: clinical significance. J Pediatr 1985;107: 276–281.
101. Miller G. Minor congenital anomalies and ataxic cerebral palsy. Arch Dis Child 1989;64:557–562.
102. Altshuler G. Some placental considerations related to neurodevelopmental and other disorders. J Child Neurol 1993;8:78–94.
103. Low JA, Robertson DM, Simpson LL. Temporal relationships of neuropathologic conditions caused by perinatal asphyxia. Am J Obstet Gynecol 1989;160:608–614.
104. Low JA, Simpson LL, Ramsay DA. The clinical diagnosis of asphyxia responsible for brain damage in the human fetus. Am J Obstet Gynecol 1992;167:11–15.
105. Scher MS, Belfan H, Maran J, Painter MJ. Destructive brain lesions of presumed fetal onset: antepartum causes of cerebral palsy. Pediatrics 1991;88:898–906.
106. Pharaoh PD, Cooke T, Rosenbloom L. Acquired cerebral palsy. Arch Dis Child 1989;64:1013–1016.
107. Ellenberg J, Nelson KB. Birthweight and gestational age in children with cerebral palsy or seizure disorders. Am J Dis Child 1979;133:1044–1048.
108. Sinha SK, D'Souza SW, Rivlin E, Chiswick ML. Ischaemic brain lesions diagnosed at birth in preterm infants: clinical events and developmental outcome. Arch Dis Child 1990;65:1017–1020.
109. Skolnick A. New ultrasound evidence appears to link prenatal brain damage, cerebral palsy. JAMA 1991;265:948–949.
110. Dykes FD, Dunbar B, Lazarra A, Ahmann PA. Posthemorrhagic hydrocephalus in high-risk preterm infants: natural history, management, and long-term outcome. J Pediatr 1989;114:611–618.
111. Skidmore MD, Rivers A, Hack M. Increased risk of cerebral palsy among very low-birthweight infants with chronic lung disease. Dev Med Child Neurol 1990; 32:325–332.
112. Perlman JM, Volpe JJ. Movement disorder of premature infants with severe bronchopulmonary dysplasia: a new syndrome. Pediatrics 1989;84:215–218.
113. Gray PH, Burns YR, Mohay HA, et al. Neurodevelopmental outcome of preterm infants with bronchopulmonary dysplasia. Arch Dis Child 1995;73:128–134.
114. Wical BS, Tomasi LG. A distinctive neurologic syndrome after induced profound hypothermia. Pediatr Neurol 1990;6:202–205.
115. Kupsky WJ, Drozd MA, Barlow CF. Selective injury of the globus pallidus in children with post–cardiac surgery choreic syndrome. Dev Med Child Neurol 1995;37:135–144.
116. Clancy RR, Sladky JT, Rorke LB. Hypoxic-ischemic spinal cord injury following perinatal asphyxia. Ann Neurol 1989;25:185–189.
117. Perlman JM, Tack ED. Renal injury in the asphyxiated newborn infant: relationship to neurologic outcome. J Pediatr 1988;113:875–889.
118. Roland EH, Hill A. Clinical aspects of perinatal hypoxic-ischemic brain injury. Semin Pediatr Neurol 1995;2:57–71.
119. Bergman I, Painter MJ, Hirsch RS. Outcome in neonates with convulsions treated in an intensive care unit. Ann Neurol 1983;14:642–647.
120. Sarnat HB, Sarnat MS. Neonatal encephalopathy following fetal distress. A clinical and electroencephalographic study. Arch Neurol 1976;33:696–705.
121. Robertson MT, Finer NN. Long-term follow-up of term neonates with perinatal asphyxia. Clin Perinatol 1993;20:483–499.
122. Hill A. Current concepts of hypoxic-ischemic cerebral injury in the term newborn. Pediatr Neurol 1991;7:317–325.
123. Holmes G, Rowe J, Hafford J, et al. Prognostic value of the electroencephalogram in neonatal asphyxia. Electroencephalogr Clin Neurophysiol 1982;53:60–72.
124. Gray PH, Tudehope DI, Masel JP, et al. Perinatal hypoxic-ischaemic brain injury: prediction of outcome. Dev Med Child Neurol 1993;35:965–983.

125. Kuenzle C, Baenziger O, Martin E, et al. Prognostic value of early MR imaging in term infants with severe perinatal asphyxia. Neuropediatrics 1994;25:191–200.
126. Younkin DP. Magnetic resonance spectroscopy in hypoxic-ischemic encephalopathy. Clin Invest Med 1993;16:115–121.
127. Gilles F. Neuropathologic Indicators of Abnormal Development. In JM Freeman (ed), Prenatal and Perinatal Factors Associated with Brain Disorders (NIH Pub. No. 85-1149). Washington, DC: U.S. Government Printing Office, 1985;53–108.
128. Larroche JC. Fetal encephalopathies of circulatory origin. Biol Neonate 1986; 50:61–74.
129. Wood JW, Johnson KG, Omori Y. In utero exposure to the Hiroshima atomic bomb. An evaluation of head size and mental retardation: twenty years later. Pediatrics 1967;39:385–392.
130. Dekaban AS. Abnormalities in children exposed to x-radiation during various stages of gestation: tentative timetable of radiation injury to the human fetus. J Nucl Med 1968;9:471–477.
131. Brent RL, Beckman DA. Environmental teratogens. Bull N Y Acad Med 1990; 66:123–163.
132. Watchko JF, Oski FA. Kernicterus in preterm newborns: past, present, and future. Pediatrics 1992;90:707–715.
133. Aiden R, Corner B, Tovey G. Kernicterus and prematurity. Lancet 1950; 1:1153–1154.
134. Hugh-Jones K, Slack J, Simpson K, et al. Clinical course of hyperbilirubinemia in premature infants. N Engl J Med 1960;263:1223–1229.
135. Coorsen EA, Msall ME, Duffy LC. Multiple minor malformations as a marker for prenatal etiology of cerebral palsy. Dev Med Child Neurol 1991;33:730–736.
136. Roland EH, Flodmark O, Hill A. Thalamic hemorrhage with intraventricular hemorrhage in the full term newborn. Pediatrics 1990;85:737–742.
137. Larroche JC, Droulle P, Delazoid AL, et al. Brain damage in monozygous twins. Biol Neonate 1990;57:261–273.
138. Scheller JM, Nelson KB. Twinning and neurologic morbidity. Am J Dis Child 1992;146:1110–1113.
139. Weig SG, Marshall PC, Abroms IF, Gauthier NS. Patterns of cerebral injury and clinical presentation in the vascular disruptive syndrome of monozygotic twins. Pediatr Neurol 1995;13:279–285.
140. Bejar R, Vigliocci G, Granajo H. Antenatal origin of neurologic damage in newborn infants: II. Multiple gestations. Am J Obstet Gynecol 1990;162:1230–1236.
141. Grether JK, Nelson KB, Cummins SK. Twinning and cerebral palsy: experience in four northern California counties, births 1983 through 1985. Pediatrics 1993; 92:854–858.
142. Petterson B, Nelson KB, Watson L, Stanley FJ. Twins, triplets, and cerebral palsy in births in Western Australia in the 1980s. Br Med J 1993;307:1239–1243.
143. Barth PG. Disorders of neuronal migration. Can J Neurol Sci 1987;14:1–6.
144. Gindoff PR, Yeh MN, Jewelewicz R. The vanishing sac syndrome. Ultrasound evidence of pregnancy failure in multiple gestations, induced and spontaneous. J Reprod Med 1986;31:322–325.
145. Landy HJ, Weiner S, Corson SL, et al. The "vanishing twin": ultrasonographic assessment of fetal disappearance in the first trimester. Am J Obstet Gynecol 1986;155:14–19.
146. Patten RM, Mack LA, Nyberg DA, Filly RA. Twin embolization syndrome: prenatal sonographic findings and significance. Radiology 1989;173:685–689.
147. Anderson RL, Golbus MS, Curry CJR, et al. Central nervous system damage and other anomalies in surviving fetus following second trimester antenatal death of co-twin. Prenat Diagn 1990;10:513–518.

193. Volpe JJ. Intraventricular hemorrhage in the premature infant: current concepts. Ann Neurol 1989;25:109–116.
194. Keeney SE, Adcock EW, McArdle CB. Prospective observations of 100 high risk neonates by high field (1.5 Tesla) magnetic resonance imaging of the central nervous system: II. Lesions associated with hypoxic-ischemic encephalopathy. Pediatrics 1991;87:431–438.
195. Krageloh-Mann I, Hagberg B, Peterson D, et al. Bilateral spastic cerebral palsy— pathogenetic aspects from MRI. Neuropediatrics 1992;23:46–48.
196. Yokochi K, Aibak K, Koduma M, Fujimoto S. Magnetic resonance imaging in cerebral palsied children. Acta Paediatr Scand 1991;80:818–823.
197. Guzzetta F, Shackelford GD, Volpe S, et al. Periventricular intraparenchymal echodensities in the premature newborn: critical determinant of neurological outcome. Pediatrics 1986;78:995–1006.
198. Gould SJ, Howard S, Hope PL, Reynolds EOR. Periventricular intraparenchymal cerebral hemorrhage in preterm infants: the role of venous infarction. J Pathol 1987;151:197–202.
199. Nelson KB. Prenatal origin of hemiparetic cerebral palsy: how often and why? Pediatrics 1991;88:1059–1062.
200. Barmada MA, Moossy J, Shuman RM. Cerebral infarcts with arterial occlusion in neonates. Ann Neurol 1979;6:495–502.
201. Miller MR, Levy SR, Abroms F, et al. Seizures and cerebral infarction in the full term newborn. Ann Neurol 1985;17:366–370.
202. Foley J. Dyskinetic and dystonic forms of cerebral palsy and birth. Acta Paediatr 1992;81:57–60.
203. Menkes JH, Curran J. Clinical and MR correlates in children with extrapyramidal cerebral palsy. Am J Neuroradiol 1994;15:451–457.
204. Barks JD, Silverstein FS, Sims K, et al. Glutamate recognition sites in human fetal brain. Neurosci Lett 1988;84:131–136.
205. Oppenheim RW. Cell death during development of the nervous system. Annu Rev Neurosci 1991;14:453–501.
206. Hillburger AC, Willis JK, Bouldin E, Henderson-Tilton A. Familial schizencephaly. Brain Dev 1993;15:234–236.
207. Haverkamp F, Zerres K, Ostertun B, et al. Familial schizencephaly: further delineation of a rare disorder. J Med Genet 1995;32:242–244.
208. Roessler E, Belloni E, Gaudenz K, et al. Mutations in human Sonic Hedgehog gene causes holoprosencephaly. Nat Genet 1996;14:357–360.
209. Dobyns WB, Andermann E, Andermann F, et al. X-linked malformations of neuronal migration. Neurology 1996;47:331–339.
210. Becker LE, Evrard P. A classification scheme for malformations of cortical development. Neuropediatrics 1996;27:59–63.
211. Rorke LB. A perspective: the role of disordered genetic control of neurogenesis in the pathogenesis of migration disorders. J Neuropathol Exp Neurol 1994; 53:105–117.
212. Dodge NN, Dobyns WV. Agenesis of the corpus callosum and Dandy-Walker malformation associated with hemimegalencephaly in the sebaceous nevus syndrome. Am J Med Genet 1995;56:147–150.
213. Rohrer H. The role of growth factors in the control of neurogenesis. Eur J Neurosci 1990;2:1005–1015.
214. Molnar GE, Gordon SU. Cerebral palsy: predictive value of clinical signs for early prognostication of motor function. Arch Phys Med Rehabil 1976;57:153–158.
215. Bleck EE. Locomotor prognosis in cerebral palsy. Dev Med Child Neurol 1975; 17:18–25.
216. da Paz AC, Burnett SM, Braga LW. Walking prognosis in cerebral palsy: a 22-year retrospective analysis. Dev Med Child Neurol 1994;36:130–134.

217. Sala DA, Grant AD. Prognosis for ambulation in cerebral palsy. Dev Med Child Neurol 1995;37:1020–1026.
218. Kudrjavcev T, Schoenberg BS, Kurland LT, Groover RV. Cerebral palsy: survival rates, associated handicaps, and distribution by clinical subtype (Rochester, MN, 1950–1976). Neurology 1985;35:900–903.
219. Evans PM, Evans SJW, Alberman E. Cerebral palsy: why we must plan for survival. Arch Dis Child 1991;65:1329–1333.
220. Crichton JU, Mackinnon M, White CP. The life expectancy of persons with cerebral palsy. Dev Med Child Neurol 1995;37:567–576.
221. Eyman RK, Grossman RK, Chaney RH, Cali TL. Survival of profoundly disabled people with severe mental retardation. Am J Dis Child 1993;147:329–336.
222. Vining PG. Cerebral palsy. A pediatric developmentalist's overview. Am J Dis Child 1976;130:643–649.
223. Taylor DC. Counselling the parents of handicapped children. Br Med J 1982;284:1027–1028.
224. Barowsky EI. Communicating Information. In G Miller, JC Ramer (eds), Static Encephalopathies of Infancy and Childhood. New York: Raven, 1992;111–118.
225. Olshansky S. Chronic sorrow: a response to having a mentally defective child. Soc Casework 1962;43:190–193.
226. Bentovim A. Handicapped pre-school children and their families—attitudes to the child. Br Med J 1972;3:579–581.
227. Palmer FB, Shapiro BK, Wachtel RC, et al. The effects of physical therapy on cerebral palsy. A controlled trial in infants with spastic diplegia. N Engl J Med 1988;318:803–808.
228. Turnbull J. Early intervention for children with or at risk for cerebral palsy. Am J Dis Child 1993;147:54–59.
229. Finnie N. Handling the Young Cerebral Palsied Child at Home. London: William Heinemann, 1974.
230. Bleck EE. Orthopaedic Management in Cerebral Palsy. Oxford: Mackeith, 1987.
231. Koop SE. Orthopedic Aspects of Static Encephalopathies. In G Miller, JC Ramer (eds), Static Encephalopathies of Infancy and Childhood. New York: Raven, 1992;95–109.
232. Cornell MS. The hip in cerebral palsy. Dev Med Child Neurol 1995;37:3–18.
233. Bleck EE. Management of the lower extremities in children who have cerebral palsy. J Bone Joint Surg 1993;72:140–144.
234. Sutherland DH, Davids JR. Common gait abnormalities of the knee in cerebral palsy. Clin Orthop 1993;288:139–147.
235. Zuromski ES. The Management of Mental Retardation. In G Miller, JC Ramer (eds), Static Encephalopathies of Infancy and Childhood. New York: Raven, 1992;119–133.
236. Dahl M, Thommessen M, Rasmussen M, Selberg T. Feeding and nutritional characteristics in children with moderate or severe cerebral palsy. Acta Paediatr 1996;85:697–701.
237. Reilly S, Skuse D, Poblete X. Prevalence of feeding problems and oral motor dysfunction in children with cerebral palsy: a community survey. J Pediatr 1996;129:877–882.
238. Stringel G, Delgado M, Guertin L, et al. Gastrostomy and Nissen fundoplication in neurologically impaired children. J Pediatr Surg 1989;24:1044–1048.
239. Spitz L, Roth K, Kiely EM, et al. Operation for gastro-oesophageal reflux associated with severe mental retardation. Arch Dis Child 1993;68:347–351.
240. Morton RE, Bonas R, Fowie B, Minford J. Videofluoroscopy in the assessment of feeding disorders of children with neurological problems. Dev Med Child Neurol 1993;35:388–395.

241. Lespargot A, Langevin MF, Muller S, Guillemont S. Swallowing disturbances associated with drooling in cerebral-palsied children. Dev Med Child Neurol 1993; 35:298–304.
242. Sellars SL. Surgery of sialorrhoea. J Laryngol Otol 1985;99:1107–1109.
243. Dunn KW, Cunningham CE, Backman JE. Self-control and reinforcement in the management of a cerebral-palsied adolescent's drooling. Dev Med Child Neurol 1987;29:305–310.
244. Reddihough D, Johnson H, Staples M, et al. Use of benzhexol hydrochloride to control drooling of children with cerebral palsy. Dev Med Child Neurol 1990; 32:985–989.
245. Siegel LK, Klingbeil MA. Control of drooling with transdermal scopolamine in a child with cerebral palsy. Dev Med Child Neurol 1991;33:1013–1014.
246. Webb K, Reddihough DS, Johnson H, et al. Long term outcome of saliva control surgery. Dev Med Child Neurol 1995;37:755–762.
247. Glenn MB, Whyte J. The Practical Management of Spasticity in Children and Adults. Philadelphia: Lea & Febiger, 1990.
248. Haslam RHA, Walcher JR, Liebman PS, et al. Dantrolene sodium in children with spasticity. Arch Phys Med Rehabil 1974;13:3–23.
249. Young RR, Delwaide PJ. Spasticity. N Engl J Med 1981;304:96–99.
250. Utili R, Biotnott JK, Zimmerman HJ. Dantrolene-associated hepatic injury. Incidence and character. Gastroenterology 1977;72:610–616.
251. Davidoff RA. Antispasticity drugs: mechanisms of action. Ann Neurol 1985; 17:107–116.
252. Terrence DY, Fromm GH. Complications of baclofen withdrawal. Arch Neurol 1981;38:588–589.
253. Albright AL. Baclofen in the treatment of cerebral palsy. J Child Neurol 1996; 11:77–83.
254. Albright AL, Cervi A, Singletary J. Intrathecal baclofen for spasticity in cerebral palsy. JAMA 1991;265:1418–1422.
255. Snow BJ, Tsui JCK, Bhatt MH, et al. Treatment of spasticity with botulinum toxin: a double blind study. Ann Neurol 1990;28:512–515.
256. Cosgrove AP, Corry IS, Graham HK. Botulinum toxin in the management of the lower limb in cerebral palsy. Dev Med Child Neurol 1994;36:386–396.
257. Korman AL, Mooney JF, Smith BP, et al. Management of spasticity in cerebral palsy with botulinum A toxin: report of a preliminary randomized double blind trial. J Pediatr Orthop 1994;14:299–303.
258. Bleck EE. Cerebral palsy hip deformities: is there a consensus? II. Botulinum-toxin A: a clinical experiment. J Pediatr Orthop 1994;14:281–282.
259. Neville B. Botulinum toxin in the cerebral palsies. Br Med J 1994;309:1526–1527.
260. Greene P, Fahn S, Diamond B. Development of resistance to botulinum toxin type A in patients with torticollis. Mov Disord 1994;9:213–217.
261. Dudgeon BJ, Libby AK, McLaughlin JF, et al. Prospective measurement of functional changes after selective dorsal rhizotomy. Arch Phys Med Rehabil 1994; 75:46–53.
262. Nishida T, Thatcher SW, Marty GR. Selective posterior rhizotomy for children with cerebral palsy: a 7 year experience. Child Nerv Syst 1995;12:1–24.
263. Speelman JD, van Manen J. Cerebral palsy and stereotactic neurosurgery: long term results. J Neurol Neurosurg Psychiatry 1989;52:23–30.

2

From Molecule to Tissue: Normal and Abnormal Brain Development

Gary D. Clark, John W. Swann, and Geoffrey Miller

In this chapter, we summarize normal and abnormal human brain formation and meld the recently described genetic aberrations that cause brain developmental disorders with pathologic descriptions of those malformations. We describe the normal development of human brain by inference from classic developmental studies in animals and from pathologic studies of human tissue. We also list the genes believed to be involved in the individual components of this development and describe the pathologic alterations involved in abnormal development attributable to gene mutations. The functions of some of the genes responsible for abnormal development can be suspected by examining the pathologic consequences. Hence, we are able to correlate genetic abnormalities with developmental neuropathology. Other genes and molecules involved in abnormal human brain formation have well-studied counterparts in animals that provide insight into their function in humans.

The study of the genetics of brain development is a rapidly growing area, and important new genes are being described. Though the information regarding human genes involved in normal and abnormal brain formation was as up-to-date as possible at the time that this chapter was written, important new insights into the genetics of human brain development have likely been made since then. We encourage the reader to visit Online Mendelian Inheritance in Man (OMIM) for the most current information (http://www3.ncbi.nlm.nih.gov/Omim/).

As it appears that general mechanisms are involved in neurodevelopment, we have attempted to anticipate some of the new advances in understanding brain formation and have provided a framework by which these advances can be understood. Given the plethora of material that could be covered in a chapter such as this, we have opted to emphasize these general mechanisms that are likely to be involved in abnormal neurodevelopment rather than to catalog all that is known about human brain formation.

Because we set out to describe the covered pathologic entities in the context of the developmental process that we believe to have gone awry, disorders previously categorized as migration abnormalities might, on the basis of new

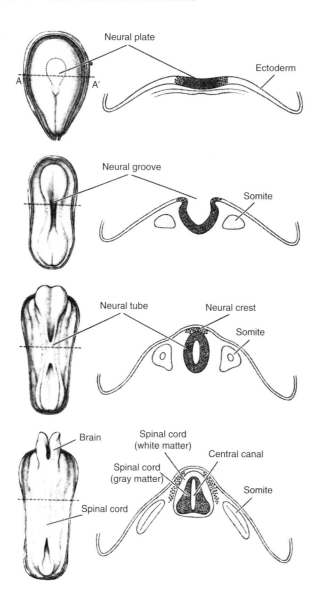

Figure 2.1 Genesis of the nervous system. The nervous system is derived from the ectoderm during the third to fourth week of gestation in the human. An external view of the ectoderm surface in early human development is shown on the left, and a cross-sectional view is shown on the right. The central nervous system begins as a thickening (a placode) in the center of the ectoderm, referred to as the *neural plate*. The plate folds laterally, and a groove intervenes. The folds appose and fuse dorsally in the region of the future cervical spinal cord. The apposition continues rostrally and caudally until a complete neural tube is formed. The central canal of this tube will form the ventricles of the brain. (Reprinted from WM Cowan. The development of the brain. Sci Am 1979;241:114. With permission from Scientific American Publishers.)

genetic insights, be found in our discussion of cellular differentiation or regional specification (segmentation). As further insights are made into human brain developmental disorders leading to the cerebral palsies, the following categorization scheme will probably have to be altered.

Human brain formation involves the sequential yet overlapping processes of neuroectoderm formation, closure of the neural tube, segmentation of the embryonic nervous system, ventral induction of the telencephalon, cellular proliferation, neuronal migration, and synapse formation (Figures 2.1–2.4). In the

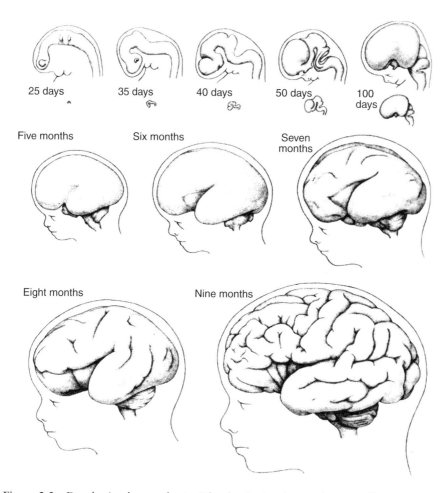

Figure 2.2 Developing human brain. The developing human brain is illustrated from a lateral perspective at the gestational ages noted on the figure. The embryonic period (primordial plexiform layer formation) is depicted to 50 days and is marked by the formation of flexures that demarcate the forebrain (prosencephalon), the midbrain (mesencephalon), and the hindbrain (rhombencephalon). Prosencephalic cleavage is an early event, occurring between 35 and 40 days; it is not well appreciated from a lateral view. The telencephalon develops into the cerebral hemispheres, which overgrow and obscure the underlying midbrain and hindbrain. Cerebral hemisphere convolutions are not apparent until 30 weeks (7 months) of gestation. (Reprinted from WM Cowan. The development of the brain. Sci Am 1979;241:116. With permission from Scientific American Publishers.)

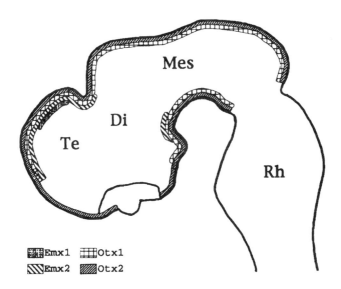

Figure 2.3 Mouse fetal brain expression of *Emx* and *Otx* genes at embryonic day 10. A compilation of in situ hybridization results is shown in this figure. Expression patterns of the individual homeobox genes are depicted by various patterns. A small checkered area anteriorly demarcates an area in which the expression pattern of *Emx2* and *Otx1* are less well defined. In all likelihood, these genes are expressed in a similar fashion in the human. (Te = telencephalon; Di = diencephalon; Mes = mesencephalon; Rh = rhombencephalon.) (Reprinted with permission from E Boncinelli, M Gulisano, F Spada, V Broccoli. *Emx* and *Otx* Gene Expression in the Developing Mouse Brain. In GR Brock, G Cardew [eds], Development of the Cerebral Cortex [Ciba Foundation Symposium 193]. Chichester, UK: Wiley, 1995;102.)

description of each of these processes, we include the timing, the molecules, and the genes involved.

OVERVIEW OF BRAIN DEVELOPMENT

As the pieces of the brain development puzzle come together, we see that certain general mechanisms tend to recur in all phases of neurodevelopment: namely, induction, cell fate determination, and cell (or cellular process) movement (migration and synapse formation). *Induction* is the process by which one group of cells determines the fate of another group of neighboring cells, probably by the release of soluble factors or inducers. These inducers act on the target cells and initiate genetic programs that determine the fates of cell lineage. Because cells in the developing nervous system rarely are born in the location in which they will finally reside, movement or migration of cells must occur. Even as cells are undergoing the process of migration, others (and perhaps even the cells that are migrating) extend processes, seek their target cells, and make precise connections, sometimes over imposing distances.

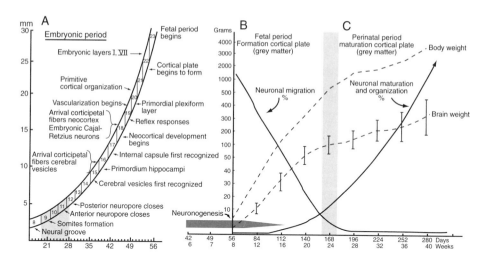

Figure 2.4 Major developmental events of human brain. This figure is reproduced from Dr. Miguel Marín-Padilla's work and represents a compilation of his observations over many years. Graphs A, B, and C represent the embryonic period (establishment of the primordial plexiform layer), the fetal period (formation of the cortical plate), and the perinatal period (differentiation; neuronal process growth of the cortical plate), respectively. Note the overlap of developmental processes involved. Segmentation of the nervous system is involved in early neural tube formation (from 3 to 8 weeks). Induction is involved in all aspects of neural development. (Reprinted from M Marín-Padilla. Ontogenesis of the pyramidal cell of the mammalian neocortex and developmental cytoarchitectonics: a unifying theory. J Comp Neurol 1992;321:223–240. Copyright © Wiley-Liss, Inc. With permission of Wiley-Liss, Inc., a subsidiary of John Wiley & Sons, Inc.)

FORMATION OF NEUROECTODERM

The human brain is formed from the *neuroectoderm*, a placode of cells that are induced by the underlying notochord to differentiate from the ectoderm beginning at 18 days of gestation (see Figures 2.1, 2.2).[1] The nature of the inducible factor(s) and the genes involved in this process remain unknown. Candidate factors include the retinoids,[2,3] follistatin, and the *Noggin* gene product.[4] The molecular action of these molecules probably is similar to that of the retinoids that likely bind to a nuclear receptor to promote or suppress specific genes.[5] This signals the fate of cells and may control differentiation of cell lineages.[6]

NEURAL TUBE CLOSURE

Primary Neurulation

The neuroectoderm develops folds in the lateral aspects that begin to approximate in the region of the future medulla and begin to fuse at approximately 22 days' gestation (see Figures 2.1, 2.2). This closure, a process known as *neurulation*, results in a tube that continues to extend by the process of approximation of the neural folds in multiple locations rostrally and caudally until a complete neural tube is formed.[7] Final closure of the neural tube occurs at 24–28 days' gestation, with the latter period marking the end of caudal neural tube closure (future spinal cord).[8,9] The rostral neural tube, which closes at approximately 24 days' gestation,[10] serves as the foundation for further brain development; at 24–26 days, it resembles a cylinder that is filled with fluid and lined by primitive neuroepithelial cells (see Figure 2.1).

Although the specific molecules and genes involved in the processes of dorsal induction or neurulation in the human are unknown, clearly a combination of genetic and environmental factors leads to disorders of these processes. Studies in mice suggest that a codeletion of *Pax1*, a gene for a *transcriptional factor* (a molecule that induces a gene to transcribe its message [i.e., turns on a gene]) that mediates notochord signaling, and *Pdgfra*, the platelet-derived growth factor alpha gene, may lead to a spina bifida–like phenotype.[11]

Certain ethnic groups experience a higher incidence of neural tube closure defects than do others,[12] and genetic disorders with an apparent autosomal recessive inheritance that include neural tube defects have been described.[13] In addition, teratogens are involved in neural tube pathology. The most notable teratogens for the pediatrician and the neurologist are the anticonvulsants valproate and carbamazepine, each of which imposes a risk of 1–6% for a neural tube defect in offspring exposed in utero to these common drugs.[14] Whereas folate supplementation appears to prevent neural tube defects in large population studies,[15] this vitamin may or may not be protective when these disorders are associated with the aforementioned anticonvulsants.[16] Given the innocuous nature of short-term treatment with folate, it seems prudent to offer this vitamin to women of childbearing age who are on anticonvulsants.

Specific Neural Tube Defects

In the human, multiple genes and factors probably are involved in the pathogenesis of disorders of neural tube formation and closure. The human disorders of neural tube closure include craniorachischisis (a complete failure of neural tube closure along the entire neuraxis), anencephaly (a failure of anterior neural tube closure), myeloschisis (a failure of posterior neural tube closure), spina bifida (myelomeningocele, a failure of closure of a portion of posterior neural tube), and encephalocele (a partial defect in anterior neural tube closure). Because this chapter deals with those brain lesions that lead to cerebral palsy, we emphasize encephaloceles, the neural tube defects that may lead to lifelong deficits in brain function.

Encephaloceles

Encephaloceles vary in location, in the amount of brain involved, and therefore, in the clinical manifestations of the lesions. In most cases, the neural tube is closed, and the gyral pattern of the protruding brain appears normal. Most encephaloceles are occipital and midline; an occasional anterior or nasal encephalocele is noted in the western hemisphere. This pattern seems to be reversed in Asia, where the frequency of anterior encephaloceles surpasses that of posterior lesions.

Meckel's Syndrome

Meckel's syndrome, an autosomal recessive disorder that involves an occipital encephalocele, microcephaly, renal dysplasia (polycystic kidneys), polydactyly, and other malformations, has been linked to 17q21–24, very near the homeobox gene *HOXB6*. Though the gene for this disorder has not yet been ascertained, Meckel's syndrome may, at least in part, be a disorder of segmentation of the developing nervous system.[17] (See the discussion in Transcriptional Factors and Homeobox Genes.)

EMBRYONIC NERVOUS SYSTEM SEGMENTATION

Flexures of the rostral neural tube delineate the primary vesicles, which are designated as the hindbrain (rhombencephalon), midbrain (mesencephalon), and forebrain (prosencephalon). These primary vesicles then further subdivide into the secondary vesicles that later will form the adult brain structures. The hindbrain consists of the metencephalon and myelencephalon; these structures will become the pons, cerebellum, and medulla oblongata of the adult. The mesencephalon will become the midbrain of the adult. The forebrain is further divided into the telencephalon and the diencephalon. The telencephalon will become the cerebral hemispheres, and the diencephalon will become the thalamus and hypothalamus of the adult (see Figures 2.2, 2.3).

Transcriptional Factors and Homeobox Genes

Regional specification of the telencephalon is an important step in central nervous system development and is likely under the control of a number of genes that encode transcriptional factors. These genes were first described in *Drosophila* and are involved in the segmentation and regional specification of this fruit fly embryo.[18] Not surprisingly, the gene function in mammals differs considerably from that in fruit flies, but the general role of these genes appears to be that of regional specification of clones of cells destined to form structures in the mature animal.

Homeobox genes encode transcriptional factors with distinct sequences that participate in DNA binding. These *homeobox sequences* are so named because they were first identified in homeotic genes in *Drosophila*. The homeobox sequence is a helix-turn-helix protein with a specific geometry that determines its specificity for DNA. In *Drosophila*, at least two transcriptional factor–encoding homeobox genes, *empty spiracles* (*ems*) and *orthodenticle* (*otd*), have been shown to specify head structures.[19,20] In the rudimentary structures of mutant flies that are devoid of *ems* or of *otd*, the genes are not characteristic of the areas of the fruit fly head that these homeobox genes seem to specify. From this finding, researchers have concluded that the homeobox genes function as transcriptional regulators of gene expression: They are directors that signal the fate of clones of cells destined to form specific structures.

These genes have been described in mouse embryo development.[20,21] Transcriptional factor genes are appreciably homologous from *Drosophila* through mouse; many such genes encode proteins that differ by only two to three amino acids.[20,21] In the mouse, these genes appear to encode important positional information to the cells that are proliferating in specific regions of developing brain. *Emx1* is confined to the dorsal telencephalon at the time that regional specification of that area takes place.[20,21] *Emx2* is more globally expressed in the ventricular zone but, at later points of development, is preferentially expressed in dorsal telencephalon and diencephalon (see Figure 2-3).[21]

The *otd* gene from the fruit fly has homologs that are expressed also in a developmental pattern in the mouse. These mouse homologous genes, *Otx1* and *Otx2*, are expressed in the developing telencephalon in both a regionally and temporally specific pattern. *Otx1* is expressed in the dorsal and ventral regions of the telencephalon and in the diencephalon.[20] Less expression is seen in the mesencephalon. *Otx2* expression encompasses the *Otx1* expression zones and is more widespread. It appears to be expressed in all dorsal and ventral regions of the telencephalon and diencephalon and in the mesencephalon. Mice with *Otx1* deletions are epileptic, owing to small brains with abnormal cortical layering in the temporal lobes and perirhinal areas; they also have small hippocampi.[22] Therefore, one wonders whether similar patterns of cortical malformations in humans are due to a similar genetic mechanism.

Other genes for transcriptional factors have been described in the mouse. *Pax3, Pax5, Pax6, Dlx1, Dlx2, Dbx*, and the *Hox* genes are found in specific brain regions. In general, the *Pax* genes tend to be expressed in midbrain and the *Dlx* genes tend to be expressed in the ventral forebrain, ventral telencephalon, and dorsal telencephalon.[23] The *Hox* genes seem to specify the rhombomeres of the hindbrain.[24]

Furthermore, in an interesting link to the ventral inductive events described later, when applied to proliferating cells at critical times in development, the protein Sonic hedgehog can alter the expression of the homeobox genes.[23] This ties the inductive proteins to the expression of homeobox genes and gives a hint as to the mechanisms involved in inductive processes.

Disorders of Segmentation

Schizencephaly (cleft in brain) has been regarded by many as a migration abnormality. We include it in disorders of segmentation because the gene that is abnormal in the more severe and familial forms is a homeobox gene, *EMX2*.[25,26] Thus, this developmental disorder, at least in the more severe cases, appears to be a result of failure of regional specification of a clone of cells that are destined to be part of the cortical mantle.

The clefts in this disorder extend from the pia to the ventricle and are lined with a polymicrogyric gray matter (see the discussion in Polymicrogyria).[27] The pia and ependyma are usually in apposition, especially in severe cases. The defect is termed *open-lipped* if the cleft walls are separated by cerebrospinal fluid. It is regarded as *closed-lipped* if the walls are in contact with one another. These clefts may be unilateral or bilateral.[28]

The severity of the clinical presentation varies with the extent of cortical involvement.[28] Bilateral schizencephaly is associated with mental retardation and spastic cerebral palsy; affected patients often are microcephalic. Seizures almost always accompany severe lesions, especially the open-lipped and bilateral schizencephalic clefts. The exact frequency of seizures in patients with the less severe lesions is uncertain. Most patients in whom schizencephaly is diagnosed undergo neuroimaging because of seizure. Therefore, a bias in favor of a universal occurrence of seizure in this disorder is noted. Hence, patients with schizencephaly who do not have epilepsy might exist, but the malformation remains undetected because no imaging is done.

Seizure type and onset may vary in this disorder. Patients may experience focal or generalized seizures. Some will present with infantile spasms. The onset varies from infancy to the early adult years. Seizures may be easily controlled or may be recalcitrant to standard anticonvulsant therapy.

Improvements in neuroimaging have enhanced the recognition of these disorders and have broadened the spectrum of the radiographic appearance of schizencephalic lesions.[27-31] The lesions may occur in isolation or may be associated with other anomalies of brain development. An especially common association is made between septo-optic dysplasia (see Disorders of Ventral Induction) and schizencephaly, because as many as 50% of patients with septo-optic dysplasia also have schizencephaly.[32]

Disorders of segmentation likely represent a heterogeneous set of abnormalities of varying etiologies. One theory holds that an early (first-trimester) destructive event disturbs subsequent formation of the cortex. Another theory is that segmental failure occurs in the formation of a portion of the germinal matrix or in the migration of primitive neuroblasts. Certainly, the finding of mutations of the *EMX2* gene in some patients with the open-lipped form of schizencephaly supports the latter hypothesis. (See the preceding discussion in Transcriptional Factors and Homeobox Genes.)

VENTRAL INDUCTION

Normal Prosencephalon Division

The telencephalon is formed by division of a single fluid-filled structure (prosencephalon); the two vesicles formed in this division become the two cerebral hemispheres. The anterior portion of this division is induced by midline facial structures. Abnormalities of this induction lead to midline abnormalities of the brain such as holoprosencephaly, septo-optic dysplasia, agenesis of the corpus callosum, and agenesis of the septum pellucidum.[33] These disruptions of normal development occur before 42 days of gestation.

At present, the molecules responsible for ventral induction are unknown. A candidate molecule would have to be Sonic hedgehog, which was described first in *Drosophila* as a soluble factor that influences dorsoventral patterning of the developing embryo.[4,34] Sonic hedgehog is expressed in the notochord (also in ventral forebrain and floor plate),[4,34] interacts through at least one identified receptor (PTCH, a human homolog of patched),[35,36] and alters the expression of transcriptional factors (homeobox and other related gene products).[4]

Other molecules of interest in this inductive process are the retinoids, which are lipids capable of crossing membranes and have been shown to exist in gradients across embryos.[37] Retinoic acid can alter the pattern of transcriptional factors in neuroepithelial cells.[4] It can also downregulate Sonic hedgehog, perhaps explaining some of the midfacial defects seen in retinoid embryopathy.[38]

Disorders of Ventral Induction

Holoprosencephaly

Holoprosencephaly is a heterogeneous disorder of ventral induction that results from a failure of the prosencephalic vesicle to cleave normally. Three forms of this disorder have been described: alobar, semilobar, and lobar.[39,40] In the alobar form, the telencephalic vesicle completely fails to divide, producing a single horseshoe-shaped ventricle, sometimes with a dorsal cyst, fused thalami, and a malformed cortex. In the semilobar form, the interhemispheric fissure is present posteriorly, but the frontal and, sometimes, parietal lobes continue across the midline.[41] In the lobar form, only minor changes may be seen: The anterior falx and the septum pellucidum usually are absent, the frontal lobes and horns are hypoplastic, and the genu of the corpus callosum may be abnormal.

Holoprosencephaly is associated with a spectrum of midline facial defects. These include cyclopia, in which there is a single central eye and a supraorbital proboscis; ethmocephali, in which the nose is replaced by a proboscis located above hypoteloric eyes; cebocephaly, in which hypotelorism and a nose with a single nostril are seen; and premaxillary agenesis, with hypotelorism, a flat nose, and a midline cleft lip.[42]

Only children who have the lobar form are known to survive for more than a few months. An infant affected with the severe form is microcephalic (unless aqueduct stenosis and hydrocephalus are present), hypotonic, and visually inattentive.[41] In infants with the less severe forms of holoprosencephaly, myoclonic seizures frequently develop and, if the infant survives, autonomic dysfunction, failure to thrive, psychomotor retardation, and atonic or spastic cerebral palsy often are present. Some infants with the lobar form may be only mildly affected and, for example, present as a relatively mild spastic diplegia. Pituitary defects may be associated with these malformations and may result in neuroendocrine dysfunction.[43]

Holoprosencephaly has been reported to be associated with maternal diabetes,[44] retinoic acid, cytomegalovirus, and rubella.[45] Chromosomal abnormalities associated with this disorder include trisomies 13 and 18; duplications in 3p, 13q, and 18q; and deletions in 2p, 7q, 13q, and 18q.[46] An autosomal dominant form exists in which the mutation is in the Sonic hedgehog gene (see earlier discussion of homeobox genes and their inducers in Transcriptional Factors and Homeobox Genes) on chromosome 7.[47] In this form, the clinical features vary. In its mildest form, presence of a single central incisor or a choroid fissure coloboma may be the only clinical manifestation of autosomal dominant holoprosencephaly.[48]

Septo-Optic Dysplasia

Septo-optic dysplasia (de Morsier syndrome) is a disorder characterized by absence of the septum pellucidum, optic nerve hypoplasia, and hypothalamic dysfunction, and may be associated with agenesis of the corpus callosum. This disorder should be considered in any patient who exhibits at least two of these brain abnormalities. Septo-optic dysplasia also appears to involve prosencephalic cleavage and development of anterior telencephalic structures.[49] As mentioned previously, 50% of these patients may have schizencephaly.[32] Magnetic resonance imaging (MRI) is the most useful neuroimaging modality for evaluating these patients, though the cortical malformation usually is detectable on computed tomographic (CT) scanning (Figure 2.5).

Patients may present with a visual disturbance (poor vision or optic nerve hypoplasia on routine ophthalmologic examination), seizures, mental retardation, hemiparesis (especially if associated with schizencephaly), quadriparesis, or hypothalamic dysfunction. Hypothalamic dysfunction may involve growth, thyroid, or antidiuretic hormone function. The consideration of septo-optic dysplasia necessitates an evaluation of the hypothalamic-pituitary axis because as many as 60% of the children with this disorder might exhibit evidence of a disturbance of this system.[50]

The etiology of this malformation is unknown. A pair of dizygotic twins with septo-optic dysplasia has been described, suggesting that the disorder might be the result of an in utero insult.[51] Numerous risk factors and teratogens have been associated with this disorder, including young maternal age, maternal diabetes,[52] and use of anticonvulsant drugs, phencyclidine, cocaine, and alcohol.

NEURONAL AND GLIAL PROLIFERATION

Normal Cell Proliferation

Lining the ventricles of the newly formed telencephalon is a single layer of pseudostratified neuroepithelium. These neuroepithelial cells will give rise to the neurons and glia of the mature brain. This primitive neuroepithelium undergoes a series of divisions until the appropriate complement of neurons and glia are formed. These divisions occur as cells move from the ventricle to the future pial

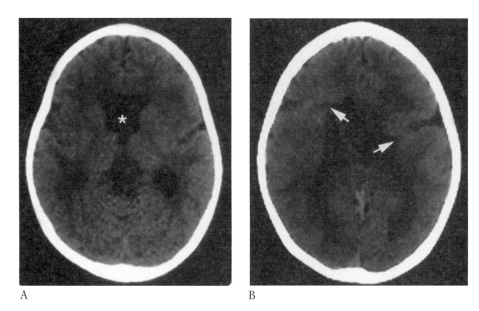

A   B

Figure 2.5 Ventral induction and segmentation defects. Axial head computed tomographic scan of patient with septo-optic dysplasia. A. Absence of the septum pellucidum. An asterisk marks the region where the septum is usually apparent. B. In the same patient, a more superior axial scan shows bilateral closed-lipped schizencephaly (*arrows*).

surface of the brain. Neuroepithelial processes extend from the ventricular surface to the pial surface, and the nuclei of the primitive neuroepithelial cells move from the cortical surface in a premitotic phase to a mitotic phase near the ventricle. Cells divide at the most ventricular aspects of the developing telencephalon and, after division, move back toward the pial surface. The pial processes of neuroepithelial cells near the ventricle often will detach from the cortical surface before a new cycle begins.

Neuroepithelial cells divide in so-called proliferative units such that each unit will undergo a specific number of divisions resulting in the appropriate number of cells for the future cortex.[53] An estimated 10–18 billion cells are generated in this process of neuronal proliferation.[54] Abnormalities in the number of proliferative units or in the total number of divisions can lead to disorders of brain manifested by abnormal brain size and, therefore, an unusually small or large head circumference. Two such disorders resulting in small head size—radial microbrain and microcephaly vera—are believed to result from abnormalities of this phase of neurodevelopment.[55] Disorders in which too many cells are generated in the proliferative phase result in megalencephaly (large brain) or, if proliferative events go awry on only one side of the developing cortex, hemimegalencephaly.

Once the appropriate complement of cells is generated in the proliferative phase, the cells that will become the neurons of the cerebral cortex become postmitotic and are referred to as *neuroblasts*. This terminology is confusing, given that cells in other parts of the body that still have mitotic capabilities are designated as *blasts*. Neuroblasts do not have a mitotic potential and, though not completely differentiated into neurons, they are destined to differentiate thus.

The genes and molecules involved in regulating the proliferative cycles in human brain formation are likely similar to those involved in other species. This cell cycle in brain can be divided into a number of distinct phases: mitosis (M), first gap (G_1), deoxyribonucleic acid synthesis (S), and second gap (G_2).[56] These phases appear to be regulated by key molecules to check the advancement of proliferation. Some cells enter a resting state (G_0) that they maintain throughout life. Others temporarily enter this phase to await a specific signal to proliferate later. Probably the G_1-S transition regulation determines the number of cell cycles and, therefore, the complement of cells that will make brain.[53]

Cyclins are proteins that appear to be involved in cell cycle control. These proteins are activating subunits of cyclin-dependent kinases. Cyclins D1, D2, D3, C, and E seem to control the key transition of a cell to the G_1-S interface; this transition is regarded as important because it commits a cell to division.[57–59] Cyclin E seems to be the gatekeeper for this transition and is essential for movement from G_1 to S phase.[60,61] The S phase of the cell cycle is regulated by cyclin A, which seems to persist well into the cellular expression of cyclins B1 and B2, markers of the G_2 phase of the cell cycle. The latter cyclins peak in expression at the G_2-M transition and, therefore, probably regulate the mitotic phase of the cell cycle. Mitosis cannot be completed until cyclins B1 and B2 have been degraded.[62,63]

These cyclins and their respective cyclin-dependent kinases are modulated by a number of molecules. The retinoblastoma protein (pRb) and p53 are known for their tumor suppressor functions; they exert these functions by regulating G_1-S transition cyclins D and E, respectively.[64–66] Mice that are deficient in pRb show defects in neuronal proliferation.[67] Proteins p21, p16, and p27 serve as cyclin-dependent kinase inhibitors. The protein p21 is activated by p53 to inhibit cyclin E–dependent kinase (G_1-S transition), whereas p27 inhibits the cyclin D–dependent kinases (M-G_1 transition).[66,68–70]

How do these cyclins respond to cues to regulate the cell cycle? Good evidence suggests that this is accomplished by cell-cell contact interactions.[71] Probably transcriptional regulation of the genes for the cyclins in part determines their expression.[72] A group of transcriptional factor–encoding genes, the *sox* family, likely plays some role in this process.[73] The cyclins are short-lived proteins that are subject to rapid degradation by proteases[74]; therefore, transcriptional regulation of the respective genes is likely to explain regional expression of the cyclins in the developing brain[75,76] and regional differences in cell cycle regulation.[77]

The number of cells that finally make up the mature nervous system is less than that generated during proliferation. Cells appear not only to be programmed to proliferate during development but to contain programs that lead to cell death.[78,79] The term *apoptosis* (from the Greek, meaning "a falling off") has been applied to this programmed loss of cells.[80] Characteristic of cells undergoing this programmed death are shrunken cell bodies, membrane vesicles, condensed DNA, and cleaved DNA.[80,81] The deliberate and orderly destruction of DNA appears to be responsible, at least in part, for denying the dying cell the opportunity to proliferate.

The genetics of apoptosis are best characterized in the simple nematode *Caenorhabditis elegans*. Approximately 10% of the cells generated during development of this worm will undergo programmed cell death. Mutations leading to smaller or larger numbers of surviving cells result in smaller or larger nematodes, respectively. The molecular characterization of these mutations has led to identification of a number of "death" genes and of genes that prevent apoptosis.[82] The mammalian counterparts of the nematode death genes encode enzymes that are cysteine aspartate–specific proteases, also known as *caspases*.[83] At least one function of such enzymes is that of an interleukin-converting enzyme. These enzymes have been shown to promote neuronal death; in addition, when an animal is produced without caspase 3, a larger than normal brain results.

Disorders of Neuronal and Glial Proliferation

Microcephaly

Although primary microcephaly may be a normal variant, in the classic symptomatic form, clinical and radiologic examinations reveal a receding forehead, flat occiput, early closure of fontanelles, and hair anomalies such as multiple hair whirls and an anterior cowlick. Neuroimaging may show small frontal and occipital lobes, open opercula, and an uncovered cerebellum.[39] The cortex may appear thickened and the white matter reduced. Histologic examination may show a reduction of cell layers in some areas and an increase in others.[84]

Neurologic findings also vary. Only mild psychomotor retardation may be noted, sometimes associated with pyramidal signs, or more severe retardation, seizures, and an atonic cerebral palsy might be evidenced. Primary microcephaly is seen in many genetic syndromes and, in its isolated form, may be autosomal recessive.[85] Autosomal dominant and X-linked transmission has also been reported.[86,87] *Microcephaly vera* is the term applied to this genetic form of microcephaly. Affected children present with a head circumference that is usually more than 4 standard deviations below the mean, hypotonia, and psychomotor retardation. They later show mental retardation, dyspraxias, motor incoordination and, sometimes, seizures. On histologic examination, neurons in layers II and III are depleted.[55]

Destructive lesions of the forming brain, such as those caused by teratogens and by infectious agents, also may result in microcephaly. Teratogens of note are alcohol, cocaine, and hyperphenylalaninemia (maternal phenylketonuria).[88] Intense radiation exposure in the first trimester can cause microcephaly.[89] Microcephaly and intracranial calcifications are likely due to well-recognized in utero infections caused by cytomegalovirus, toxoplasmosis, or the human immunodeficiency virus.[10]

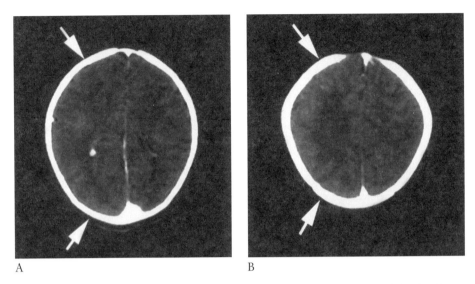

A   B

Figure 2.6 Hemimegalencephaly. Axial computed tomographic scans of the head in a patient presenting with a spastic left hemiparesis and seizures early in life. A. Arrows point to a larger right hemisphere with a thickened, disordered cortical mantle. B. A more superior axial scan of the same patient depicted in A.

Megalencephaly and Hemimegalencephaly

The terms *megalencephaly* and *hemimegalencephaly* refer to disorders in which the brain volume is greater than normal (not owing to the abnormal storage of material); usually, the enlarged brain is accompanied by macrocephaly, or a large head. Although considered by some to be a migration disorder, the increase in brain size in these disorders appears to be attributable to errors in neuroepithelial proliferation, as the microscopical appearance of the brain is that of an increase in number of cells (both neurons and glia) and in cell size.[27,90–93]

Typically, patients are noted to have large heads at birth and may manifest an accelerated head growth in the first few months of life.[94,95] Children with megalencephaly or hemimegalencephaly may come to medical attention when presenting with seizures, a developmental disorder (mental retardation), hemihypertrophy, or a hemiparesis (opposite the affected hemisphere). Seizures vary both in onset and in type and usually are the most problematic symptom, sometimes necessitating hemispherectomy or callosotomy (Figure 2.6).[93]

Approximately 50% of patients with linear sebaceous nevus syndrome have hemimegalencephaly.[96–98] Many patients with hypomelanosis of Ito also have hemimegalencephaly.[99] The neuropathologic and clinical pictures in these conditions appear to be identical to the isolated hemimegalencephalies.

Microscopical examination of the affected brain usually reveals an increase in cellularity, large bizarre neurons, enlarged glia, cortical lamination defects, and heterotopias. The cortex usually is thickened, and malformed neurons are noted. Interestingly, the cytologic basis for the increase in brain size may be the abundant cytoplasm of individual cells.[91] The genetic basis of these disorders remains poorly understood, but they appear to be sporadic in occurrence.

NEURONAL DIFFERENTIATION

Normal Differentiation

At the time of neuronal differentiation the neural tube consists of four consecutive layers: (1) the ventricular zone, the innermost layer, which gives rise to neurons and all the glia of the central nervous system; (2) the subventricular zone, which is the adjacent, more superficial layer and is the staging area from which postmitotic neuroblasts begin to differentiate and to migrate; (3) the intermediate zone, which is the contiguous, more superficial zone and which is destined to become the cortical plate and the future cerebral cortex; and (4) the marginal zone, which is the outermost zone and is composed of the cytoplasmic extensions of ventricular neuroblasts, corticopetal fibers, and the terminal processes of radial glia (which, at this time, are completely spanning the neural tube).

Differentiation of neuroepithelial cells begins in the subventricular layer at approximately gestational day 26. The neuroepithelial cells were destined to become neurons at the time of the final mitotic division of the neuroepithelial cell precursor, before moving to the subventricular zone, the staging area for neuronal migration. At this point, these neuroblasts lack electrically polarized membranes as would commonly be seen in neurons.[100] The fate of the neuroblast probably is determined before this final mitosis has occurred, as the postmitotic neuroblast has the properties of many neuron types.[101] The older, larger pyramidal cells are the first cells to be born and probably differentiate early in order to act as targets in the migration of the nervous system.[102]

No disorders of neuronal differentiation have yet been identified, though some disorders may be found to fit into this category. For instance, premature neuroblast differentiation could result in an inability of these cells to migrate and thus could be manifest as a migration abnormality. The megalencephaly and hemimegalencephaly syndromes may yet be found to be the results of disturbances in differentiation, as discussed earlier.

Disorders such as tuberous sclerosis, in which both tumor development and areas of migration abnormalities are seen, also might be a differentiation disorder. The brain manifestations of this disorder include hamartomas of the subependymal layer (tubers), areas of cortical migration abnormalities (cortical dysgenesis), and the development of giant-cell astrocytomas in upwards of 5% of patients.[103] Two genes for tuberous sclerosis have been identified: TSC1 (encodes for Hamartin) has been localized to 9q34[104] and TSC2 (encodes for Tuberin) has been localized to 16p13.3.[105] TSC2 has been cloned and is a putative growth-suppressing gene that encodes a 175-kd protein known as *Tuberin*.[106] TSC1 encodes a 130-kd protein, Hamartin, the function of which is unknown.[107] The frequency of gene abnormalities in tuberous sclerosis patients has been estimated to be almost equally distributed between TSC1 and TSC2.

NEURONAL MIGRATION

Normal Migration

At the most rostral end of the neural tube in the 40- to 41-day-old fetus, the first mature neuron begins the complex trip to the cortical surface. These first neurons are the *Cajal-Retzius cells*, which are the major neurons of the cortex by day 43. Cajal-Retzius cells, along with corticopetal nerve fibers, form a so-called preplate.[108] These cells will be the major cell type of the most superficial layer of the cerebral cortex, layer I. At the same time that the Cajal-Retzius cells are arriving at the most superficial layer of cortex, other pioneering neurons differentiate and form a so-called subplate.[109] These subplate neurons receive input from thalamic structures. Some researchers propose that these thalamic inputs define areas of cortex for specific functions (e.g., visual, motor). The pioneering neurons of the subplate and the preplate act as the police officers of the developing nervous system and define the limits of the developing cortical plate. Most of the cells of the subplate will die postnatally in a programmed cell death (see earlier discussion of apoptosis).[110,111]

Near the end of the proliferative phase of neurodevelopment, billions of neuroblasts are poised to begin the trip to the cortical surface and to form the cortical plate. This tremendous number of neurons accomplishes this task by attaching to and migrating along radial glial in a process known as *radial migration* (Figure 2.7).[112] The radial glia extend from the ventricle to the cortical surface. In the process of migration, the deepest layer of the cortical plate forms before the other layers. Therefore, the first neurons to arrive at the future cortical plate are layer VI neurons. More superficial layers of cortex then are formed such that the neurons of layer V migrate and pass the neurons of layer VI; the same process occurs for layers IV, III, and II. The cortex therefore is formed in an inside-out fashion.[110,112,113]

The molecules and the interactions between neurons and glia are extremely important in this process of neuronal migration. Reelin, the protein involved in the migration mouse mutant, reeler, appears to be one such important molecule. Reelin appears to promote an attachment of neurons to glia and, when abnormal, as in the mouse mutant reeler, it leads to an inverted cortex such that the most superficial neurons are the first to arrive and the later-arriving neurons are deeper. This mouse mutant cortex appears to be due to an abnormally adhesive interaction between neurons and glia.[108] Additional molecules that appear to act in an adhesive manner are laminin, astrotactin, L1 antigen, fibronectin, neural cell adhesion molecules (NCAM), and adhesion molecule on glia (AMOG).[114]

The molecular mechanisms for the movement of cells in the process of migration are now being elucidated. Neuroblast movement on radial glia involves an extension of a leading process, a neural outgrowth having an orderly

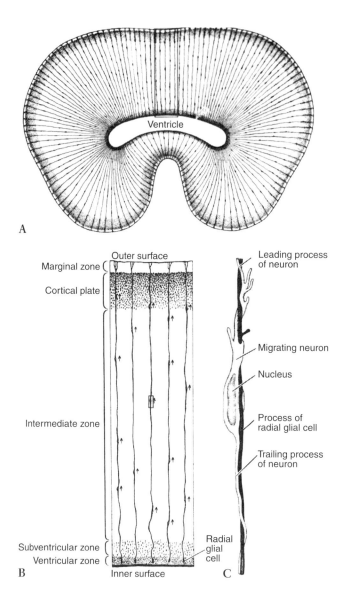

Figure 2.7 Neuronal migration. A. A Golgi-stained, thick transverse section of a fetal monkey brain showing the radially directed, spoke-like glia (radial glia). B. Column from the transverse section depicted in A (demarcated with a rectangle and magnified) that shows more cellular detail. Neuroblasts are seen to be migrating radially from the subventricular zone, through the intermediate zone, to the cortical plate. Note the paucity of cells in the marginal zone (layer I) and the well-defined boundary between the cortical plate and that zone. C. Neuroblast (demarcated by a rectangle in the previous figure and magnified) in close apposition to a radial glial process. (Reprinted from WM Cowan. The development of the brain. Sci Am 1979;241:124. With permission from Scientific American Publishers.)

arrangement of microtubules. *Microtubules* are cytoskeletal elements with a polymerizing (positive) end and a depolymerizing (negative) end. They serve as the major structural element that gives shape to long neural processes. When microtubules depolymerize, or slide, long neural processes are shortened. Shortening of the leading process of migrating neurons has been associated with forward movement of the soma of migrating neurons in vitro. Cytoskeletal changes in leading processes have been purported to be responsible for this shortening and somal movement.

A possible mode of movement in neuronal migration on glia would be the attachment of the neuroblast to a matrix secreted by either the glia or the neuroblasts. This matrix is likely to consist of the aforementioned adhesion molecules. The attachment of the neuroblast would be through *integrin* receptors, cytoskeletal-linking membrane-bound recognition sites for adhesion molecules. That attachment serves as a stronghold for the leading process and soma of the neuroblast. Shortening of the leading process owing to depolymerization or shifts of microtubules results in movement of the soma relative to the attachment points. This theory of movement of neuroblasts also must include a phase of detachment from the matrix at certain integrin receptors, so that the neuroblast can navigate successfully along as much as 6 cm of developing cortex (the maximum estimated distance of radial migration of a neuroblast in the human). Finally, the movement of cells must stop at the appropriate location, the boundary between layer I and the forming cortical plate. Therefore, some stop signal must be given in order for the migrating neuroblast to detach from the radial glia and begin to differentiate into a cortical neuron.

Other forms of neuronal migration occur in brain development. Some evidence exists for a tangential migration of neurons in the cortex and in the early granule cell migration in the cerebellum. A so-called chain migration of neurons on other neurons occurs in the formation of the olfactory bulbs.[115] In this chain migration, neuroblasts from the subventricular zone of the lateral ventricle migrate to the olfactory bulb through a sheath of glial cells, but the actual migration occurs on other neurons.

Migration Disorders

Many clinical entities are associated with neuronal migration disorders. In some, abnormalities are limited to the nervous system but, in others, malformations involving other organs also are present. In this section, we briefly review some of the syndromes in both categories. The responsible gene has been identified in some of these disorders, and new genes are being identified regularly. Though the role of the gene product in producing many of these migration disorders may not yet be entirely clear, the disorders provide important clues to mechanisms that are responsible for normal brain development.

Advanced neuroimaging techniques, particularly MRI, have allowed the recognition of major migration disorders. Some of these disorders are associated with typical clinical features that might alert the clinician to the presence of such abnormalities even before imaging is obtained. In other disorders, the clinical features are so varied that a strong correlation between imaging and clinical presentation does not exist. In this section, we review syndromes that have a recognizable imaging or clinical picture.

Lissencephaly

Lissencephaly (smooth brain) refers to the external appearance of the cerebral cortex in those disorders in which a neuronal migration aberration leads to an improper number of neurons at the surface of the cortex (see Figure 2.2). Gyri and sulci do not form because the cortical-cortical attractive forces that result from strong associations are decreased, owing to improper axon pathways (i.e., the targets for synapses are malpositioned). At least two types of lissencephaly have been identified: type I, or classic, lissencephaly and type II, or cobblestone, lissencephaly. This classification is based on both the external appearance of the brain and the underlying histology.

Type I (Classic) Lissencephaly Type I lissencephaly most often accompanies the *Miller-Dieker syndrome*.[116–119] In this disorder, an interruption of radial migration of neurons appears to take place at approximately 15–17 weeks of gestation. The cortex is described as being composed of a four-layer sequence,[120–122] consisting of an outer molecular layer (layer 1), which is similar to normal layer I; a cellular layer (layer 2) (similar to layers II–VI of the normal cortical plate); a cell-sparse zone (layer 3); and a heterotopic zone of neurons that have been arrested in neuronal migration (layer 4).[120,122,123] The most extensive layer in this lissencephalic sequence is layer 4, the heterotopic zone. The neurons and cells of this zone have the appearance of cells that would normally be in layers II–IV of the normal cortical plate. Therefore, the later waves of neuronal migration that form the outer cortical plate appear to be those most affected by the migration abnormality in this disorder. The cortex is very orderly in its appearance and resembles the fetal cortex at approximately 13–15 weeks of gestation; the brain remains in this configuration throughout life.

Hallmarks on imaging are a lack of opercularization (covering of the sylvian fissure), large ventricles with colpocephaly (fetal-like configuration of the occipital horns), and agyria or pachygyria (Figure 2.8).[124] The corpus callosum is almost never absent, and the posterior fossa has a normal appearance on neuroimaging. Head size typically is in the low-normal range at birth, but patients develop microcephaly owing to a decreased rate of brain growth over the first year of life. Most patients with this disorder will develop seizures within this first year, and more than 80% of them will have infantile spasms. This seizure frequency is far greater than that seen in other neuronal migration disorders.[119]

In the Miller-Dieker syndrome, facial dysmorphism, cardiac abnormalities (40%), sacral abnormalities (70%), deep palmar creases and, in male patients, genital abnormalities (70%) may be seen. The sacral abnormalities include deep sacral dimples, sacral pits, and sacral tracks.[119] Facial abnormalities include upturned nares, a short nose, a thin, "pouty" upper lip, a long philtrum, micrognathia, and bitemporal hollowing. Though the bitemporal hollowing may be the result of the underlying brain abnormality and thus a conformation of the skull to the underlying malformed brain, the other facial features would be difficult to explain on the basis of the brain abnormality alone. Therefore, these abnormalities are believed to result from deficits of genes near the lissencephaly gene on the seventeenth chromosome.[125] Larger deletions of the distal short arm of chromosome 17 appear to result in the full

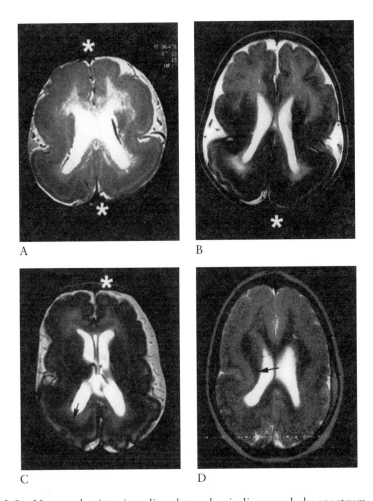

Figure 2.8 Neuronal migration disorders: classic lissencephaly spectrum. Representative axial T$_2$-weighted head magnetic resonance imaging scans from patients with brain malformations in the classic or type I lissencephaly spectrum. A. Grade 2, type I lissencephaly in a male patient with hypotonic cerebral palsy, profound mental retardation, and seizures that were difficult to control. Asterisks are near areas of agyria and thickened cellular layers. This patient has no apparent deletion of *LIS1* by fluorescent in situ hybridization. B. Grade 3, type I lissencephaly in a male patient with hypotonic cerebral palsy, profound mental retardation, infantile spasms, and a known *LIS1* deletion. Note that the agyria and the thickened cellular layers are worse posteriorly (*asterisk*). C. Grade 5, type I lissencephaly spectrum in a male patient with hypotonic cerebral palsy, mental retardation, and no apparent deletion of *LIS1*. Diffuse pachygyria is evident, with a thickened cellular layer that is worse anteriorly (*asterisk*) and a subcortical band posteriorly (*black arrow*). D. Grade 6, type I lissencephaly, or subcortical band heterotopia (double cortex), in a female patient with partial seizures and mental retardation. The black arrow points to a subcortical band. The cortical surface appears to be malformed in this patient.

Miller-Dieker phenotype, whereas microdeletions of just the lissencephaly gene, *LIS1* result in isolated lissencephaly.[126,127] Therefore, a deletion in the lissencephaly gene appears to be sufficient for the brain abnormalities, but perhaps other genes must be deleted for the full phenotypic manifestations of the Miller-Dieker syndrome to be seen.

Miller-Dieker lissencephaly is one of the migration disorders of brain in which the responsible genetic defect has been identified. By both molecular and cytogenetic techniques, deletions in the terminal portion of one arm of chromosome 17 can be found in approximately 90% of Miller-Dieker lissencephaly cases.[128] These patients typically have dysmorphic features and other congenital anomalies (see earlier discussion). The deletions of the terminal part of chromosome 17 in these cases have included microdeletions,[128–130] ring 17 chromosome,[131] pericentric inversions,[132] and a partial monosomy of 17p13.3.[128,133] These genetic abnormalities often are the result of an inherited unbalanced translocation from a parent with a balanced translocation involving this region of chromosome 17; multiple mechanisms of inheritance similar to this have been described for this disorder.[128] Of course, a parent with a balanced translocation is at a greatly increased risk of having another child with Miller-Dieker lissencephaly. In families that are affected in this manner, screening with amniocentesis can be performed in subsequent pregnancies.

To enhance detection of microdeletions for this lissencephaly locus, *fluorescent in situ hybridization* (FISH) techniques have been developed with markers for chromosome 17 and for the region near this gene for lissencephaly. By this technique, a conserved region near the centromere on chromosome 17 is labeled with a fluorescent marker, and another fluorescent marker is used to label the lissencephaly region. In patients with lissencephaly due to deletions of the chromosome 17 gene, FISH may reveal lack of fluorescence at the lissencephaly locus.

Some patients with *isolated lissencephaly* (no facial, skeletal, or cardiac abnormalities) also have deletions (often submicroscopical) of the terminal portion of the short arm of chromosome 17.[134,135] Therefore, some researchers suspected that within one deleted region of chromosome 17 was a gene that, when deleted, was sufficient to result in the lissencephaly phenotype. In 1993, the human gene for this form of lissencephaly was identified as *LIS1*.[125] As microdeletions of one arm of chromosome 17 appear to be sufficient to result in isolated lissencephaly, this disease most likely is caused by a haplo-insufficiency of this gene and its protein product.

The protein encoded by *LIS1* has 99% homology to a 45-kD subunit of a bovine brain platelet-activating factor acetylhydrolase.[136,137] Subsequently, depletion of this protein has been demonstrated in the brains of patients with Miller-Dieker syndrome and with isolated lissencephaly.[138] Interestingly, whereas the message for *Lis1* is expressed ubiquitously, the *LIS1* protein product has been localized to the neuropile, Cajal-Retzius cells, and ventricular neuroepithelium at the time of human neuronal migration.[139]

Therefore, this form of lissencephaly appears to be the result of a deficiency of a brain enzyme that hydrolyzes and inactivates platelet-activating factor. At this point, the manner in which a deficiency of a component of this enzyme and, therefore, a probable accumulation or elevated level of platelet-activating factor during neurodevelopment leads to a migration abnormality is not understood. Hints of a role for platelet-activating factor in this disorder come from observations of this messenger promoting neurite outgrowth in neurohybrid cells and causing growth cone collapse and neurite withdrawal in primary hippocampal and cerebellar cultures.[140,141] Given these effects, this lipid messenger probably somehow is linked to intracellular signaling systems, such as the nonreceptor kinases (tyrosine or serine-threonine) and phosphatases, which have been shown to participate in morphologic changes in developing neural processes.[142] Platelet-activating factor also might activate genes that are important in the process of neuronal migration, as do the retinoids (see Ventral Induction). Candidate genes for induction would be such adhesion molecules as astrotactin and NCAM.

X-linked lissencephaly looks nearly identical to the *LIS1* deletion form of this disorder: Patients have classic lissencephaly, and the neurologic presentation is the same. However, the skeletal and other anomalies seen in the Miller-Dieker syndrome are not noted in this form of lissencephaly. In addition, X-linked lissencephaly occurs mostly in boys.[86,143] Girls who are heterozygous for the same gene have band heterotopia. Women with band heterotopia have been noted to give birth to boys with lissencephaly.[144]

The *X-linked lissencephaly–band heterotopia syndrome* has been linked to Xq22.3.[145,146] In female patients, the less severe phenotype probably is attributable to random lyonization of the X chromosome, such that in a variable percentage of cells, normal gene expression is seen and, in the remaining cells, the gene for lissencephaly is expressed. Whether the abnormal X chromosome is expressed in the radial glia or in the migratory neuroblasts is not yet clear, but it appears that this is a cell-autonomous disorder. In other words, the cell expressing the abnormal X chromosome manifests aberrant migration or disturbed substrate on which cells can migrate.

The band heterotopia or double-cortex syndrome is a unique form of a neuronal migration defect that almost exclusively occurs in girls.[147,148] In this disorder, a circumferential, thick band of tissue is isointense with cerebral gray matter located within what should be the white matter of the hemispheres (see Figure 2.8). This band is most obvious in the frontocentroparietal regions. The inner and outer margins at its interface with the adjacent white matter usually are smooth. The overlying gyral appearance may vary from normal cortex to a thickened layer. This anomaly represents incomplete neuronal migration. The exact mechanism is unclear, but possibilities include a lack of separation of the migrating neuron from the radial fiber or an arrest on the path to a normal cortical location. Other possible mechanisms might be a block of migrating neurons by other neurons or a failure of chemotaxis. A brain biopsy performed in one patient showed well-preserved lamination in cortical layers I–IV.[148] Layers V–VI were not clearly separated and layer VI merged with the underlying U-fibers of the white matter. Beneath the white matter was a coalescent cluster of large, nonlaminated, well-differentiated neurons.

Patients with band heterotopia typically present with seizures and a developmental disorder. The seizure type is variable, and the onset of epilepsy usually is between 2 months and 11 years of age. Patients may present with infantile spasms or, even though the migration abnormality is diffuse, some patients may present with focal seizures. Control of the epilepsy varies, some patients being controlled with monotherapy and others being entirely refractory to all agents.[148,149]

Most patients with the X-linked lissencephaly–band heterotopia syndrome have impaired intellectual development that ranges from severe retardation to low-normal IQs; one girl had an IQ of 91.[148] Generally, individuals with this syndrome are less impaired than are patients with other diffuse neuronal migration defects such as lissencephaly. Patients in whom seizures are of later onset generally have less developmental impairment. Neurologic findings include mild dysarthria and mild bilateral pyramidal syndromes.[86,143,144]

Type II (Cobblestone) Lissencephaly In type II lissencephaly, the brain may have a smooth appearance or may exhibit polymicrogyria and pachygyria. The underlying cortical histology is that of a bizarre arrangement of neurons. Typically, in the most affected areas, normal cortical plate formation is not evident. Rather, bizarre whirls of cells are found. In addition, cells seem to penetrate the molecular layer and may spill into the subarachnoid space. This deposition of neurons in the subarachnoid space imparts a cobblestone street–like appearance to the brain surface; thus, the term *cobblestone lissencephaly* has been used to describe the cortex in these disorders. Whereas, in type I lissencephaly, neurons appear to begin to obey the rules of neuronal migration but then fail to accomplish their task, in type II lissencephaly no rules seem to be obeyed.

Despite the widespread cortical abnormalities, only one-third of patients develop seizures. The typical presentation is that of a child with marked hypotonia, macrocephaly, and eye abnormalities. Depending on the brain and muscle involvement, this disorder may or may not be compatible with life. Long-term survival is rare.

Syndromes accompanying type II lissencephaly include the Walker-Warburg syndrome, HARD±E (*h*ydrocephalus, *a*gyria, *r*etinal *d*ysplasia, with or without *e*ye [anterior chamber] abnormalities) syndrome, muscle-eye-brain disease, and Fukuyama muscular dystrophy. These disorders have been suspected of being the result of a single genetic defect with varying phenotypes, perhaps even among family members. However, some evidence points to a depletion of muscle merosin in Fukuyama muscular dystrophy and, though the muscle merosin depletion is not a primary deficiency, its presence in the Walker-Warburg patients perhaps finally distinguishes these syndromes as distinct entities.[150]

All these syndromes probably are accompanied by muscle abnormalities; the most extreme muscle involvement is in the Fukuyama muscular dystrophy patients. In the Walker-Warburg syndrome, the muscle abnormalities may or may not be apparent.[151]

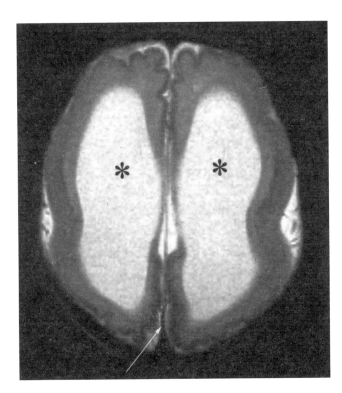

Figure 2.9 Neuronal migration disorders: cobblestone lissencephaly. T_2-Weighted axial head magnetic resonance imaging scan from a patient with Walker-Warburg syndrome. Note the massive hydrocephalus (*asterisks*), smooth cortical surface, and thickened falx (*white arrow*). If one were to look at this brain pathologically, the surface would appear pebbled. (Scan LP97-063 courtesy of Dr. William B. Dobyns and the Lissencephaly Project.)

The Walker-Warburg, muscle-eye-brain, and HARD±E syndromes are likely all varying degrees of the same entity. Abnormalities that may or may not be seen in these disorders include muscle aberrations (as just mentioned), ocular anterior chamber abnormalities, retinal dysplasias (abnormal electroretinogram and visual evoked responses), hydrocephalus (usually of an obstructive type), and encephaloceles. The Walker-Warburg syndrome might be diagnosed even if the ocular examination and muscle biopsies are normal. On MRI, an abnormal white matter signal and a thickened falx suggest the Walker-Warburg diagnosis (Figure 2.9). Neuroimaging of the muscle-eye-brain disorders might reveal focal white matter abnormalities.

Fukuyama muscular dystrophy is distinguished from the Walker-Warburg–like syndromes by the severity of the muscular dystrophy. This disorder is seen more often in Japan than in the Western hemisphere, probably because it is the result of a founder mutation. Patients typically present with evidence of a neuronal migration defect, hypotonia, and depressed reflexes.

To date, no gene for type II lissencephaly has been identified. A depletion of merosin (laminin type II alpha), an extracellular matrix glycoprotein with a possible role in neural adhesion, has been described in muscle of patients with Fukuyama muscular dystrophy who may have type II lissencephaly. However, this depletion might be a consequence of the dystrophic process and not a primary abnormality related to the disease. Nonetheless, the merosin depletion seems to distinguish Fukuyama muscular dystrophy from the Walker-Warburg–like syndromes,[150] all of which are associated with type II lissencephaly. Furthermore, genetic linkage of Fukuyama muscular dystrophy to 9q31–33 should lead to a final distinction between this disorder and Walker-Warburg–like syndromes.[152,153]

Kallmann Syndrome

The Kallmann syndrome is an X-linked disorder characterized by anosmia and a defect in gonad development.[154] Patients with this disorder may have other neurologic signs and symptoms, including cerebellar dysfunction and eye movement abnormalities.[155,156] Therefore, abnormalities in other areas of brain, especially cerebellum, have been suspected in this disorder. Gonadal dysfunction is thought to result from a deficiency in gonadotropin-releasing hormone.[157] Because the neurons that produce gonadotropin-releasing hormone are derived from the olfactory plate and actually migrate back into the forebrain via the olfactory nerve, the abnormality of this hormone is likely due to an arrest in migration of the gonadotropin-releasing hormone neurons.[158]

The gene for Kallmann syndrome has been localized to the X chromosome and has been cloned. This gene appears to encode a fibronectin type III–like molecule. Because fibronectin type III has been proposed to be a neural adhesion molecule, the gene for Kallmann syndrome probably also encodes a neural adhesion molecule.[159]

Zellweger Syndrome

Zellweger syndrome is an autosomal recessive, peroxisomal disorder characterized by neuronal migration abnormalities, hepatomegaly, renal cysts, and stippled calcification of the patella. The neuronal migration defects include pachygyria and polymicrogyria, with underlying abnormalities best characterized as a nonlayered appearance of the cortex. Migration abnormalities are also noted in the cerebellum and in the brain stem in this disorder.[160,161] Children with Zellweger syndrome present in the neonatal period with severe hypotonia, characteristic facies, hepatomegaly, and seizures.[162] A mouse model of Zellweger syndrome has been produced; migration abnormalities were noted in the cerebellum and cortex, despite normal-appearing radial glia.[163] Disturbed maturation of neurons and apoptotic neurons also are noted in this mouse model; perhaps similar mechanisms are operative in the comparable human disorder.[163,164]

Zellweger syndrome results from the body's inability to make peroxisomes owing to a deficiency of the peroxisome-targeting receptor gene (*PXR1*)[163] or the peroxisome assembly factor–1 (*PAF1*) gene, among others.[165] A number of peroxisomal enzymes are abnormal and lead to the accumulation of very-long-chain fatty acids.[166] Therefore, testing for this disorder includes an assay of very-long-chain fatty acids. An additional fatty acid that may be depleted in this disorder is platelet-activating factor.[167] This potential depletion links platelet-activating factor, the lipid that is abnormally regulated in Miller-Dieker lissencephaly, to the pathogenesis of Zellweger syndrome.

Polymicrogyria

Polymicrogyria (many small gyri) is a disorder often considered to be a neuronal migration disorder, but alternate theories exist regarding its pathogenesis.[27,29,31] The microscopic appearance of the lesion is that of too many small abnormal gyri. The gyri may be shallow and separated by shallow sulci, which may be associated with an apparent increased cortical thickness. The multiple small convolutions may not have intervening sulci, or the sulci may be bridged by fusion of overlying molecular layer, which may give a smooth appearance to the brain's surface; alternatively, the brain may appear to have pachygyria.

Polymicrogyria takes two distinct histologic forms, four-layered and unlayered. The four-layer form consists of an outer layer, a neuronal layer, a cell-sparse layer, and a deeper neuronal layer. One theory is that the lower cell-sparse layer of the four-layer types represents a glial scar from a laminar necrosis. On the basis of examination of fetuses in which the occurrence of the insult causing the malformation has been accurately timed, this pattern is believed to occur as a result of insults late in the first or early in the second trimester.[27] Others believe that this is a postmigration insult resulting from distorted migration of cells through an injured area, the outcome of which is the cell-sparse layer. A cell-sparse layer between the upper and lower neuronal layers is absent from the unlayered form. Insults that occur early in the second trimester before migration is completed are believed to be the origin of unlayered microgyria. The common association of congenital cytomegalovirus infection with polymicrogyria supports the hypothesis that a destructive process is involved in these disorders.[168]

Polymicrogyria has also been associated with genetic and chromosomal disorders. It is found in disorders of peroxisomal metabolism such as Zellweger syndrome and neonatal adrenal leukodystrophy. It has also been associated with the Bloch-Sulzberger syndrome, Meckel-Gruber syndrome, thanatophoric dysplasia, and Fukuyama congenital muscular dystrophy. Familial bilateral frontal polymicrogyria and bilateral perisylvian polymicrogyria have been reported.[168] Therefore, if no identifiable cause of the polymicrogyric malformation is found, the recurrence risk may be that of an autosomal recessive disorder (25%). A bilateral parasagittal parieto-occipital polymicrogyria has also been described.[169]

The clinical picture varies depending on the location, extent, and etiology of the abnormality. Microcephaly with severe developmental delay and hypertonia may result when polymicrogyria is diffuse. When polymicrogyria is unilateral, focal deficits might be seen. Epilepsy often is present, characterized by partial-complex seizures or partial seizures that secondarily generalize. The age at presentation and severity of seizures depends on the extent of the associated pathology.

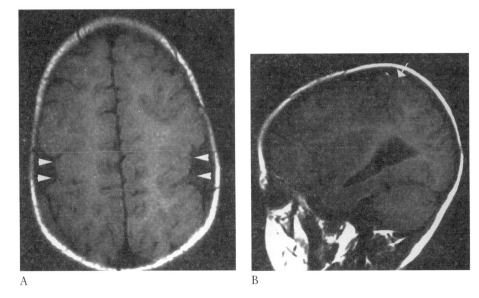

A   B

Figure 2.10 Neuronal migration disorders: bilateral polymicrogyria. T_2-Weighted, axial and saggital head magnetic resonance imaging (MRI) scans of two patients with spastic cerebral palsy, swallowing difficulties, and mental retardation. A. Axial MRI scan shows a large, uncovered sylvian fissure. Irregular, thickened gray matter (the appearance of polymicrogyria on a thick axial MRI) is noted in the area of the sylvian fissure (*arrows*). B. A saggital view of another patient with this disorder. Arrow points to a sylvian fissure that extends too superiorly to the top of the convexity. (Scans LP97-081 and LP97-087 courtesy of Dr. William B. Dobyns and the Lissencephaly Project.)

The lesions are most clearly recognized by MRI and are best noted sagittally. They often are recognized by the rough appearance of the surface of the cortex on a thin-cut T_2-weighted image. If MRI cuts are thick, these lesions may be confused with pachygyria.[168] Because the genetic implications of pachygyria and polymicrogyria differ considerably, distinguishing between these two conditions is important.

Congenital Bilateral Perisylvian Syndrome

Advances in neuroimaging have led to the recognition of the congenital bilateral perisylvian syndrome, also known as the *Foix-Chavanay-Marie syndrome*.[170–173] MRI demonstrates bilateral abnormalities in the opercular and perisylvian regions. The cortex is irregular, and the sylvian fissure may be noted to extend to the top of the convexity (Figure 2.10).

Striking clinical features include a pseudobulbar palsy with abnormal tongue movements, dysarthria, dysphasia, mental retardation, absent or hyperactive gag reflex, drooling, and pyramidal signs in more than 70% of the reported cases. These patients may be mentally retarded, and nearly all have severe language disorders. Dysphagia can impair proper nutrition. Seizures are present in more than 85% of patients. The onset of epilepsy is between 1 month and 14 years of age. Several patients have had infantile spasms during the first year of life. Seventy percent of the patients experience seizures before the age of 10.[171,173]

The etiology of this syndrome remains unknown, although hints of a genetic mechanism exist. Detailed chromosomal analyses have revealed no abnormalities. Monozygotic twins and siblings with this disorder have been described, suggesting a possible autosomal recessive mechanism. Some speculate that this is a disorder of regional specification, given the bilateral, symmetric nature of the lesions.

Heterotopias

Heterotopias are collections of normal-appearing neurons in an abnormal location secondary to a disturbance in radial migration. The exact mechanism of the migration aberration has not been established. Various hypotheses include damage to the radial glial fibers, premature transformation of radial glial cells into astrocytes, or a deficiency of specific molecules on the surface of neuroblasts or of the radial glial cells (or the receptors for those molecules) that results in disruption of the normal migration process.[27,174] Heterotopias often occur as isolated defects that may result in only epilepsy. However, when they are multiple, heterotopias might also be associated with a developmental disorder and cerebral palsy (usually spastic). In addition, if other migration defects such as gyral abnormalities are present, the clinical syndrome may be more profound. Usually, no cause is apparent. Occasionally, heterotopias may be found in a variety of syndromes, including neonatal adrenal leukodystrophy, glutaric aciduria type II, GM_2 gangliosidosis, neurocutaneous syndromes, multiple congenital anomaly syndromes, chromosomal abnormalities, and fetal toxic exposures.[168]

Heterotopias may be classified by their location: subpial, within the cerebral white matter, and in the subependymal region. Leptomeningeal heterotopias often contain astrocytes mixed with ectopic neurons and may resemble a gliotic scar. They may be related to discontinuities in the external limiting membrane and often are associated with type II lissencephaly. These *subarachnoid heterotopias* are responsible for the pebbled appearance of the surface of the brain. *White matter heterotopias* may be focal, subcortical, or diffuse. They may cause distortion of the ventricles and may be associated with diminished white matter in the surrounding area. When diffuse, they may take the form of a circumferential subcortical layer of heterotopic gray matter, which has been called *band heterotopia* or the *double-cortex syndrome* (see previous discussion in Type I [Classic] Lissencephaly). Laminar heterotopia may consist of sheets of ectopic gray matter that may be split into elongated islands. A central ovoid mass of white matter may be present within the band. Patients with this form of subcortical heterotopia have a high prevalence of developmental delay, hemiplegia, and seizures. Nodular subcortical heterotopias may be seen in association with subependymal heterotopias.

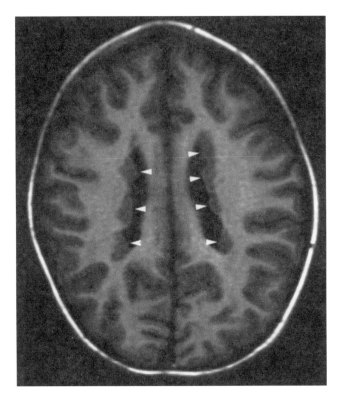

Figure 2.11 Periventricular nodular heterotopia. An axial T$_1$-weighted head magnetic resonance imaging (MRI) scan of a girl with a seizure disorder. Arrowheads point to periventricular heterotopias demonstrating the same MRI signal characteristics as those of gray matter. (Scan LP97 courtesy of Dr. William B. Dobyns and the Lissencephaly Project.)

Subependymal heterotopias often are associated only with epilepsy. Most patients will have normal intelligence and no motor deficits. These heterotopias are located just beneath and abut the ependymal lining of the lateral ventricles. They may be either bilateral or unilateral and are located most often adjacent to the occipital horns and trigones and, less commonly, within the temporal horns and frontal horns (Figures 2.11, 2.12). Seizure onset in patients with subependymal heterotopias is relatively late, often in the second decade, and more often affects women. The seizures may be partial-complex, tonic-clonic, or focal motor. Subependymal heterotopias have been identified as an X-linked dominant syndrome linked to markers in the distal Xq28 locus.[175] This gene may represent an important epilepsy susceptibility locus. An increased incidence of spontaneous abortions and a much higher than expected incidence of female offspring are noted in affected women, suggesting that inheritance of the gene for this form of periventricular heterotopia is lethal for male embryos. A syndrome marked by periventricular heterotopia, mental retardation, and syndactyly has recently been described in male patients.[176]

Patients with diffuse gray matter heterotopias, whether subependymal or in the white matter, usually are candidates for medical treatment of the epilepsies present. Occasionally, patients who are refractory to medical management

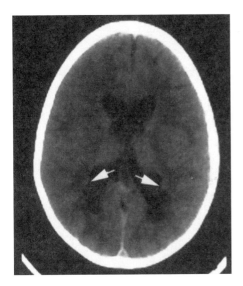
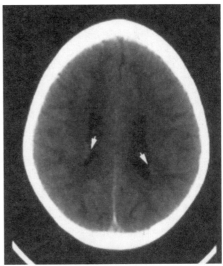

Figure 2.12 Periventricular nodular heterotopia. An axial head computed tomographic scan of a male patient with mental retardation and no seizures. Arrows point to periventricular nodules.

may be considered for hemispherectomies or focal cortical resections. In the case of bilateral temporal lobe periventricular heterotopias, the prognosis for a surgical cure may be poor.

Cortical Dysgenesis

Cortical dysgenesis refers to disorders of cortical formation. In general, many of the disorders just discussed are considered to be within the spectrum of this entity. In this section, we emphasize those focal macroscopic lesions that do not fit into the preceding classifications.

The terms *cortical dysplasia* and *cortical dysgenesis* often are used synonymously for migration disorders. Included in these terms are not only the obvious malformations such as smooth gyri and clefts but also lesions classified as focal cortical dysplasias and microdysgenesis. Focal cortical dysplasia may involve a major part of a lobe and may be characterized by the congregation of large, bizarre neurons and abnormal glial cells in the subadjacent white matter (Figure 2.13).[177] *Microdysgenesis*, by definition, can be detected only histologically and is beyond the imaging capability of current MRI scans. It consists of unipolar and bipolar neurons under the pia, increased neurons in the first layer of the cortex, indistinct boundaries between the first and second layers of the cortex, neuronal glial heterotopias in the pia, persistence of columnar architecture of the cortex, and an increased number of neurons in the white matter. Patients with microdysgenesis are reported only in series of patients undergoing epilepsy surgery. Microdysgenesis is

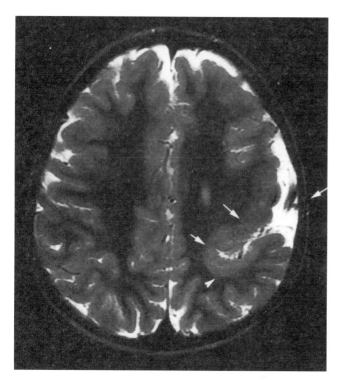

Figure 2.13 Focal cortical dysplasia. An axial T_2-weighted head magnetic resonance imaging scan of a patient presenting with a right hemiparesis and new onset of seizures. Arrows point to an area of focal cortical dysplasia in the left parietal area.

not detected in patients with controlled epilepsy and thus the incidences of migration disorders and of microdysgenesis responsible for epilepsy are unknown.

Microdysgenesis was the most common migration disorder noted in a series of pathologic examinations of brain tissue removed from epileptic patients.[178] Malformations of this type were found in 14% of epileptic brains; the frequency of other abnormalities in epileptic brains was microgyria, 4.7%, heterotopia, 15%, and pachygyria, 8%. In patients with microdysgenesis, seizure onset occurs between 2 and 20 years of age.

A surprisingly high incidence of microdysgenesis has been reported in brain tissue removed from adults to treat recalcitrant seizures.[179] The lesions noted included ectopic neurons within the subcortical white matter in 42% of the specimens and neuronal clustering in 28%; in addition, bare areas were present within layers II–VI. Similar findings have been reported in epilepsy surgical specimens from children.[180] Polymicrogyria, heterotopia, and various cortical dysplasias were found in resected tissues. Examination of the tissue revealed increased thickness of the cortical ribbon and blurring of the gray and white matter interface. Thus, microscopic abnormalities have been found in 20–40% of specimens from patients undergoing surgical therapy for intractable epilepsy, the most common lesions being microdysgenesis and cortical dysplasias.

As mentioned earlier, MRI has been useful in detecting migration abnormalities and generally has been found to be more sensitive than CT scanning. MRI-apparent migration abnormalities have been detected in as many as 50% of patients who underwent epilepsy surgery.[181] Of those patients with epilepsy alone, 6.7% had migration abnormalities; in those who had both mental retardation and epilepsy, such abnormalities were found in 13.7%. The abnormalities included pachygyria or polymicrogyria or both, schizencephaly, heterotopias, and hemimegalencephaly. Of 222 adults with temporal lobe epilepsy studied by MRI, 7.2% were found to have malformations of the temporal lobe.[182] These malformations consisted of heterotopias, focal neocortical dysgenesis, hippocampal malformations, or a combination of various lesions.

Cortical dysgenesis has also been associated with hippocampal sclerosis, leading some to believe that hippocampal sclerosis is a disorder of brain formation. Raymond and colleagues[183] studied 100 patients with hippocampal sclerosis diagnosed by histologic examination or MRI and found that 15 of the patients also had cortical dysgenesis. The most common abnormality was subependymal heterotopia.[183] The cortical dysplasia was, at times, contralateral to the hippocampal sclerosis.

Clearly, migration aberrations need not be manifested by abnormal motor function; rather, epilepsy and mental retardation might be the only clinical symptoms in these disorders.

The severity of the migration disorder correlates with clinical symptoms. Patients with milder forms of neuronal migration defects (i.e., focal cortical dysplasias, heterotopias, microdysgenesis) may appear normal. Most often, migration disorders are diagnosed in patients with epilepsy, as neuroimaging is performed for seizure. These patients generally have partial seizures and normal life expectancies. Some patients with these disorders will have developmental delays, mild intellectual deficits, or spastic or atonic cerebral palsy. Profound defects are associated with more severe symptoms.

Children presenting with intractable epilepsy, significant mental retardation, and neurologic signs more often have diffuse migration abnormalities on MRI scanning. Therefore, not surprisingly, the degree of abnormality on MRI scans correlates well with the degree of neurologic involvement. The age of onset of seizures varies from early childhood to young adult life. Generally, the severity of the seizures and the severity of the pathology correlate positively.[184] Severe abnormalities are associated with seizures in the first year of life, whereas microdysgenesis may be associated with adult onset of seizures. Later-onset seizures also tend to correlate with subependymal heterotopias.

Although the pathogenic mechanisms involved in focal dysgenesis remain poorly understood, mechanisms similar to those involved in global or more extensive migration disorders probably are operative. Therefore, definition of the pathogenic mechanisms causing these disorders is important.

PROCESS OUTGROWTH
AND SYNAPSE FORMATION

Normal Synapse Formation

Even as neurons are arriving in the cortical plate, important neural out-growths and synapses are forming. The process by which neurons sprout new extensions (neurites) that grow impressive distances to make precise synaptic connections is remarkable and has been well studied, though it is still being elucidated. During development, many more synapses are made than are needed; these subsequently are pruned to improve precision of synaptic connections. Such pruning occurs while other synapses are strengthened. Pruning may be a phenomenon peculiar to the developing nervous system, but synapse strengthening probably continues throughout life.

Most early neurites will form axons. The distance and the terrain that a forming axon must negotiate to reach its target is often formidable, yet this process occurs with little error. Neurites consist of a long shaft of dynamic cytoskeletal elements that terminate in a growth cone, a highly motile structure capable of responding to chemical cues.

The nature of the chemical cues that guide growth cones and, thus, developing axons are threefold: adhesive, chemoattractive, and chemorepulsive.[185,186] Adhesive molecules, such as those in the NCAM family, line projection pathways; integrin receptors on growth cones and neurites link the internal cytoskeleton of these structures with the extracellular adhesive molecules. These adhesive molecules provide a substrate on which the motile growth cone and neurite can respond to the chemical cues that determine the final synaptic target.

Diffusible cues appear to provide a trophic influence on developing axons through a chemoaffinity mechanism. One hypothesis is that gradients of chemotactic substances, emitted at the targets for synapse formation, interact with receptors on the growth cone that steer the growth cone toward the target.[187-189]

In addition to the chemotactic substances, chemorepulsive molecules participate in growth cone guidance to synaptic targets.[190,191] Molecules such as collapsin and platelet-activating factor,[141] the lipid implicated in Miller-Dieker lissencephaly, appear to be chemorepulsive agents that induce growth cone collapse in vitro. A collapse of a growth cone in effect steers that structure away from the chemorepulsive source. Hence, a combination of chemoattractant and chemorepellant cues probably aid the developing neurites in negotiating the adhesive molecule pathways to make proper synaptic connections, even over distances as far as that from the motor cortex to the anterior horn cells of the lower spinal cord.

The specificity of synapse connections appears to be related to the presynaptic neuronal type, and functional synapses are noted within moments of growth cone contact with the appropriate postsynaptic cell.[192,193] This early synaptic activity does not appear to be critical in the formation of synapses, as pharmacologic blockade of postsynaptic responses does not prevent synapse formation.[194,195]

Although it appears not to play a role in the early stages of synapse formation, synaptic activity is critical for subsequent remodeling. Pathways apparently are overrepresented often in early postnatal life, and "exuberant" projections of axons must be appropriately pruned. This occurs in a use-dependent fashion such that pathways used for neural activity are retained and those not used are eliminated.[186,196] The classic studies of Hubel and Wiesel[197] have demonstrated that this process is critical in the formation of the proper synaptic connections of the visual cortex. In their studies, the eyelid of one kitten eye was closed temporarily. The eye deprived of light was underrepresented, whereas the eye that remained open was overrepresented in the visual cortex. This phenomenon is noted in children who have significant amblyopia (so-called lazy eye). If this amblyopia is not recognized during a critical period of synapse remodeling, these children can be cortically blind in the affected eye.

Throughout life, significant synaptic plasticity persists. Memory is believed to result from a strengthening of heavily used synapses, a phenomenon known as *long-term potentiation*.[198] Considering the lessons learned about the role neuronal activity plays in the remodeling of connectivity in sensory systems, one wonders whether early life experiences, such as seizures, could also alter local circuit remodeling for the recurrent axon collaterals of hippocampal pyramidal cells. Hence, during hippocampal development, if repeated seizures occurred, the synchronous discharging of pyramidal cells might prevent axonal remodeling that normally takes place, and so an excess in axonal branching present in early life could be maintained into adulthood. In turn, this consolidation could result in an imbalance between recurrent excitation and inhibition and lead to the production of a chronic epileptic focus in hippocampus.

To explore this idea, an animal model is needed in which hippocampal seizures can be experimentally induced during the critical period of pronounced seizure susceptibility. Ideally, the seizures should occur frequently throughout the critical period during which network remodeling is believed to take place. If a pharmacologic agent is used to induce seizures, its effects should normally persist for 5–10 days; thereafter, its efficacy should be greatly reduced or eliminated so the consequences of the seizures themselves can be assessed in the absence of the convulsant agent. Such a model was developed, and indeed an epileptic tendency persists in animals made epileptic during a critical period.[199]

Disorders of Process Outgrowth

The disorders of process outgrowth probably are poorly recognized, given the current limitations of neuroimaging. Many children with cerebral palsy and normal neuroimaging scans likely have disorders involving dendritic branching and axonal growth. Here we briefly discuss three disorders in which abnormalities of neuronal processes have been demonstrated, though other diseases of this phase of neurodevelopment probably exist.

Down Syndrome

Down syndrome (trisomy 21) includes a static encephalopathy characterized by mental retardation and hypotonia. The major neuropathologic changes in Down syndrome are a reduction in both the dendritic spines and the number of synapses.[200–202]

Rett Syndrome

Rett syndrome is apparently a progressive disorder that affects girls. After a normal gestation, normal birth, and normal first 6 months of development, regression in intellect and motor function is seen. Girls affected with this disorder develop a gait and a truncal apraxia, loss of purposeful hand movements, stereotypic hand movements, progressive spasticity, autismlike social withdrawal, and mental retardation. Accompanying this decline is a deceleration in head growth, which occurs during a time that brain development mainly involves glial proliferation and neuronal process outgrowth (Figure 2.14). Although patients typically have normal head sizes at birth, they become microcephalic during the time of their decline in function.

Pathologic examinations of the brains of patients with Rett syndrome support a disturbance in neuronal process outgrowth. The size of individual neurons is reduced, which is accompanied by an increase in packing density in the cerebral cortex, thalami, and basal ganglia.[203,204] Abnormal dendritic branching has been noted in affected brain; this is especially prominent in layers III and V neurons of the frontal, motor, and temporal cortices.[205,206] Because dendritic branching is believed to occur in response to axonal innervation, an examination of Rett syndrome brains for axonal aberrations was undertaken. This examination revealed significantly lower numbers of axons entering cortex as compared to normal.[207,208]

Fragile X Syndrome

Fragile X syndrome is the most common nonchromosomal, genetic form of mental retardation seen in boys and men. The disorder results from the disturbance of the *FMR1* gene on the long arm of the X chromosome by a tripli-

Figure 2.14 ➤ Pyramidal neuron prenatal development. A drawing based on Golgi studies of human (A) and cat (B) layer V neurons. Note the apical dendrite and its interaction with layer I. In the maturation and structural differentiation of the pyramidal neuron, dendrites sprout and the cell body enlarges. Dendritic sprouting probably occurs in response to axon innervation. Well-defined layering in the cortical plate is not apparent until near term in the human. Most of prenatal brain growth after 24 weeks is due to glial proliferation and neuronal process outgrowth. (Reprinted from M Marín-Padilla. Ontogenesis of the pyramidal cell of the mammalian neocortex and developmental cytoarchitectonics: a unifying theory. J Comp Neurol 1992;321:223–240. Copyright © Wiley-Liss, Inc. With permission of Wiley-Liss, Inc., a subsidiary of John Wiley & Sons, Inc.)

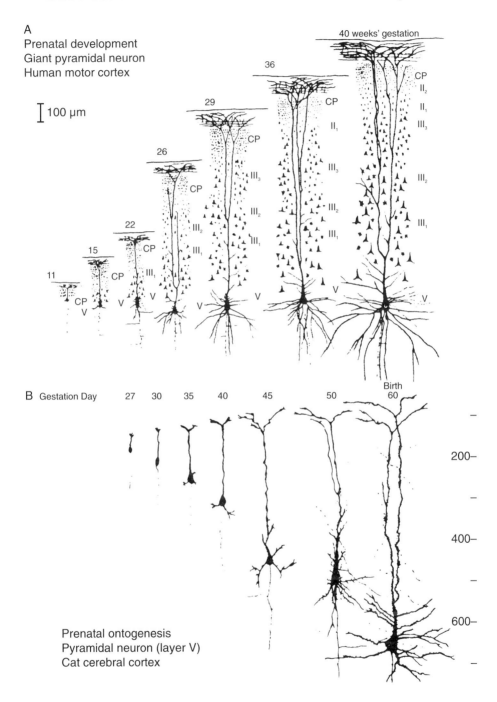

A
Prenatal development
Giant pyramidal neuron
Human motor cortex

100 μm

B Gestation Day

Prenatal ontogenesis
Pyramidal neuron (layer V)
Cat cerebral cortex

cate repeat.[209] The brain in this disorder appears normal but, on microscopic examination, dendritic spine abnormalities are apparent.[210]

REFERENCES

1. Lemire R, Loeser J, Leech R, et al. Normal and Abnormal Development of the Human Nervous System. New York: Harper & Row, 1975.
2. Thaller C, Eichele G. Isolation of 3,4-didehydroretinoic acid, a novel morphogenetic signal in the chick wing bud. Nature 1990;345:815–819.
3. Brockes J. Reading the retinoid signals. Nature 1990;345:766–768.
4. Scotting PJ, Rex M. Transcription factors in early development of the central nervous system. Neuropathol Appl Neurobiol 1996;22:469–481.
5. Mangelsdorf DJ, Ong ES, Dyck JA, et al. Nuclear receptor that identifies a novel retinoic acid response pathway. Nature 1990;345:224–229.
6. Eichele G. Retinoids and vertebrate limb pattern formation. Trends Genet 1989;5:246–251.
7. Geelan JA, Langman J. Closure of the neural tube in the cephalic region of the mouse embryo. Anat Rec 1977;189:625–640.
8. Marín-Padilla M. Cephalic axial skeletal-neural dysraphic disorders: embryology and pathology. Can J Neurol Sci 1991;18:153–169.
9. Marín-Padilla M. Ontogenesis of the pyramidal cell of the mammalian neocortex and developmental cytoarchitectonics: a unifying theory. J Comp Neurol 1992;321:223–240.
10. Volpe J. Neurology of the Newborn. Philadelphia: Saunders, 1995.
11. Helwig U, Imai K, Schmahl W, et al. Interaction between undulated and Patch leads to an extreme form of spina bifida in double-mutant mice. Nat Genet 1995;11:60–63.
12. Nakano KK. Anencephaly: a review. Dev Med Child Neurol 1973;15:383–400.
13. Cohen MMJ, Lemire RJ. Syndromes with cephaloceles. Teratology 1983;25:161–172.
14. Lindhout D, Omtzigt JG, Cornel MC. Spectrum of neural-tube defects in 34 infants prenatally exposed to antiepileptic drugs. Neurology 1992;42:119–125.
15. MRC Vitamin Study Research Group. Prevention of neural tube defects: results of the Medical Research Council Vitamin Study. Lancet 1991;338:131–137.
16. Hansen JW, Ardinger HH, DiLiberti JH. Effects of valproic acid of the fetus. Pediatr Res 1984;18:306.
17. Paavola P, Salonen R, Weissenbach J, et al. The locus for Meckel syndrome with multiple congenital anomalies maps to chromosome 17q21–q24. Nat Genet 1995;11:213–215.
18. Garcia-Bellido A, Lawrence PA, Morata G. Compartments in animal development. Sci Am 1979;241:102–110.
19. Dalton D, Chadwick R, McGinnis W. Expression and embryonic function of empty spiracle: a *Drosophila* homeobox gene with two patterning functions on the anterior-posterior axis of the embryo. Genes Dev 1989;3:1940–1956.
20. Boncinelli E, Gulisano M, Broccoli V. *Emx* and *Otx* homeobox genes in the developing mouse brain. J Neurobiol 1993;24:1356–1366.
21. Gulisano M, Broccoli V, Pardini C, et al. *Emx1* and *Emx2* show different patterns of expression during proliferation and differentiation of the developing cerebral cortex in the mouse. Eur J Neurosci 1996;8:1037–1050.
22. Acampora D, Mazan S, Avantaggiato V, et al. Epilepsy and brain abnormalities in mice lacking the *Otx1* gene. Nat Genet 1996;14:218–222.
23. Nakagawa Y, Kaneko T, Ogura T, et al. Roles of cell-autonomous mechanisms for differential expression of region-specific transcription factors in neuroepithelial cells. Development 1996;122:2449–2464.

24. Keynes R, Krumlauf R. Hox genes and regionalization of the nervous system. Annu Rev Neurosci 1994;17:109–132.
25. Hillburger AC, Willis JK, Bouldin E, et al. Familial schizencephaly. Brain Dev 1993;15:234–236.
26. Brunelli S, Faiella A, Capra V, et al. Germline mutations in the homeobox gene *EMX2* in patients with severe schizencephaly. Nat Genet 1996;12:94–96.
27. Barth P. Disorders of neuronal migration. Can J Neurol Sci 1987;14:1–16.
28. Barkovich A, Kjos B. Schizencephaly: correlation of clinical findings with MR characteristics. AJNR Am J Neuroradiol 1992;13:85–94.
29. Barkovich A, Chuang S, Norman D. MR of neuronal migration anomalies. AJNR Am J Neuroradiol 1987;8:1009–1017.
30. Brodtkorb E, Nilsen G, Smevik O, et al. Epilepsy and anomalies of neuronal migration: MRI and clinical aspects. Acta Neurol Scand 1992;86:24–32.
31. Kuzniecky R. Magnetic resonance imaging in developmental disorders of the cerebral cortex. Epilepsia 1994;35(suppl 6):S44–S56.
32. Aicardi J, Goutieres F. The syndrome of absence of the septum pellucidum with porencephalies and other developmental defects. Neuropediatrics 1981;12:319–329.
33. Leech R, Shuman R. Midline telencephalic dysgenesis: report of three cases. J Child Neurol 1986;1:224–232.
34. Smith J. Hedgehog, the floor plate, and the zone of polarizing activity. Cell 1994;76:193–196.
35. Johnson RL, Rothman AL, Xie J, et al. Human homolog of patched, a candidate gene for the basal cell nevus syndrome. Science 1996;272:1668–1671.
36. Stone DM, Hynes M, Armanini M, et al. The tumour-suppressor gene patched encodes a candidate receptor for Sonic hedgehog. Nature 1996;384:129–134.
37. Conlon RA. Retinoic acid and pattern formation in vertebrates. Trends Genet 1995;11:314–319.
38. Helms JA, Kim CH, Hu D, et al. Sonic hedgehog participates in craniofacial morphogenesis and is down-regulated by teratogenic doses of retinoic acid. Dev Biol 1997;187:25–35.
39. Dobyns WB. Cerebral Dysgenesis: Causes and Consequences. In G Miller, JC Ramer (eds), Static Encephalopathies of Infancy and Childhood. New York: Raven, 1992;235–248.
40. Barkovich AJ. Imaging Aspects of Static Encephalopathies. In G Miller, JC Ramer (eds), Static Encephalopathies of Infancy and Childhood. New York: Raven, 1992;45–94.
41. Nyberg DA, Mack LA, Bronstein A, et al. Holoprosencephaly: prenatal sonographic diagnosis. AJNR Am J Neuroradiol 1987;149:1051–1058.
42. Souza JP, Siebert JR, Beckwith JB. An anatomic comparison of cebocephaly and ethmocephaly. Teratology 1990;42:347–357.
43. Romshe CA, Sotos JF. Hypothalamic-pituitary dysfunction in siblings of patients with holoprosencephaly. J Pediatr 1973;83:1088–1090.
44. Barr M, Hansen JW, Currey K, et al. Holoprosencephaly in infants of diabetic mothers. J Pediatr 1983;102:565–568.
45. Cohen MM. Perspectives on holoprosencephaly: I. Epidemiology, genetics and syndromology. Teratology 1989;40:211–235.
46. Munke M. Clinical, cytogenetic, and molecular approaches to the genetic heterogeneity of holoprosencephaly. Am J Med Genet 1989;34:237–245.
47. Roessler E, Belloni E, Gaudenz K, et al. Mutations in the human Sonic hedgehog gene cause holoprosencephaly. Nat Genet 1996;14:357–360.
48. Berry SA, Pierpont ME, Gorlin RJ. Single central incisor in familial holoprosencephaly. J Pediatr 1984;104:877–880.
49. Ouvier R, Billson F. Optic nerve hypoplasia: a review. J Child Neurol 1986;1:181–188.

50. Costin G, Murphree AL. Hypothalamic-pituitary function in children with optic nerve hypoplasia. Am J Dis Child 1985;139:249–254.
51. Benner JD, Presian MW, Gratz E, et al. Septo-optic dysplasia in two siblings. Am J Ophthalmol 1990;109:632–637.
52. Patel H, Tze WJ, Crichton JU, et al. Optic nerve hypoplasia with hypopituitarism: septo-optic dysplasia with hypopituitarism. Am J Dis Child 1975;129:175–180.
53. Caviness VS, Takahashi T. Proliferative events in the cerebral ventricular zone. Brain Dev 1995;17:159–163.
54. Blinkov S, Glezer II. The Human Brain in Figures and Tables. Translated by B Haign. New York: Basic Books, 1968.
55. Evrard P, De Saint-Georges P, Kadhim H, et al. Pathology of Prenatal Encephalopathies. In JH French, S Harel, P Casaer (eds), Child Neurology and Development Disabilities. Baltimore: Paul H Brookes, 1989;153–176.
56. Ross ME. Cell division and the nervous system: regulating the cycle from neural differentiation to death. Trends Neurosci 1996;19:62–68.
57. Pardee AB. G1 events and regulation of cell proliferation. Science 1989;246:603–608.
58. Meyerson M, Harlow M. Identification of G1 kinase activity for cdk6, a novel cyclin D partner. Mol Cell Biol 1994;14:2077–2086.
59. Matsushime H, Quelle DE, Shurtleff SA, et al. D-type cyclin-dependent kinase activity in mammalian cells. Mol Cell Biol 1994;14:2066–2076.
60. Sherr CJ. G1 phase progression: cycling on cue. Cell 1994;79:551–555.
61. Dulic V, Lees E, Reed SI. Association of human cyclin E with a periodic G1-S phase protein kinase. Science 1992;257:1958–1961.
62. Murray AW, Solomon MJ, Kirschner MW. The role of cyclin synthesis and degradation in the control of maturation promoting factor activity. Nature 1989;339:280–286.
63. Amon A, Irniger S, Naysmyth K. Closing the cell cycle circle in yeast: G2 cyclin proteolysis initiated at mitosis persists until the activation of G1 cyclins in the next cycle. Cell 1994;77:1037–1050.
64. Kato J, Matsushime H, Hiebert SW, et al. Direct binding of cyclin D to the retinoblastoma gene product (pRb) and pRb phosphorylation by the cyclin D–dependent kinase CDK4. Genes Dev 1993;7:331–342.
65. Harper JW, Adami GR, Wei N, et al. The p21 cdk-interacting protein Cip1 is a potent inhibitor of G1 cyclin-dependent kinases. Cell 1993;75:805–816.
66. el-Deiry WS, Tokino T, Velculescu VE, et al. WAF1, a potential mediator of p53 tumor suppression. Cell 1993;75:817–825.
67. Lee EY-HP, Chang C-Y, Hu N, et al. Mice deficient for Rb are nonviable and show defects in neurogenesis and haematopoiesis. Nature 1992;359:288–294.
68. Polyak K, Lee MH, Erdjument-Bromage H, et al. Cloning of p27Kip1, a cyclin-dependent kinase inhibitor and a potential mediator of extracellular antimitogenic signals. Cell 1994;78:59–66.
69. Hannon GJ, Beach D. p15INK4B is a potential effector of TGF-beta-induced cell cycle arrest. Nature 1994;371:257–261.
70. Toyoshima H, Hunter T. p27, a novel inhibitor of G1 cyclin-Cdk protein kinase activity, is related to p21. Cell 1994;78:67–74.
71. Gao W-Q, Heintz N, Hatten ME. Cerebellar granule cell neurogenesis is regulated by cell-cell interactions in vitro. Neuron 1991;6:705–715.
72. Matsushime H, Roussel MF, Ashmun RA, et al. Colony-stimulating factor 1 regulates novel cyclins during the G1 phase of the cell cycle. Cell 1991;65:701–713.
73. Uwanogho D, Rex M, Cartwright E, et al. Embryonic expression of the chicken Sox2, Sox3, and Sox11 genes suggests an interactive role in neuronal development. Mech Dev 1995;49:23–36.
74. Glotzer M, Murray AW, Kirschner MW. Cyclin is degraded by the ubiquitin pathway. Nature 1991;349:132–138.

75. Ross ME, Riskin M. MN20, a D2 cyclin found in brain, is implicated in neural differentiation. J Neurosci 1994;14:6384–6391.
76. Ross ME, Carter M, Lee J. MN20, a D2 cyclin, is transiently expressed in selected neural populations during embryogenesis. J Neurosci 1996;16:210–219.
77. Dehay C, Giroud P, Berland M, et al. Modulation of the cell cycle contributes to the parcellation of the primate visual cortex. Nature 1993;366:464–466.
78. Clarke PG. Developmental cell death: morphological diversity and multiple mechanisms. Anat Embryol 1990;181:195–213.
79. Schwartz LM, Smith SW, Jones MEE, et al. Do all programmed cell deaths occur via apoptosis? Proc Natl Acad Sci U S A 1993;90:980–984.
80. Kerr JFR, Wyllie AH, Currie AR. Apoptosis: a basic biological phenomenon with wide-ranging implications in tissue kinetics. Br J Cancer 1972;26:239–257.
81. Wyllie AH, Kerr JFR, Currie AR. Cell death: the significance of apoptosis. Int Rev Cytol 1980;68:251–306.
82. Driscoll M, Chalfie M. Developmental and abnormal cell death in *C. elegans*. Trends Neurosci 1992;15:15–19.
83. Alnemri ES, Livingston DJ, Nicholson DW, et al. Human ICE/CED-3 protease nomenclature [letter]. Cell 1996;87:171.
84. Warkany J, Lemire RJ, Cohen MM. Mental Retardation and Congenital Malformations of the Central Nervous System. Chicago: Year Book, 1981;13–40.
85. Optiz JM, Holt MC. Microcephaly: general considerations and aids to nosology. J Craniofac Genet Dev Biol 1990;10:175–204.
86. Renier WO, Gabreels FJM, Jasper HH, et al. An X-linked syndrome with microcephaly, severe mental retardation, spasticity, epilepsy and deafness. J Ment Defic Res 1982;26:27–40.
87. Haslam R, Smith DW. Autosomal dominant microcephaly. J Pediatr 1979; 95:701–705.
88. Lenke RR, Levy HL. Maternal phenylketonuria and hyperphenylalaninemia. N Engl J Med 1980;303:1202–1208.
89. Yamazaki JN, Schull WJ. Perinatal loss and neurological abnormalities among children of the atomic bomb. Nagasaki and Hiroshima revisited, 1949 to 1989. JAMA 1990;264:605–609.
90. Barkovich A, Chuang S. Unilateral megalencephaly: correlation of MR imaging and pathologic characteristics. AJNR Am J Neuroradiol 1990;11:523–531.
91. DeRosa MJ, Secor DL, Barsom M, et al. Neuropathologic findings in surgically treated hemimegalencephaly: immunohistochemical, morphometric and ultrastructural study. Acta Neuropathol 1992;84:250–260.
92. Rintahaka P, Chugani H, Messa C, et al. Hemimegalencephaly: evaluation with positron emission tomography. Pediatr Neurol 1993;9:21–28.
93. Renowden S, Squier M. Unusual magnetic resonance and neuropathological findings in hemi-megalencephaly: report of a case following hemispherectomy. Dev Med Child Neurol 1994;36:357–369.
94. DeMyer W. Megalencephaly: types, clinical syndromes, and management. Pediatr Neurol 1986;2:321–328.
95. DeMyer W. Megalencephaly in children. Clinical syndromes, genetic patterns, and differential diagnosis from other cases of megalencephaly. Neurology 1972;22:634–643.
96. Sakuta R, Aikawa H, Takashima S, et al. Epidermal nevus syndrome with hemimegalencephaly: neuropathological study. Brain Dev 1991;13:260–265.
97. Hager BC, Dyme IZ, Guertin SR, et al. Linear nevus sebaceous syndrome: megalencephaly and heterotopic gray matter. Pediatr Neurol 1991;7:45–49.
98. Pavone L, Curatolo P, Rizzo R, et al. Epidermal nevus syndrome: a neurologic variant with hemimegalencephaly, gyral malformation, mental retardation, seizures, and facial hemihypertrophy. Neurology 1991;41:266–271.

99. Jelinek JE, Bart RS, Schiff GM. Hypomelanosis of Ito ("incontinentia pigmenti achromians"): report of three cases and review of the literature. Arch Dermatol 1973;107:596–601.
100. Smart I. Proliferative characteristics of the ependymal layer during the early development of the spinal cord in the mouse. J Anat 1992;111:365–380.
101. Turner D, Cepko C. Cell lineage in the rat retina: a common progenitor for neurons and glia persists late in development. Nature 1987;328:131–136.
102. Lamborghini J. Rohon-Beard cells and other large neurons in *Xenopus* embryos originate during gastrulation. J Comp Neurol 1980;189:323–333.
103. Gomez M. Tuberous Sclerosis. New York: Raven, 1979.
104. Haines JL, Short MP, Kwiatkowski DJ, et al. Localization of one gene for tuberous sclerosis within 9q32–9q34, and further evidence for heterogeneity. Am J Hum Genet 1991;49:764–772.
105. Green AJ, Smith M, Yates JR. Loss of heterozygosity on chromosome 16p13.3 in hamartomas from tuberous sclerosis patients. Nat Genet 1994;6:193–196.
106. European Chromosome 16 Tuberous Sclerosis Consortium. Identification and characterization of the tuberous sclerosis gene on chromosome 16. Cell 1993;75:1305–1315.
107. van Slegtenhorst M, de Hoogt R, Hermans C, et al. Identification of the tuberous sclerosis gene TSC1 on chromosome 9q34. Science 1997;277:805–808.
108. Ogawa M, Miyata T, Nakajima K, et al. The reeler gene–associated antigen on Cajal-Retzius neurons is a crucial molecule for laminar organization of cortical neurons. Neuron 1995;14(suppl):899–912.
109. Allendoerfer K, Shatz C. The subplate, a transient neocortical structure: its role in the development of connections between thalamus and cortex. Annu Rev Neurosci 1994;17:185–218.
110. Aicardi J. The place of neuronal migration abnormalities in child neurology. Can J Neurol Sci 1994;21:185–193.
111. McConnell S. The control of neuronal identity in the developing cerebral cortex. Curr Opin Neurobiol 1992;2(1):23–27.
112. Sidman R, Rakic P. Neuronal migration, with special reference to developing human brain: a review. Brain Res 1973;62:1–35.
113. Angevine J, Sidman R. Autoradiographic study of cell migration during histogenesis of cerebral cortex of the mouse. Nature 1961;192:766–768.
114. Liesi P, Seppala I, Trenkner E. Neuronal migration in cerebellar microcultures is inhibited by antibodies against a neurite outgrowth domain of laminin. J Neurosci Res 1992;33:170–176.
115. Lois C, Garcia-Verdugo J, Alvarez-Buylla A. Chain migration of neuronal precursors. Science 1996;271:978–981.
116. Miller J. Lissencephaly in 2 siblings. Neurology 1963;13:841–850.
117. Daube J, Chou S. Lissencephaly: two cases. Neurology 1966;16:179–191.
118. Dieker H, Edwards RH, Zu Rhein G. The lissencephaly syndrome. Birth Defects 1969;5:53.
119. Jones KL, Gilbert EF, Kaveggia EG, et al. The Miller-Dieker syndrome. Pediatrics 1980;66:277–281.
120. Stewart R, Richman D, Caviness V. Lissencephaly and pachygyria. Acta Neuropathol 1975;31:1–12.
121. Takashima S, Becker LE, Chan, Takada K. A Golgi study of the cerebral cortex in Fukuyama-type congenital muscular dystrophy, Walker-type "lissencephaly," and classical lissencephaly. Brain Dev 1987;9:621–626.
122. Takada K, Becker LE, Chan F. Aberrant dendritic development in the human agyric cortex: a quantitative and qualitative Golgi study of two cases. Clin Neuropathol 1988;7:111–119.
123. Bordarier C, Robain O, Rethore M, et al. Inverted neurons in agyria. A Golgi study of a case with abnormal chromosome 17. Hum Genet 1986;73:374–378.

124. Garcia CA, Dunn D, Trevor R. The lissencephaly (agyria) syndrome in siblings. Computerized tomographic and neuropathologic findings. Arch Neurol 1978;35: 608–611.

125. Reiner O, Carrozzo R, Shen Y, et al. Isolation of a Miller-Dieker lissencephaly gene containing G protein–subunit-like repeats. Nature 1993;364:717–721.

126. Lo Nigro C, Chong SS, Smith ACM, et al. Point mutations and an intragenic deletion in LIS1, the lissencephaly causative gene in isolated lissencephaly sequence and Miller-Dieker syndrome. Hum Mol Genet 1997;6:157–164.

127. Chong SS, Pack SD, Roschke AV, et al. A revision of the lissencephaly and Miller-Dieker syndrome critical regions in chromosome 17p13.3. Hum Mol Genet 1997;6:147–155.

128. Ledbetter SA, Kuwano A, Dobyns WB, Ledbetter, DH. Microdeletions of chromosome 17p13 as a cause of isolated lissencephaly. Am J Hum Genet 1992;50:182–189.

129. Dhellemmes C, Girard S, Dulac O, et al. Agyria—pachygyria and Miller-Dieker syndrome: clinical, genetic and chromosome studies. Hum Genet 1988;79:163–167.

130. Kohler A, Hain J, Müller U. Clinical and molecular genetic findings in five patients with Miller-Dieker syndrome. Clin Genet 1995;47:161–164.

131. Sharief N, Craze J, Summers D, et al. Miller-Dieker syndrome with ring chromosome 17. Arch Dis Child 1991;66:710–712.

132. Greenberg F, Stratton R, Lockhart L, et al. Familial Miller-Dieker syndrome associated with pericentric inversion of chromosome 17. Am J Med Genet 1986;23:853–859.

133. Dobyns WB, Stratton RF, Parke JT, et al. Miller-Dieker syndrome: lissencephaly and monosomy 17p. J Pediatr 1983;102:552–558.

134. de Rijk–van Andel JF, Catsman-Berrevoets CE, Halley DJJ, et al. Isolated lissencephaly sequence associated with a microdeletion at chromosome 17p13. Hum Genet 1991;87:509–510.

135. Norman M, Roberts M, Sirois J, et al. Lissencephaly. Can J Neurol Sci 1976;3:39–46.

136. Hattori M, Arai H, Inoue K. Purification and characterization of bovine brain platelet-activating factor acetylhydrolase. J Biol Chem 1993;268:18748–18753.

137. Hattori M, Adachi H, Tsujimoto M, et al. Miller-Dieker lissencephaly gene encodes a subunit of brain platelet-activating factor acetylhydrolase. Nature 1994;370:216–218.

138. Mizuguchi M, Takashima S, Kakita A, et al. Localization in the central nervous system and loss of immunoreactivity in Miller-Dieker syndrome. Am J Pathol 1995;147:1142–1151.

139. Clark GD, Mizuguchi M, Antalffy B, et al. Predominant localization of the LIS family of gene products to Cajal-Retzius cells and ventricular neuroepithelium in the developing human cortex. J Neuropathol Exp Neurol 1997;56:1044–1052.

140. Kornecki E, Ehrlich Y. Neuroregulatory and neuropathological actions of the ether-phospholipid platelet-activating factor. Science 1988;240:1792–1794.

141. Clark G, McNeil R, Bix G, et al. Platelet-activating factor produces neuronal growth cone collapse. Neuroreport 1995;6:2569–2575.

142. Merrick SE, Trojanowski JQ, Lee VM. Selective destruction of stable microtubules and axons by inhibitors of protein serine/threonine phosphatases in cultured human neurons. J Neurosci 1997;17:5726–5737.

143. Dobyns WB, Andermann E, Andermann F, et al. X-linked malformations of neuronal migration. Neurology 1996;47:331–339.

144. Pinard JM, Motte J, Chiron C, et al. Subcortical laminar heterotopia and lissencephaly in two families: a single X-linked dominant disorder. J Neurol Neurosurg Psychiatry 1994;57:914–920.

145. Ross ME, Allen KM, Srivastava AK, et al. Linkage and physical mapping of X-linked lissencephaly/SBH (XLIS)—a gene causing neuronal migration defects in human brain. Hum Mol Genet 1997;6:555–562.

146. des Portes V, Pinard JM, Smadja D, et al. Dominant X-linked subcortical laminar heterotopia and lissencephaly syndrome (XSCLH/LIS): evidence for the occurrence

of mutation in males and mapping of a potential locus in Xq22. J Med Genet 1997;34:177–183.

147. Barkovich A, Jackson D, Boyar R. Band heterotopias: a newly recognized neuronal migration anomaly. Radiology 1989;171:455–458.

148. Palmini A, Andermann F, Aicardi J, et al. Diffuse cortical dysplasia, or the "double cortex" syndrome: the clinical and epileptic spectrum in 10 patients. Neurology 1991;41:1656–1662.

149. Palmini A, Andermann F, Olivier A, et al. Focal neuronal migration disorders and intractable partial epilepsy: a study of 30 patients. Ann Neurol 1991;30:741–749.

150. Voit T, Sewry CA, Meyer K, et al. Preserved merosin M-chain [or laminin-alpha(2)] expression in skeletal muscle distinguishes Walker-Warburg syndrome from Fukuyama muscular dystrophy and merosin-deficient congenital muscular dystrophy. Neuropediatrics 1995;26:148–155.

151. Dobyns WB, Patton MA, Stratton RF, et al. Cobblestone lissencephaly with normal eyes and muscle. Neuropediatrics 1996;27:70–75.

152. Toda T, Miyake M, Kobayashi K, et al. Linkage-disequilibrium mapping narrows the Fukuyama-type congenital muscular dystrophy (FCMD) candidate region to less than 100 kb. Am J Hum Genet 1996;59:1313–1320.

153. Toda T, Kanazawa I, Nakamura Y. Localization of a gene responsible for Fukuyama type congenital muscular dystrophy to chromosome 9q31–33 by linkage analysis [abstract]. Hum Gen Map Wkshp 1993;93:20.

154. Kallmann F, Schoenfeld W, Barrera S. The genetic aspects of primary eunuchoidism. Am J Ment Defic 1944;48:203–236.

155. Schwankhaus J, Currie J, Jaffe M, et al. Neurologic findings in men with isolated hypogonadotropic hypogonadism. Neurology 1989;39:223–226.

156. Sunohara N, Sakuragawa N, Satoyoshi E, et al. A new syndrome of anosmia, ichthyosis, hypogonadism, and various neurological manifestations with deficiency of steroid sulfatase and arylsulfatase C. Ann Neurol 1986;19:174–181.

157. Naftolin F, Harris G, Bobrow M. Effect of purified luteinizing hormone releasing factor on normal and hypogonadotropic anosmic men. Nature 1971;232:496–497.

158. Schwanzel-Fukuda M, Bick D, Pfaff D. Luteinizing hormone–releasing hormone (LH-RH)–expressing cells do not migrate normally in an inherited hypogonadal (Kallmann) syndrome. Mol Brain Res 1989;6:311–326.

159. Rugarli E, Lutz B, Kuratani S, et al. Expression pattern of the Kallmann syndrome gene in the olfactory system suggests a role in neuronal targeting. Nat Genet 1993;4:19–26.

160. Powers JM. The pathology of peroxisomal disorders with pathogenetic considerations. J Neuropathol Exp Neurol 1995;54:710–719.

161. Powers JM, Tummons RC, Caviness VS, et al. Structural and chemical alterations in the cerebro-hepato-renal (Zellweger) syndrome. J Neuropathol Exp Neurol 1989;48:270–289.

162. Volpe J, Adams R. Cerebro-hepato-renal syndrome of Zellweger: an inherited disorder of neuronal migration. Acta Neuropathol 1972;20:175–198.

163. Baes M, Gressens P, Baumgart E, et al. A mouse model for Zellweger syndrome. Nat Genet 1997;17:49–57.

164. Faust P, Hatten ME. Production of a mouse model for Zellweger syndrome, a neuronal migration disorder [abstract]. J Neuropathol Exp Neurol 1996;55:630.

165. Shimozawa N, Tsukanoto T, Surubi Y, et al. A human gene responsible for Zellweger's syndrome that affects peroxisome assembly. Science 1992;255:1132–1134.

166. van den Bosch H, Schrakamp G, Hardeman D, et al. Ether lipid synthesis and its deficiency in peroxisomal disorders. Biochimie 1993;75:183–189.

167. Sturk A, Schaap MCL, Prins A, et al. Age-related deficiency of synthesis of platelet activating factor by leukocytes from Zellweger patients. Blood 1987;70:460–463.

168. Dobyns WB, Truwit CL. Lissencephaly and other malformations of cortical development: 1995 update. Neuropediatrics 1995;26:132–147.
169. Guerrini R, Dubeau F, Dulac O, et al. Bilateral parasagittal parietooccipital polymicrogyria and epilepsy. Ann Neurol 1997;41:65–73.
170. Kuzniecky R, Berkovic S, Andermann F, et al. Focal cortical myoclonus and Rolandic cortical dysplasia; clarification by magnetic resonance imaging. Ann Neurol 1988;23:317–325.
171. Kuzniecky R, Andermann F, Guerrini R, et al. Congenital bilateral perisylvian syndrome: study of 31 patients. Lancet 1993;341:608–612.
172. Kuzniecky R, Andermann F. The congenital bilateral perisylvian syndrome: imaging findings in a multicenter study. AJNR Am J Neuroradiol 1994;15:139–144.
173. Kuzniecky R, Andermann F, Guerrini R. The epileptic spectrum in the congenital bilateral perisylvian syndrome. Neurology 1994;44:379–385.
174. Raymond AA, Fish D, Sisodiya S, et al. Abnormalities of gyration, heterotopias, tuberous sclerosis, focal cortical dysplasia, microdysgenesis, dysembryoplastic neuroepithelial tumour and dysgenesis of the archicortex in epilepsy: clinical, EEG and neuroimaging features in 100 adult patients. Brain 1995;118:629–660.
175. Eksioglu YZ, Scheffer IE, Cardenas P, et al. Periventricular heterotopia: an X-linked dominant epilepsy locus causing aberrant cerebral cortical development. Neuron 1996;16:77–87.
176. Dobyns WB, Guerrini R, Czapansky-Beilman DK, et al. Bilateral periventricular nodular heterotopia with mental retardation and syndactyly in boys: a new X-linked mental retardation syndrome. Neurology 1997;49:1042–1047.
177. Armstrong D. The neuropathology of temporal lobe epilepsy. J Neuropathol 1993;52:433–443.
178. Meencke HJ, Veith G. Migration disturbances in epilepsy. Mol Neurobiol Epilepsy 1992;9:31–40.
179. Hardiman O, Burke T, Phillips J, et al. Microdysgenesis in resected temporal neocortex: incidence and clinical significance in focal epilepsy. Neurology 1988;38:1041–1047.
180. Farrell MA, DeRosa MJ, Curran JG, et al. Neuropathologic findings in cortical resections (including hemispherectomies) performed for the treatment of intractable childhood epilepsy. Acta Neuropathol 1992;83:246–259.
181. Kuzniecky R, Garcia J, Faught E, et al. Cortical dysplasia in temporal lobe epilepsy magnetic resonance imaging correlations. Ann Neurol 1991;29:293–298.
182. Lehericy S, Dormont D, Semah F, et al. Developmental abnormalities of the medial temporal lobe in patients with temporal lobe epilepsy. AJNR Am J Neuroradiol 1995;16:617–626.
183. Raymond A, Fish D, Stevens J, et al. Association of hippocampal sclerosis with cortical dysgenesis in patients with epilepsy. Neurology 1994;44:1841–1845.
184. Mischel P, Nguyen L, Vinters H. Cerebral cortical dysplasia associated with pediatric epilepsy: review of neuropathologic features and proposal for a grading system. J Neuropathol Exp Neurol 1995;54:137–153.
185. Sanes JR. Topographic maps and molecular gradients. Curr Opin Neurobiol 1993;3:67–74.
186. Goodman CS, Shatz CJ. Developmental mechanisms that generate precise patterns of neuronal activity. Cell 1993;10:77–98.
187. O'Leary DDM, Heffner CD, Kutka L, et al. A target-derived chemoattractant controls the development of the corticopontine projection by a novel mechanism of axon targeting. Development 1991;2(suppl):123–130.
188. Sperry RW. Chemoaffinity in the orderly growth of nerve fiber patterns and connections. Proc Natl Acad Sci U S A 1963;50:703–710.
189. Tessier-Lavigne M. Axon guidance by molecular gradients. Curr Opin Neurobiol 1992;2:60–65.

190. Raper JA, Kapfhammer JP. The enrichment of a neuronal growth cone collapsing activity from embryonic chick brain. Neuron 1990;2:21–29.
191. Fan J, Raper JA. Localized collapsing cues can steer growth cones without inducing their full collapse. Neuron 1995;14:263–274.
192. Haydon PG, Zoran MJ. Formation and modulation of chemical connections: evoked acetylcholine release from growth cones and neurites of specific identified neurons. Neuron 1989;2:1483–1490.
193. Xie A-P, Poo M-M. Initial events in the formation of neuromuscular synapse: rapid induction of acetylcholine release. Proc Natl Acad Sci U S A 1986;83:7069–7073.
194. Furshpan EJ, Potter DD. Seizure-like activity and cellular damage in rat hippocampal neurons in cell culture. Neuron 1989;3:199–207.
195. Segal MM. Epileptiform activity in microcultures containing one excitatory hippocampal neuron. J Neurophysiol 1991;65:761–770.
196. Constantine-Paton M, Cline HT, Debski E. Patterned activity, synaptic convergence, and the NMDA receptor in developing visual pathways. Annu Rev Neurosci 1990;13:129–154.
197. Hubel DH, Wiesel TN. The period of susceptibility to the physiological effects of unilateral eye closure in kittens. J Physiol 1970;206:419–436.
198. Kato K, Clark GD, Bazan NG, et al. Platelet-activating factor as a potential retrograde messenger in CA1 hippocampal long-term potentiation. Nature 1994;367:175–179.
199. Gomez-Di Cesare C, Smith KL, Rice FL, et al. Axonal remodeling during postnatal maturation of CA3 hippocampal pyramidal neurons. J Comp Neurol 1997;384:165–180.
200. Marín-Padilla M. Structural abnormalities of the cerebral cortex in human chromosomal aberrations: a Golgi study. Brain Res 1972;44:625–629.
201. Becker LE, Armstrong DL, Chan F. Dendritic atrophy in children with Down's syndrome. Ann Neurol 1986;20:520–526.
202. Armstrong DD, Antalffy B, Dunn JK. Quantitative Golgi studies of dendrites in Rett syndrome and trisomy 21 [abstract]. J Neuropathol Exp Neurol 1996;55:630.
203. Bauman ML, Kemper TK, Arin DM. Microscopic observations of the brain in Rett syndrome. Neuropediatrics 1995;26:105–108.
204. Bauman ML, Kemper TK. Pervasive neurological abnormalities of the brain in Rett syndrome: a second case. J Neuropathol Exp Neurol 1992;51:340.
205. Armstrong D, Dunn JK, Antalffy B, et al. Selective dendritic alterations in the cortex of Rett syndrome. J Neuropathol Exp Neurol 1995;54:195–201.
206. Armstrong DD. Review of Rett syndrome. J Neuropathol Exp Neurol 1997;56:843–849.
207. Belichenko PV, Oldfors A, Hagberg B, et al. Rett syndrome: 3-D confocal microscopy of cortical pyramidal dendrites and afferents. Neuroreport 1994;5:1509–1513.
208. Belichenko PA, Hagberg B, Dahlstrom A. Morphological study of neocortical areas in Rett syndrome. Acta Neuropathol 1997;93:50–61.
209. Verkerk AJMH, Pieretti M, Sutcliffe JS, et al. Identification of a gene (FMR-1) containing a CGG repeat coincident with a breakpoint cluster region exhibiting length variation in fragile X syndrome. Cell 1991;65:905–914.
210. Hinton VJ, Brown WT, Wisniewski K, et al. Analysis of neocortex in three males with the fragile X syndrome. Am J Med Genet 1991;41:289–294.

3

The Value of Cranial Ultrasonography in Predicting Cerebral Palsy

Linda S. de Vries

When cranial ultrasonography was introduced in the late 1970s, no one could foresee the impact that the data collected via this new technique would have on future management of infants, especially preterm infants in the neonatal intensive care unit (NICU). The first ultrasound (US) machines were of the linear array type. The scanner head, when placed on the temporal bone, provided an axial view through the brain with a 5-MHz transducer.[1] Within 1 year, a better acoustic window—the anterior fontanelle—was identified.[2,3] Use of the anterior fontanelle provided a clearer picture as the sound now was passing only through the skin rather than through bone and skin. The linear-array US machine allowed a view of the lateral ventricles but permitted almost no visualization of periventricular white matter (Figure 3.1A).[3] When the first cases of intraventricular hemorrhages (IVH) in infants were identified in vivo by ultrasonography they were followed up for several weeks. On follow-up, posthemorrhagic ventricular dilatation could be visualized, and the diameter of the lateral ventricles could be measured.[4,5]

The early 1980s heralded the introduction of mechanical-sector scanners, which offer an improved field of view, especially when the angle of insonation is 90 instead of 60 degrees. A pie-shaped area of the brain, including the periventricular white matter, could be seen with these devices. At approximately the same time, transducers with better resolution (7.5 + 10 MHz) became available (Figure 3.1B,C), enabling recognition of cystic lesions in children with periventricular leukomalacia (PVL); these cysts often were missed or were poorly recognized using only a 5-MHz transducer.[6–8] Many prospective US studies performed in the early 1980s provided an enormous amount of information about the neonatal brain, information that previously had been recognized in vivo in only a few computed tomography (CT) studies.[9] Before the introduction of mechanical-sector US scanners, most of our knowledge of the neonatal brain had come from postmortem studies. Ultrasonography allowed practitioners to learn that even a large IVH could be present in a child

83

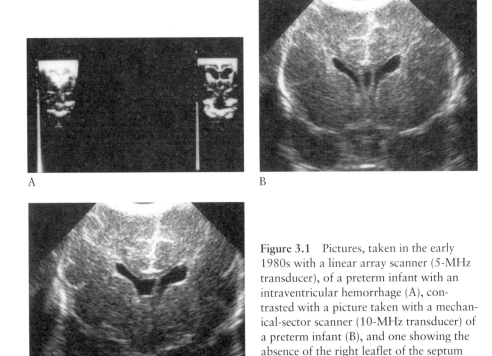

A

B

C

Figure 3.1 Pictures, taken in the early 1980s with a linear array scanner (5-MHz transducer), of a preterm infant with an intraventricular hemorrhage (A), contrasted with a picture taken with a mechanical-sector scanner (10-MHz transducer) of a preterm infant (B), and one showing the absence of the right leaflet of the septum pellucidum (C). (Photograph A courtesy of Professor MI Levene, Leeds, UK.)

who exhibited no obvious clinical signs and that some infants with large parenchymal lesions demonstrated few or no adverse neurologic sequelae; such findings at follow-up were exciting and suggestive of brain plasticity.[10] Prospective US studies provided us with information about the incidence of germinal matrix hemorrhages (GMH) and IVH, which, in the early 1980s, was approximately 40–50% in infants younger than 32 weeks' gestational age. Performing cranial ultrasonography at 6-hour intervals, we were able to identify risk factors for GMH-IVH, the most important factors in most of these studies being gestational age and ventilation for respiratory distress syndrome.[11,12] Awareness of these risk factors coincided with a gradual lowering of the incidence of GMH-IVH in subsequent years.[13,14]

Many studies were performed in which several drugs were used to prevent the occurrence of GMH-IVH. Studies of the use of phenobarbital,[15] ethamsylate,[16] and indomethacin[17,18] received the most attention. Except for indomethacin, which is used prophylactically in many neonatal hospital units in the United States, no drugs are used routinely in most neonatal units. Better antenatal care and particularly the use of corticosteroids have helped to reduce the incidence of GMH-IVH, which continues to diminish worldwide.[19]

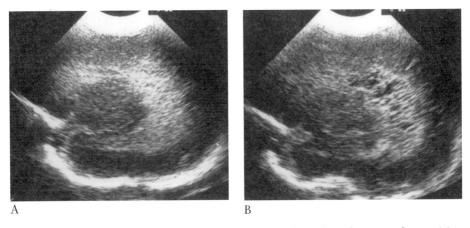

A   B

Figure 3.2 Preterm infant, born at 31 weeks, admitted on day 8 because of necrotizing enterocolitis. Parasagittal views on admission (A) and after 2 weeks (B) show marked echogenicity that, over time, developed into cysts.

PERIVENTRICULAR LEUKOMALACIA

In the mid-1980s, the periventricular white matter became a focus of attention for the medical community. PVL, especially in its cystic form, was discovered to be of major importance in regard to neurodevelopmental outcome and usually carried a worse prognosis than did large IVH.[20,21] Visualization of the cysts required use of a mechanical-sector scanner with a wide field of view and a transducer with sufficiently high resolution (7.5 MHz).[22] In addition to these two factors, sequential studies were discovered to be essential for making the diagnosis, as longitudinal US studies revealed a stepwise development of the disease, from an early echogenic phase to a cystic phase, in some cases after 2–3 weeks (Figures 3.2, 3.3).[6,7] These cystic lesions tended to resolve some weeks after the preterm infants had reached full-term age.

Prospective US studies that attempted to identify the risk factors for cystic PVL provided disappointingly varied results. Some risk factors, such as antepartum hemorrhage and hypocapnia, were identified in several studies, but hypotension, surprisingly, could not always be identified as a risk factor.[23–26] In some studies, large GMH-IVH tended to occur in less mature preterm infants than did cystic PVL, but this finding was not confirmed by other studies.[27] GMH-IVH tended to occur soon after delivery, generally within the first 72 hours and rarely beyond the first week of life, whereas cystic PVL could be present at birth or could develop many weeks after delivery.[28]

Once cystic PVL was recognized ultrasonographically, periventricular echogenicity (PVE), sometimes referred to as *flares*, became apparent in some cases; this condition resolved without subsequent cystic evolution. PVE now is recognized by many groups as the milder end of the spectrum of PVL (Figure 3.4).[22,29–31] The terminology, however, differs from one study to the next, some

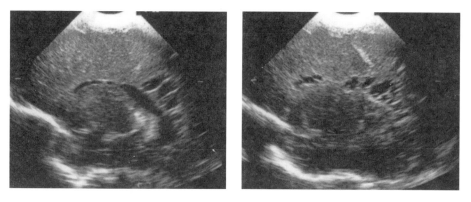

Figure 3.3 Same infant as in Figure 3.2, showing more extensive cysts at 5 weeks of age.

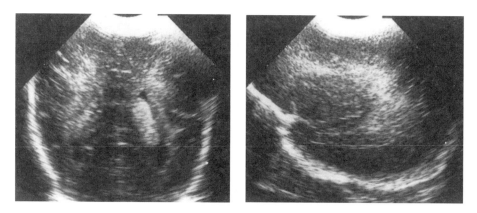

Figure 3.4 Preterm infant born at 30 weeks. Despite a rather uncomplicated neonatal course, marked periventricular echogenicity was noted during the first 2 weeks. No cystic evolution occurred. The child developed a mild spastic diplegia and is delayed globally.

authors stressing the degree of echogenicity (as dense as the choroid plexus or patchy rather than homogeneous) and others stressing the duration of the densities (at least 7 days or more than 14 days).[32] In addition, the demonstration of PVE tends to differ from one machine to the next, making it difficult to compare data from different groups.[32] Correlation between PVE and histologic confirmation of leukomalacia varies from very poor[33] (with a sensitivity as low as 28%) to quite good[31] (with a sensitivity of 85%).

In a small number of cases, the presence of PVE is followed by evolution into a few small localized cysts, which usually are located in the frontoparietal white matter (Figure 3.5). These cysts cannot be recognized using a 5-MHz transducer, tend to be present for 1–2 weeks only, and therefore are at risk for going unnoticed, either because of early referral back to a level 2 hospital or

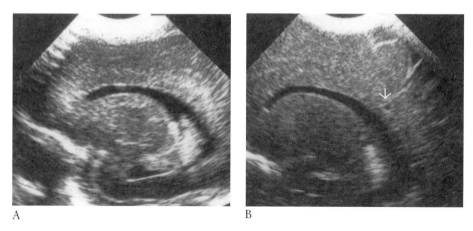

A   B

Figure 3.5 Preterm infant, born at 27 weeks' gestation, colonized with group B strepto-coccus, one of monozygous twins. Parasagittal views show marked periventricular echogenicity on day 2 (A), evolving into localized cysts (*arrow*), best seen with a 10-MHz transducer 2 weeks later (B).

because of insufficient repetition of the US scans. In our experience,[34] approximately 65% of infants with small localized cysts, compared to approximately 10% with PVE, develop spastic diplegia. The performance of sequential US scans on a weekly basis for as long as the PVE is present is essential. The degree of cerebral palsy is least severe in those infants with PVE; almost all affected infants with diplegia managed to walk unaided by the age of 24–30 months. More severe cases of cerebral palsy were seen in infants with localized cysts, who were likely to be wheelchair-bound.

HYPOXIC-ISCHEMIC ENCEPHALOPATHY

Few data are available in the literature about the the use of cranial ultrasonography in the full-term infant who has sustained hypoxic-ischemic encephalopathy (HIE). Most studies performed in this group of infants are disappointing and suggest that CT scans or, preferably, magnetic resonance imaging (MRI) might be more useful modalities.[35,36] Unlike in the preterm infant, in whom the lesions are present mainly in the germinal matrix or the periventricular white matter, lesions in the full-term infant with HIE are present in the thalami or basal ganglia, in the subcortical white matter, and in the cortex. The first two areas can be visualized with a 5- or, preferably, a 7.5-MHz transducer, though lesions in the cortex will be missed using a transducer with this level of resolution. Use of a 10-MHz transducer usually permits identification of such changes in the cortex as laminar necrosis (Figure 3.6).[37] Use of the small posterior fontanelle as a second acoustic window affords a better view of the occipital subcortical and cortical areas.[38] Cranial US findings and histologic data are well

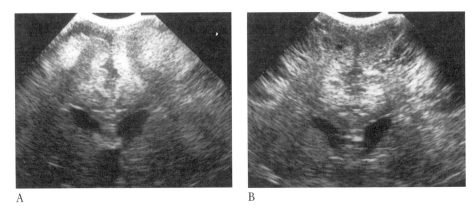

A   B

Figure 3.6 Preterm infant, born at 34 weeks. Hypotensive episode at 46 weeks' postmenstrual age. Coronal view 3 days later shows echogenicity of the cortex and the subcortical white matter (10-MHz transducer) (A), and cystic breakdown is noted 10 days later (B).

correlated both for lesions in the thalami and basal ganglia and for lesions in the cortex and subcortical white matter.[39]

Comparison of ultrasonography and neonatal MRI has been undertaken by several groups. In one study involving 40 cases of HIE, all infants who had a poor neurologic outcome were identified by these imaging modalities.[40] In all studies, however, lesions in the basal ganglia and the cortex were better visualized using MRI. None of the studies used a 10-MHz transducer.

NEONATAL STROKE

Neonatal stroke occurs especially in the full-term, but also in the preterm, infant.[41–43] In its best-recognized form, neonatal stroke is an infarct in the vascular distribution of one of the main cerebral arteries, most commonly the middle cerebral artery, and more often on the left. An anterior or posterior cerebral artery infarct can occur but is less common. Most articles dealing with this condition refer to full-term infants who present with hemiconvulsions, sometimes after a normal delivery but in other cases after a complicated delivery with subsequent neonatal encephalopathy.[43,44] A wedge-shaped area of increased echogenicity is noted to develop gradually, becoming increasingly obvious during the first week of life (Figure 3.7).[45] In some cases, the echogenicity remains very mild and the infarct will pass unnoticed by ultrasonography. CT or MRI, the latter being preferred, will have to be performed to make the diagnosis (see Figure 3.7C). In other affected infants, in whom hemorrhage is present in the area of infarction, the lesion is more easily recognized owing to the patchy echogenicity within the area of infarction. Doppler studies can be useful to find either decreased or increased pulsations in the affected area. Subsequent US studies several weeks

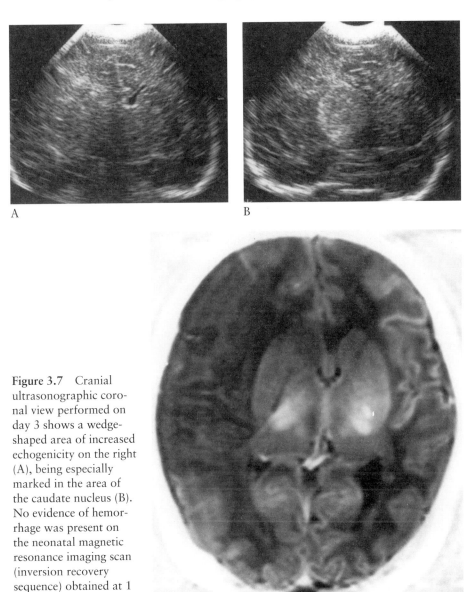

A   B

C

Figure 3.7 Cranial ultrasonographic coronal view performed on day 3 shows a wedge-shaped area of increased echogenicity on the right (A), being especially marked in the area of the caudate nucleus (B). No evidence of hemorrhage was present on the neonatal magnetic resonance imaging scan (inversion recovery sequence) obtained at 1 week (C).

later will show ex vacuo dilatation on the affected side and cystic evolution of the infarcted area (Figure 3.8). Often, the cystic conversion is more obvious on MRI, and the true extent of the lesion is better appreciated (see Figure 3.8C). Wallerian degeneration can also be recognized on MRI in those infants developing a contralateral hemiplegia (Figure 3.8D).[46] Recognition of posterior cerebral

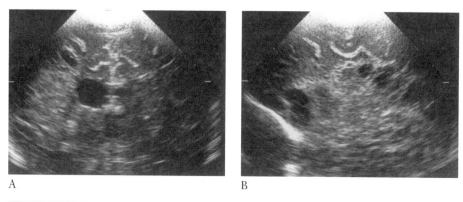

A   B

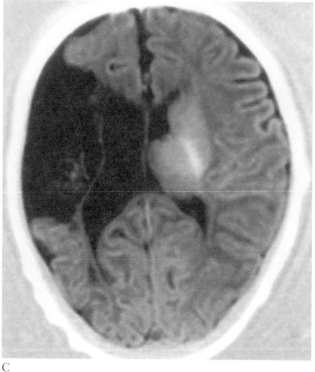

C

Figure 3.8 Cranial ultrasonography at 3 months shows ex vacuo dilatation of the right ventricle and cystic evolution on coronal (A) and parasagittal (B) views, which is better delineated on magnetic resonance imaging (C). Wallerian degeneration at the level of the mesencephalon is also noted (D).

artery infarcts can be difficult using ultrasonography, but scanning through the posterior fontanelle can sometimes be helpful (Figure 3.9).[38]

Although in full-term infants the main branch of the middle cerebral artery usually is occluded, possibly only a cortical branch or some of the perforating lenticulostriatal branches will be involved. Involvement of only these branches can occur in both full-term and preterm infants and is comparable to the lacunar infarct seen in children and adults.[47]

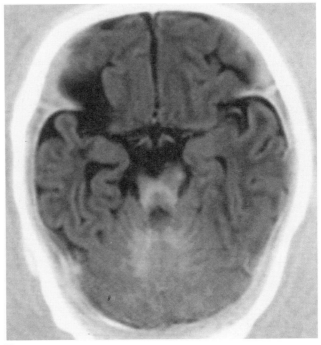

D

We have seen a number of preterm infants with these so-called lacunar infarcts, in which the blood flow through the lenticulostriatal arteries appeared to be affected (Figure 3.10).[47] Areas of increased echogenicity were seen initially by the end of the first week and cystic conversion was not obligatory, with some lesions remaining echogenic until the infants had reached full-term age, even though a cystic lesion by then was apparent on MRI. Of the 13 preterm infants with lacunar infarct for whom we cared, the infarct was associated with an IVH in two infants and cystic PVL in two others.

In contrast to other studies,[43] we were unable to identify any full-term infants who had a middle cerebral artery infarct affecting the main branch and who suffered *no* adverse neurologic sequelae at follow-up. Aside from the development of a contralateral hemiplegia, hypsarrhythmia occurred in some of the infants, and cognition sometimes was impaired.

Nonetheless, in our preterm infants with more localized infarcts in this region, only 5 of 12 had motor sequelae. Except for the pathologic study by Paneth and coworkers,[48] no data are available about this type of lesion in preterm infants.

Although a neonatal stroke can be found after a difficult delivery and a thromboembolism can sometimes be shown postmortem, the etiology is unknown in most cases. Attention has been drawn to associated coagulopathy, especially the roles of proteins C and S; factor V Leiden also appears to be important.[49]

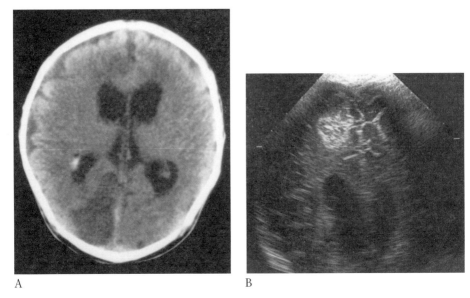

A   B

Figure 3.9 Full-term infant. After extracorporeal membrane oxygenation, a posterior cerebral artery infarct was seen on a computed tomography scan performed because of convulsions (A). This lesion was missed initially by ultrasonography but could, in fact, be recognized on a scan performed through the posterior fontanelle (B). (Reproduced with permission from LS de Vries, P Eken, E Beek, et al. The posterior fontanelle: a neglected acoustic window. Neuropediatrics 1996;26:101–104.)

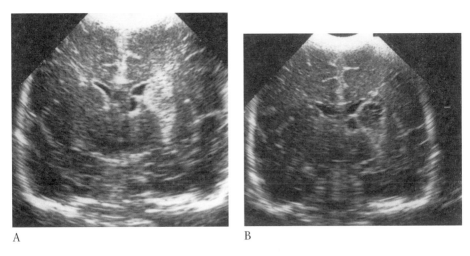

A   B

Figure 3.10 Cranial ultrasonographic coronal views show the evolution of a lacunar infarct, with a wedge-shaped echogenic area at the level of the caudate nucleus and the striate on day 14 (A) and subsequent cystic evolution on day 28 (B). (Reproduced with permission from LS de Vries, P Eken, F Groenendaal, et al. Infarcts in the vascular distribution of the middle cerebral artery in preterm and full-term infants. Neuropediatrics 1997;28:88–96.)

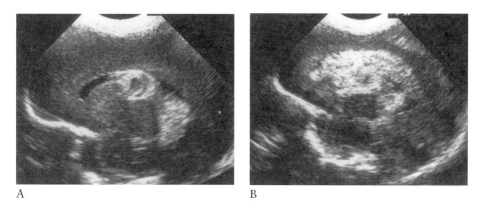

A   B

Figure 3.11 Cranial ultrasonographic parasagittal view of a preterm infant, born at 27 weeks by emergency cesarean section because of placental abruption. A very large clot in the left ventricle, worse on day 2 (B) than on day 1 (A), caused acute ventricular dilatation.

CEREBRAL PALSY

Soon after cranial ultrasonography was introduced, the possibility of predicting cerebral palsy in at least some cases was recognized, especially those cases exhibiting extensive lesions in the brain parenchyma.[21,50]

Some intracranial lesions that do not appear to affect the brain parenchyma are also commonly associated with the development of cerebral palsy during infancy. Knowledge of this fact is especially relevant in those children who develop infantile hydrocephalus after a large IVH without obvious parenchymal involvement (Figure 3.11).[51–54] According to the results of the Ventriculomegaly Trial Group,[51,52] 55% of the infants in whom no parenchymal involvement was recorded had neurologic impairment with loss of function. Others made similar findings, although no differentiation was made concerning parenchymal involvement in the study by Fernell and colleagues,[54] in which 67% of infants who had a shunt developed cerebral palsy. Among 33 infants with ventriculomegaly after a moderate to severe hemorrhage, 19 (57%) had sequelae[53]: Of the 33 infants, 23 required a shunt, but the neurodevelopmental outcome between those with and without a shunt did not differ. The most important predictor of motor and mental outcome was the degree of ventricular decompression after shunt insertion.

In our own NICU, we cared for 44 infants with a large IVH, 25 (57%) of whom survived. Only 3 (12%) of the survivors developed cerebral palsy in infancy. Of the 25 survivors, 8 (32%) required insertion of a ventriculoperitoneal shunt, but none of these developed cerebral palsy.

An explanation for this difference between our findings and the studies by the Ventriculomegaly Trial Group and others[51–54] is not readily defined, especially as the number of surviving infants is small. Possibly, withdrawal of intensive care from some patients who had both severe acute dilatation at the time of the hemorrhage and severe PVE is responsible for the different outcomes, as

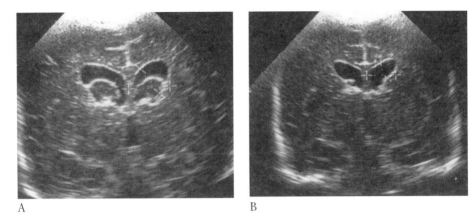

A   B

Figure 3.12 Cranial ultrasonographic coronal view on day 21 shows resolving clots in dilated ventricles before (A) and after (B) a lumbar puncture. Note that the diagonal shape especially has almost normalized.

intensive care might have been continued in other hospitals. The ventriculomegaly trial was performed in the early 1980s; hence, associated PVL might not have been noted on ultrasonography or might not have been recorded after trial entry, as the trial researchers themselves suggest.[51,52] The difference in outcome also could be related to earlier intervention: In our unit, lumbar punctures were begun as soon as clear progression in ventricular size was noted, such progression being associated with a balloon shape of the ventricle (Figure 3.12).[55] This same intervention was undertaken later in the ventriculomegaly trial, only after ventricular size exceeded the ninety-seventh percentile plus 4 mm (according to Levene[4]). We also prefer to insert a subcutaneous reservoir instead of performing ventricular taps in those infants with noncommunicating hydrocephalus, because of the risk of damage from needle tracks (Figure 3.13).

Parenchymal Lesions in Preterm Infants

Hemorrhagic Lesions

In the early 1980s, parenchymal hemorrhages were first recognized during life, using both CT scanning and ultrasonography. Sequential US studies sometimes showed that infants who had an IVH on 1 day showed unilateral parenchymal involvement 1–2 days later (Figure 3.14).[56] This parenchymal involvement was considered initially to be an extension of the IVH. More recently, several postmortem studies involving venous angiography[57,58] have suggested that this unilateral hemorrhagic lesion is most likely due to impaired drainage of veins passing through the periventricular white matter.[57,58] This type of lesion now is called *venous infarction* by some groups, although others still include it in the spectrum of PVL.

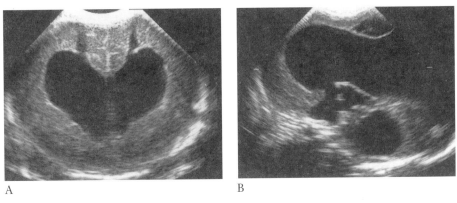

A   B

Figure 3.13 Cranial ultrasonography, day 26, shows bilateral needle tracks after ventricular taps (A). Lumbar punctures were unsuccessful, probably due to the normally rapid rate of cerebrospinal fluid formation and obstruction at the outlet of the fourth ventricle, which has become very dilated (B).

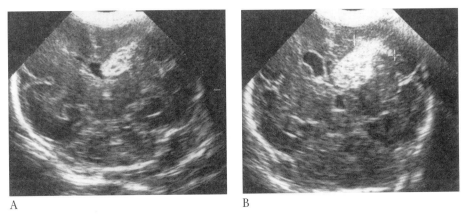

A   B

Figure 3.14 Preterm infant at 27 weeks' gestation with a large intraventricular hemorrhage with a very small area of periventricular echogenicity 2 hours after delivery (A). Twenty-four hours later, a large left-sided, wedge-shaped venous infarct, in communication with the lateral ventricle, can be seen (B).

A power Doppler study by Taylor[59] also supported the role of impaired venous drainage. In a group of 56 infants with unilateral hemorrhagic lesions, we were able to show that the parenchymal lesion could be large, globular, and in complete or partial communication with the lateral ventricle. After several weeks, resolution of the clot became apparent, eventually resulting in a porencephalic cyst.[60] In a large number of cases, however, the unilateral lesion in the parenchyma was echogenic and wedge-shaped but remained separate from the lateral ventricle.

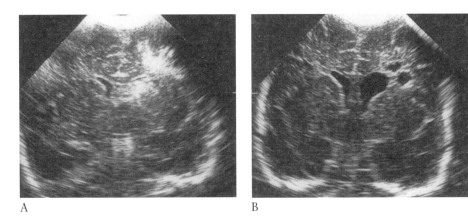

A   B

Figure 3.15 Preterm infant at 34 weeks' gestation, admitted because of apneic spells. Coronal views on day 2 (A) and day 28 (B) show a left-sided intraventricular hemorrhage associated with a wedge-shaped echogenic area separate from the lateral ventricle, with subsequent cystic evolution. (Reproduced with permission from KJ Rademaker, F Groenendaal, GH Jansen, et al. Unilateral hemorrhagic parenchymal lesions in the preterm infant: shape, site and prognosis. Acta Paediatr 1994;83:602–608.)

On follow-up of unilateral hemorrhagic lesions with repeated ultrasonography, a few small cystic lesions could be identified in this previously echogenic area (Figure 3.15). In a few cases, the lesion could be seen, on subsequent scans, to evolve from wedge-shaped and separate to globular and communicating, findings that support the theory of a continuity of one type of lesion. Prediction of the subsequent development of cerebral palsy depended mainly on the site of the parenchymal lesion. The more anterior the lesion (best seen on a parasagittal view), the less likely was development of cerebral palsy in the child.[60] Similar conclusions were drawn by others.[61]

In our study,[60] 15 of the 30 survivors with unilateral hemorrhagic lesions underwent MRI later in infancy. Correlation between neonatal US findings and later MRI scans was good. Separation seen initially on ultrasonography could still be recognized on MRI. Gliosis usually was present around the porencephalic cyst but was less diffuse than in those infants suffering cystic PVL. In those infants who had a contralateral hemiplegia, wallerian degeneration was evident, sometimes only at a level of the brain stem but usually also in the internal capsule.[46] Hemosiderin breakdown products were present only in those infants scanned before the end of the first year of life.[46]

Ischemic Lesions

As soon as more sophisticated US equipment made possible the recognition of cystic PVL, researchers learned that this type of parenchymal lesion had an enormous impact on subsequent neurodevelopmental outcome.[20,21,62] The first short-term follow-up studies reported on small groups of infants and noted that all or nearly all infants had adverse neurologic sequelae.[23,63] Several prospective studies have now shown that cerebral visual impairment, in addition to severe motor impairment, commonly is present among these infants, in contrast to those children with large hemorrhages.[64] However, subsequent studies involving larger groups of infants have identified some infants who did not develop cerebral palsy, despite extensive cysts in the brain parenchyma.[65] As with the unilateral parenchymal lesions mentioned previously, several groups have observed that the more posterior the cysts, the more likely is the development of motor problems in the child. That infants affected with cystic PVL fare so much worse than those infants with a unilateral hemorrhagic parenchymal lesion is easy to understand, because cystic PVL is usually a bilateral, although not necessarily a symmetric, lesion. Unilateral venous hemorrhagic infarction, however, can occur together with cystic PVL.

Many MRI studies performed later in infancy have shown the long-term effect of this extensive cystic form of PVL.[44,66–68] All such studies have pointed out that the ventricles usually are mildly dilated and irregular in shape. Furthermore, delayed myelination and extensive gliosis commonly are present, especially affecting those areas in which the cysts were seen initially. The corpus callosum is also affected, being both abnormally shaped and thin, which correlates well with the degree of motor impairment.[69] The degree of involvement of the optic radiation as well as the visual cortex was noted to be related to the presence of cerebral visual impairment.[70,71]

Subsequent studies involved not only infants with extensive cystic PVL but infants with localized cysts (usually located in the frontoparietal white matter) and infants with PVE. Although cerebral palsy does occur in children with this milder form of PVL, the disorder in such children is less common and often less severe.[34,62,72] Comparison of the degree of PVL diagnosed using cranial ultrasonography and later MRI findings revealed a good correlation, with more ventricular dilatation and more extensive gliosis among the infants with the more extensive US abnormalities.[34]

Several groups have now researched infants with PVE only and have shown that transient tone abnormalities can be seen during the first year of life in up to half of the cases, whereas up to 10% of the infants developed mild spastic diplegia.[72–74] Long-term follow-up studies have shown that the duration of PVE was important with regard to the development of perceptual-motor incompetence.[75]

A slightly different form of white matter disease may be present in the extremely low-birth-weight preterm infant. Paneth and colleagues[76] reported on autopsy findings in 22 preterm infants who died after 5 days. Although 15 of them had white matter necrosis, only 3 had the classic changes of PVL, initially described by Banker and Larroche,[77] indicating that the condition may be different and apparently more diffuse in very preterm infants. In some of these cases, only mild ventriculomegaly becomes apparent after several weeks, without preceding evidence of PVE. Wheater and Rennie[78] reported on 47 infants who were ventilated for more than 27 days. Only 10 of the 27 survivors did not sustain a major handicap. The presence of the handicap could be explained by US abnor-

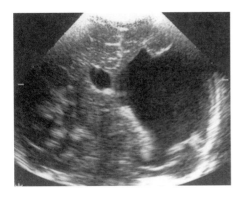

Figure 3.16 Cranial ultrasonographic coronal view, showing a left-sided porencephalic cyst in an infant born at 36 weeks, who was affected by neonatal alloimmune thrombocytopenia.

malities in only 9 of 17 cases. These authors therefore suggested that prolonged and repetitive hypoxic spells could affect the white matter in these infants, changes that were not revealed by repeated ultrasonography.

Another ischemic lesion seen in preterm but especially in full-term infants is an infarct in the vascular distribution of a major cerebral artery. See the section Neonatal Stroke.

Antenatal Onset

Both hemorrhagic and ischemic lesions can occur antenatally. In a small number of cases, a large hemorrhage or, more often, posthemorrhagic ventricular dilatation is recognized on an antenatal US scan. Maternal trauma,[79,80] coagulopathy (e.g., neonatal alloimmune thrombocytopenia),[81] or the death of a monozygous cotwin can be held responsible for some of these lesions.[82–84] Neurologic signs often are not obvious or may even be absent in the neonatal period. Figure 3.16 is an example of a child born at 36 weeks who was affected by neonatal alloimmune thrombocytopenia. A large porencephalic cyst was present on the left side of the brain in this child, and remains of a clot were present in the right ventricle. Figure 3.17 is an example of the severe sequelae that occurs in approximately 25% of the cases in which the monozygous cotwin dies. In this set of twins, a bradycardia of one twin was noted in the clinic at 29 weeks. The mother was referred to the university hospital, but the twin had died before her arrival. When the other twin was born only 2 weeks later, extensive cysts were seen throughout the parieto-occipital white matter.

Performing cranial ultrasonography as soon as possible after admission of preterm infants will help to determine how often severe lesions occur antenatally, an important piece of information given the ever-increasing number of medicolegal cases entering our justice system. In a study by Murphy and associates,[85] who studied a cohort of 83 very preterm infants who died, 57% had evidence of cerebral damage, and this was considered to be of antenatal onset in 31%. Bejar and colleagues,[86] who prospectively studied 127 preterm infants with a gestational age of less than 36 weeks to determine the incidence of white matter necrosis, found a very high incidence—10.3% of the children had cysts by day 3.

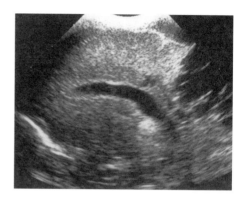

Figure 3.17 Cranial ultrasonographic parasagittal view shows extensive cysts in the parieto-occipital white matter in a preterm infant born at 31 weeks, 2 weeks after the death of his monozygous cotwin.

Parenchymal Lesions in the Full-Term Infant with Hypoxic-Ischemic Encephalopathy

As discussed earlier, lesions in the full-term infant with HIE are seen mainly in the thalami and basal ganglia or in the cortex and subcortical white matter.

Thalami and Basal Ganglia

Abnormalities seen in the thalami and basal ganglia gradually appear during the first week of life. If mild, the abnormalities are not very striking on ultrasonography. The increased echogenicity usually is more striking in the thalamus than in the basal ganglia but, when echogenicity is present in both areas, the internal capsule may be seen as an area of lower echogenicity between these organs, giving what sometimes is called an *onion-peel appearance* (Figure 3.18).[87] In a small number of cases, hemorrhagic conversion occurs, such that the abnormalities are more easily recognized using cranial ultrasonography.

The outcome in affected children varies and depends on associated brain lesions. When lesions are restricted to the basal ganglia, a dystonic type of cerebral palsy is most likely to develop, with a variable degree of mental retardation. At a later stage, MRI sometimes reveals small cystic lesions in the lentiform nuclei.[88] Associated damage in the central gyrus usually coexists in this pattern of acute brain injury, but this damage will invariably be missed on US scanning and will be recognized only on MRI (Figure 3.19).

Subcortical White Matter

Increased echogenicity alone or together with the changes just mentioned can develop also in the subcortical white matter (Figure 3.20). Usually, these affected infants start off with slitlike ventricles. After several days, patchy echogenicity is noted, coinciding with opening of the lateral ventricles. After 10–14 days, cysts (known as *subcortical cysts*) can develop in these previously echogenic areas. In some infants, these cysts involve most of the white matter

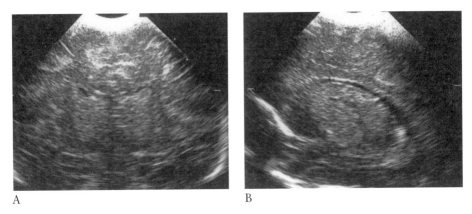

A   B

Figure 3.18 Cranial ultrasonography performed on day 4. Coronal (A) and parasagittal (B) views show increased echogenicity in thalami and basal ganglia; the internal capsule has a relatively low echogenicity.

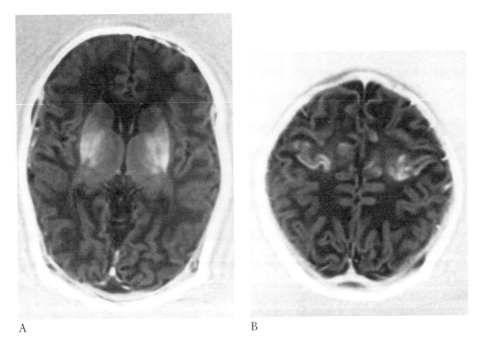

A   B

Figure 3.19 Magnetic resonance imaging (inversion recovery sequence), which was done at the age of 1 week, confirmed lesions in the basal ganglia (A) and showed an abnormal signal in the central gyrus (B).

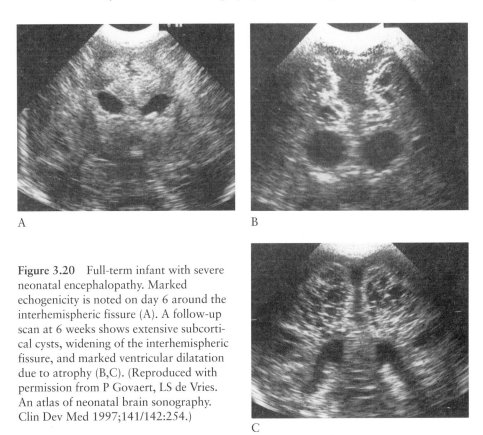

A   B

C

Figure 3.20 Full-term infant with severe neonatal encephalopathy. Marked echogenicity is noted on day 6 around the interhemispheric fissure (A). A follow-up scan at 6 weeks shows extensive subcortical cysts, widening of the interhemispheric fissure, and marked ventricular dilatation due to atrophy (B,C). (Reproduced with permission from P Govaert, LS de Vries. An atlas of neonatal brain sonography. Clin Dev Med 1997;141/142:254.)

and are then classified as *multicystic encephalomalacia*. These larger cysts seen in subcortical leukomalacia or multicystic encephalomalacia rarely disappear and can be visualized as long as the fontanelle remains open. The outcome in these children is extremely poor, most being afflicted with severe microcephaly, mental retardation, quadriplegia, and cerebral visual impairment.[89,90]

Necrosis of the Cortex

All full-term infants with HIE should be examined with a 10-MHz transducer in an attempt to visualize the surface of the brain. In a small number of infants, increased echogenicity will be noted in the cortex several days after birth (see Figure 3.6). In some of the infants who die, cortical laminar necrosis is diagnosed by histology. In others who survive, cystic lesions develop in the markedly echogenic areas, and changes suggestive of ulegyria are noted on MRI performed later in infancy. In some of these infants, the abnormalities are most marked in the occipital region, which is first noted when scanning is accomplished through the posterior fontanelle.[38] In the few survivors with only this type of US abnormality, mental retardation is marked at follow-up.

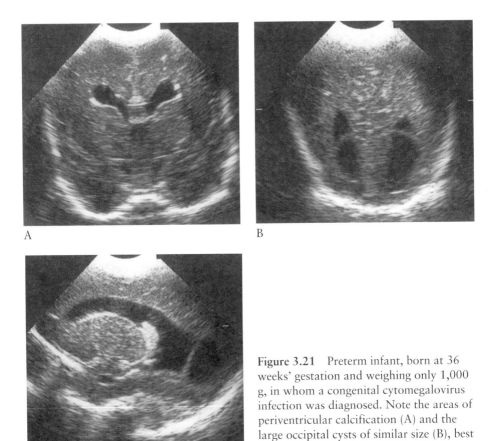

Figure 3.21 Preterm infant, born at 36 weeks' gestation and weighing only 1,000 g, in whom a congenital cytomegalovirus infection was diagnosed. Note the areas of periventricular calcification (A) and the large occipital cysts of similar size (B), best seen on the parasagittal view (C).

Infective Fetopathy

Parenchymal damage can occur in infants who present with a congenital infection. Cyst formation in the germinal matrix, calcification that surrounds the ventricular wall (cytomegalovirus) or that is more widespread throughout the parenchyma (toxoplasmosis), and vasculitis (appearing as dense lines along the striatal arteries in the thalami, the so-called candlestick appearance) are most common.[91] Cysts in the occipital white matter may be seen in infants with a congenital cytomegalovirus infection (Figure 3.21).[92] Other types of infection, such as an echovirus encephalitis[93] or a herpetic infection (which can cause cystic encephalomalacia[94]), can lead to extensive damage of the white matter.

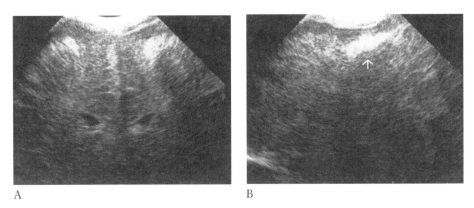

A   B

Figure 3.22 Preterm infant, born at 36 weeks' gestation, with a late-onset group B streptococcal meningitis. Cranial ultrasonographic coronal (A) and parasagittal (B) views, obtained with a 10-MHz transducer, showing a layer of echogenicity just below the brain surface, which was confirmed at postmortem to be areas of infection and necrosis.

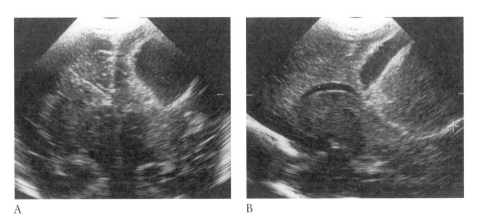

A   B

Figure 3.23 Full-term infant admitted at 2 weeks. Ultrasonographic coronal (A) and parasagittal (B) views showing a large abscess with a level of debris. Group A hemolytic streptococci were cultured. (Reproduced with permission from P Govaert, LS de Vries. An atlas of neonatal brain sonography. Clin Dev Med 1997;141/142:323.)

Neonatal Bacterial Cerebral Infections

Bacterial meningitis or ventriculitis can lead to extensive damage of the white matter. Hemorrhagic necrosis can occur in fulminating gram-positive (hemolytic streptococci group B) or, more often, gram-negative (*Escherichia coli, Proteus*) brain infections, which often are fatal (Figure 3.22). A brain abscess is another rare finding (Figure 3.23). It begins as a focal infarct caused by thrombophlebitis in the white matter.[95] Debris either can fill the whole cavity or can form a level within a fluid-filled encapsulated cavity. Temporary drainage may sometimes be required.

Congenital Malformations

It is beyond the scope of this chapter to discuss the role of ultrasonography with regard to congenital malformations. Today, some of these malformations are already identified antenatally. Some milder problems, such as agenesis of the corpus callosum or absence of the septum pellucidum, will be identified in preterm infants who are scanned routinely after admission to a neonatal ICU. In some of these infants, a chromosomal abnormality or a syndrome will be diagnosed at an early stage, whereas in other infants, no diagnosis will be made and this apparently incidental finding may be of major concern to the parents. MRI will provide additional information about disorders in migration, which can only rarely be identified on ultrasonography.[96–98]

REFERENCES

1. Johnson ML, Mack LA, Rumack CM, et al. B-mode echo-encephalography in the normal and high risk infant. AJR Am J Roentgenol 1979;133:375–381.
2. Pape KE, Cusick G, Houang MTW, et al. Ultrasound detection of brain damage in preterm infants. Lancet 1979;2:1261–1264.
3. Levene MI, Wigglesworth JS, Dubowitz V. Cerebral structure and intraventricular hemorrhage in the neonate: a real-time ultrasound study. Arch Dis Child 1981; 56:416–424.
4. Levene MI. Measurement of the growth of the lateral ventricles in preterm infants with real-time ultrasound. Arch Dis Child 1981;56:900–904.
5. Levene MI, Starte DR. A longitudinal study of post-hemorrhagic ventricular dilatation in the newborn. Arch Dis Child 1981;56:905–910.
6. Bowerman RA, Donn SM, DiPietro MA, et al. Periventricular leukomalacia in the preterm infant: sonographic and clinical features. Radiology 1984;151:383–388.
7. Dolfin T, Skidmore MB, Fong KW, et al. Diagnosis and evolution of periventricular leukomalacia: a study with real-time ultrasound. Early Hum Dev 1984;9:105–109.
8. Levene MI, Wigglesworth JS, Dubowitz V. Hemorrhagic periventricular leukomalacia in the neonate: a real-time ultrasound study. Pediatrics 1983;71:794–797.
9. Papile L, Burstein J, Burstein R, et al. Incidence and evaluation of subependymal hemorrhage: a study of children with birth weights less than 1,500 gm. J Pediatr 1978;92:529–534.
10. Fawer C-L, Levene MI, Dubowitz LMS. Intraventricular hemorrhage in a preterm neonate: discordance between clinical course and ultrasound scan. Neuropediatrics 1983;14:242–244.
11. Levene MI, Fawer C-L, Lamont RF. Risk factors in the development of intraventricular hemorrhage in the preterm neonate. Arch Dis Child 1982;57:410–417.
12. Thorburn RJ, Lipscomb AP, Stewart AL, et al. Timing and antecedents of periventricular hemorrhage and of cerebral atrophy in very preterm infant. Early Hum Dev 1982;7:221–238.
13. Batton DG, Holtrop P, Dewitte D, et al. Current gestational age–related incidence of major intraventricular hemorrhage. J Pediatr 1994;125:623–625.
14. Philip AGS, Allan WC, Tito AM, et al. Intraventricular hemorrhage in preterm infants: declining incidence in the 1980s. Pediatrics 1989;84:797–801.

15. Donn SM, Roloff DW, Goldstein GW. Prevention of intraventricular hemorrhage in preterm infants with phenobarbital. Lancet 1981;2:215.
16. The EC Ethamsylate Trial Group. The EC randomised controlled trial of prophylactic ethamsylate for very preterm neonates: early mortality and morbidity. Arch Dis Child 1994;70:F201–F205.
17. Ment LR, Oh W, Ehrenkranz RA, et al. Low-dose indomethacin and prevention of intraventricular hemorrhage: a multicenter randomized trial. Pediatrics 1994;93:543–550.
18. Fowlie, PW. Prophylactic indomethacin: systematic review and meta-analysis. Arch Dis Child 1996;74:F81–F87.
19. Garland JS, Buck S, Leviton A. Effect of maternal glucocorticoid exposure on risk of severe intraventricular hemorrhage in surfactant-treated preterm infants. J Pediatr 1995;126:272–279.
20. de Vries LS, Dubowitz LMS, Dubowitz V, et al. Predictive value of cranial ultrasound: a reappraisal. Lancet 1985;2:137–140.
21. Graham M, Levene MI, Trounce JQ, et al. Prediction of cerebral palsy in very low birth weight infants: prospective ultrasound study. Lancet 1987;2:593–596.
22. de Vries LS, Eken P, Dubowitz LMS. The spectrum of leukomalacia using cranial ultrasound. Behav Brain Res 1992;49:1–6.
23. Calvert SA, Hoskins EM, Fong KW. Etiological factors associated with the development of periventricular leukomalacia. Acta Paediatr Scand 1987;76:254–259.
24. Trounce JQ, Shaw OE, Levene MI, et al. Clinical risk factors and periventricular leukomalacia. Arch Dis Child 1988;63:17–22.
25. Graziani L, Spitzer AR, Mitchell DG, et al. Mechanical ventilation in preterm infants: neurosonographic and developmental studies. Pediatrics 1992;90:515–522.
26. Fujimoto S, Togari H, Yamaguchi N, et al. Hypocarbia and cystic periventricular leukomalacia in preterm infants. Arch Dis Child 1994;71:F107–F110.
27. de Vries LS, Regev R, Dubowitz LMS, et al. Perinatal risk factors for the development of extensive cystic leukomalacia. Am J Dis Child 1988;42:732–735.
28. de Vries LS, Regev R, Dubowitz LMS. Late onset cystic leukomalacia. Arch Dis Child 1986;61:298–299.
29. McMenamin JB, Shackelford GD, Volpe JJ. Outcome of neonatal IVH with periventricular echodense lesions. Ann Neurol 1984;15:285–290.
30. Fawer C-L, Calame A, Perentes E, Anderegg A. Periventricular leukomalacia: a correlation study between real-time ultrasound and autopsy findings. Neuroradiology 1985;27:292–300.
31. Trounce JQ, Rutter N, Levene MI. Periventricular leukomalacia and intraventricular hemorrhage in the preterm neonate. Arch Dis Child 1986;61:1196–1202.
32. Dammann O, Leviton A. Duration of transient hyperechoic images of white matter in very-low-birthweight infants: a proposed classification. Dev Med Child Neurol 1997;39:2–5.
33. Hope PL, Gould SJ, Howard S, et al. Ultrasound diagnosis of pathologically verified lesions in the brains of very preterm infants. Dev Med Child Neurol 1988; 30:457–471.
34. de Vries LS, Eken P, Groenendaal F, et al. Correlation between the degree of periventricular leukomalacia diagnosed using cranial ultrasound and MRI later in infancy in children with cerebral palsy. Neuropediatrics 1993;24:263–268.
35. Gray PH, Tudehope DI, Masel JP, et al. Perinatal hypoxic-ischemic brain injury: prediction of outcome. Dev Med Child Neurol 1993;35:965–973.
36. Rollins NK, Morriss MC, Evans D, et al. The role of early MR in the evaluation of the term infant with seizures. AJNR Am J Neuroradiol 1994;15:239–248.
37. Couture A, Veyrac C, Baud C, et al. New imaging of cerebral ischemic lesions. High frequency probes and pulsed Doppler. Ann Radiol 1987;30:452–461.

38. de Vries, LS, Eken P, Beek E, et al. The posterior fontanelle: a neglected acoustic window. Neuropediatrics 1996;27:101–104.

39. Eken P, Jansen GH, Groenendaal F, et al. Intracranial lesions in the full-term infant with hypoxic ischemic encephalopathy: ultrasound and autopsy correlation. Neuropediatrics 1994;25:301–307.

40. Rutherford MA, Pennock JM, Dubowitz LMS. Cranial ultrasound and magnetic resonance imaging in hypoxic-ischemic encephalopathy: a comparison with outcome. Dev Med Child Neurol 1994;36:813–825.

41. Barmada MA, Moossy J, Shuman RM. Cerebral infarcts with arterial occlusion in neonates. Ann Neurol 1979;6:495–502.

42. Mannino FL, Trauner DA. Stroke in neonates. J Pediatr 1983;102:605–610.

43. Estan J, Hope P. Unilateral neonatal cerebral infarction in full term infants. Arch Dis Child 1997;76:F88–F93.

44. Mercuri E, Cowan F, Rutherford M, et al. Ischemic and hemorrhagic brain lesions in newborns with seizures and normal Apgar scores. Arch Dis Child 1995;73:F67–F74.

45. Hill A, Martin DJ, Danemann A, et al. Focal ischemic cerebral injury in the newborn: diagnosis by ultrasound and correlation with computed tomographic scans. Pediatrics 1983;71:790–793.

46. Bouza H, Dubowitz LMS, Rutherford M, et al. Prediction of outcome in children with congenital hemiplegia: a magnetic resonance imaging study. Neuropediatrics 1994;25:60–66.

47. de Vries LS, Eken P, Groenendaal F, et al. Infarcts in the vascular distribution of the middle cerebral artery in preterm and full-term infants. Neuropediatrics 1997;28:88–96.

48. Paneth N, Rudelli R, Kazam E, et al. Associated pathologic lesions: cerebellar hemorrhage, pontosubicular necrosis, basal ganglia necrosis. Clin Dev Med 1994;131:163–170.

49. Nowak-Göttl U, Sträter R, Dübbers A, et al. Ischemic stroke in infancy and childhood: role of the Arg[506] to Gln mutation in the factor V gene. Blood Coagul Fibrinolysis 1996;7:684–688.

50. Pinto-Martin JA, Riolo S, Cnaan A, et al. Cranial ultrasound prediction of disabling and nondisabling cerebral palsy at age two in a low birth weight population. Pediatrics 1995;95:249–254.

51. Ventriculomegaly Trial Group. Randomised trial of early tapping in neonatal posthemorrhagic ventricular dilatation. Arch Dis Child 1990;65:3–10.

52. Ventriculomegaly Trial Group. Randomised trial of early tapping in neonatal posthemorrhagic ventricular dilatation: results at 30 months. Arch Dis Child 1994; 70:F129–F136.

53. Shankaran S, Koepke T, Woldt E, et al. Outcome after posthemorrhagic ventriculomegaly in comparison with mild hemorrhage without ventriculomegaly. J Pediatr 1989;114:109–114.

54. Fernell E, Hagberg G, Hagberg B. Infantile hydrocephalus in preterm, low-birthweight infants: a nationwide Swedish cohort study 1979–1988. Acta Paediatr 1993;82:45–48.

55. Sauerbrei EE, Digney M, Harrison PB, et al. Ultrasonic evaluation of neonatal intracranial hemorrhage and its complications. Radiology 1981;139:677–685.

56. Levene MI, de Vries LS. Extension of neonatal intraventricular hemorrhage. Arch Dis Child 1984;59:631–636.

57. Gould SJ, Howard S, Hope PL, et al. Periventricular intraparenchymal cerebral hemorrhage in preterm infants: the role of venous infarction. J Pathol 1987;151: 197–202.

58. Takashima S, Takashi M, Ando Y. Pathogenesis of periventricular white matter hemorrhage in preterm infants. Brain Dev 1986;8:25–30.

59. Taylor GA. Effect of germinal matrix hemorrhage on terminal vein position and patency. Pediatr Radiol 1995;25:S37–S40.
60. Rademaker KJ, Groenendaal F, Jansen GH, et al. Unilateral hemorrhagic parenchymal lesions in the preterm infant: shape, site and prognosis. Acta Paediatr 1994;83: 602–608.
61. Blackman JA, McGuinness GA, Bale JF, et al. Large postnatally acquired porencephalic cysts: unexpected developmental outcomes. J Child Neurol 1991;6:58–64.
62. Fawer CL, Diebold P, Calame A. Periventricular leukomalacia and neurodevelopmental outcome in preterm infants. Arch Dis Child 1987;62:30–36.
63. Bozynski ME, Nelson MN, Matalon TAS, et al. Cavitary periventricular leukomalacia: incidence and short term outcome in infants weighing <1200 grams at birth. Dev Med Child Neurol 1985;27:572–577.
64. Eken P, van Nieuwenhuizen O, van der Graaf Y, et al. Correlation between neonatal cranial ultrasound abnormalities and cerebral visual impairment in infancy. Dev Med Child Neurol 1994;36:3–15.
65. Graziani LJ, Pasto M, Stanley C, et al. Neonatal neurosonographic correlates of cerebral palsy in preterm infants. Pediatrics 1987;78:88–95.
66. Flodmark O, Lupton B, Li D, et al. MR imaging of periventricular leukomalacia in childhood. Am J Neuroradiol 1989;10:111–118.
67. Koeda T, Suganama I, Kohno Y, et al. MR imaging of spastic diplegia. Comparative study between preterm and term infants. Neuroradiology 1990;32: 187–190.
68. Yokochi K, Aiba K, Horie M, et al. Magnetic resonance imaging in children with spastic diplegia: correlation with the severity of their motor and mental abnormality. Dev Med Child Neurol 1991;33:18–25.
69. Iai M, Tanabe Y, Goto M, et al. A comparative magnetic resonance imaging study of the corpus callosum in neurologically normal children and children with spastic diplegia. Acta Paediatr 1994;83:1086–1090.
70. Cioni G, Fazzi B, Ipata AE, et al. Correlation between cerebral visual impairment and magnetic resonance imaging in children with neonatal encephalopathy. Dev Med Child Neurol 1996;38:120–132.
71. Uggetti C, Egitto MG, Fazzi E, et al. Cerebral visual impairment in periventricular leukomalacia: MR correlation. AJNR Am J Neuroradiol 1996;17:979–985.
72. de Vries LS, Regev R, Pennock JM, et al. Ultrasound evolution and later outcome of infants with periventricular densities. Early Hum Dev 1988;16:225–233.
73. Appleton RE, Lee REJ, Hey EN. Neurodevelopmental outcome of transient neonatal intracerebral echodensities. Arch Dis Child 1990;65:27–29.
74. Ringelberg J, van de Bor M. Outcome of transient periventricular echodensities in preterm infants. Neuropediatrics 1993;24:269–273.
75. Jongmans M, Meruri E, de Vries LS, et al. Minor neurological signs and perceptual-motor difficulties in prematurely born children. Arch Dis Child 1997;76: F9–F14.
76. Paneth N, Rudelli R, Monte W, et al. White matter necrosis in very low birth weight infants: neuropathologic and ultrasonographic findings in infants surviving six days or longer. J Pediatr 1990;116:975–984.
77. Banker BQ, Larroche J-L. Periventricular leukomalacia in infancy: a form of neonatal anoxic encephalopathy. Arch Neurol 1962;7:386–410.
78. Wheater M, Rennie JM. Poor prognosis after prolonged ventilation for bronchopulmonary dysplasia. Arch Dis Child 1994;71:F210–F211.
79. Larroche JC. Fetal encephalopathies of circulatory origin. Biol Neonate 1986;50: 61–74.
80. Murdoch Eaton DG, Ahmed Y, et al. Maternal trauma and cerebral lesions in preterm infants. Br J Obstet Gynecol 1991;98:1292–1294.

81. Dean LM, McLeary M, Taylor GA. Cerebral hemorrhage in alloimmune thrombocytopenia. Pediatr Radiol 1995;25:444–445.
82. Fusi L, McParland P, Fisk N, Wigglesworth J. Acute twin-twin transfusion: a possible mechanism for brain-damaged survivors after intrauterine death of a monochorionic twin. Obstet Gynecol 1991;78:517–520.
83. Larroche JC, Droullé P, Delezoide AL, et al. Brain damage in monozygous twins. Biol Neonate 1990;57:261–278.
84. Szymonowicz W, Preston H, Yu VYH. The surviving monozygotic twin. Arch Dis Child 1986;61:454–458.
85. Murphy DJ, Squier MV, Hope PL, et al. Clinical associations and time of onset of cerebral white matter damage in very preterm babies. Arch Dis Child 1996;75: F27–F32.
86. Bejar R, Wozniak P, Allard M, et al. Antenatal origin of neurologic damage in newborn infants: I. Preterm infants. Am J Obstet Gynecol 1988;159:357–363.
87. Voit T, Lemburg P. Damage of thalamus and basal ganglia in asphyxiated full-term neonates. Neuropediatrics 1987;18:176–181.
88. Rutherford MA, Pennock J, Murdoch-Eaton D, et al. Athetoid cerebral palsy with cysts in the putamen after hypoxic-ischemic encephalopathy. Arch Dis Child 1992; 67:846–850.
89. de Vries LS, Connell JA, Dubowitz LMS, et al. Electrophysiological, neurological and MRI abnormalities in infants with extensive cystic leukomalacia. Neuropediatrics 1987;18:61–66.
90. Eken P, de Vries LS, van Nieuwenhuizen O, et al. Early predictors of cerebral visual impairment in infants with cystic leukomalacia. Neuropediatrics 1996;27:16–25.
91. Shaw DWW, Cohen WA. Viral infections of the CNS in children: imaging features. AJR Am J Roentgenol 1993;160:125–133.
92. Boesch C, Issakainen G, Kewitz R, et al. Magnetic resonance imaging of the brain in congenital cytomegalovirus infection. Pediatr Radiol 1989;19:91–93.
93. Haddad J, Messer J, Gut JP, et al. Neonatal echovirus encephalitis with white matter necrosis. Neuropediatrics 1990;21:215–217.
94. Gray PH, Tudehope DI, Masel J. Cystic encephalomalacia and intrauterine herpes simplex virus infection. Pediatr Radiol 1992;22:529–532.
95. Ries M, Deeg K-H, Heininger U, et al. Brain abscesses in neonates—report of three cases. Eur J Pediatr 1993;152:745–746.
96. Trounce JQ, Fagan DG, Young ID, et al. Disorders of neuronal migration: sonographic features. Dev Med Child Neurol 1986;28:467–471.
97. Pellicer A, Cabanas F, Perez-Higueras A, et al. Neural migration disorders studied by cerebral ultrasound and colour Doppler flow imaging. Arch Dis Child 1995;73: 55–61.
98. Govaert P, de Vries LS. An atlas of neonatal brain sonography. Clin Dev Med 1996;141/142:39–109.

4

Neuroradiologic Evaluation of the Cerebral Palsies

Patrick D. Barnes and Richard L. Robertson

Cerebral palsy (CP) is a symptom complex related to a group of nonprogressive, but often changing, motor impairment syndromes secondary to lesions or anomalies arising in the early stages of brain development.[1,2] CP is classified according to the clinical distribution of motor involvement (i.e., monoplegia, hemiplegia, diplegia, or quadriplegia) and the type of neurologic impairment (i.e., spasticity, hypotonia, dystonia, athetosis, or combined). Several other dysfunctions often might accompany CP and include epilepsy, visual impairment, cognitive disorder, and extrapyramidal abnormalities.[2] The clinical manifestations of CP often differ in terms of gestational age of the causative insult, the chronologic age, lesion distribution, and the underlying disease.

This chapter is designed to provide guidelines for the imaging evaluation of static encephalopathies and their differentiation from progressive neurologic disorders of childhood. Disorders of the developing brain that may be associated with, or may complicate, the static encephalopathies of CP include (1) congenital and developmental disorders, (2) hydrocephalus, (3) neurovascular disease, (4) trauma, and (5) infectious and inflammatory processes. By definition, progressive disorders (e.g., metabolic, degenerative, and neoplastic) are not included but occasionally must be ruled out.

GENERAL GUIDELINES

Imaging modalities may be classified as structural or functional.[3–9] Structural imaging modalities provide spatial resolution based primarily on anatomic or morphologic data (e.g., computed tomography [CT]). Functional imaging modalities provide spatial resolution based on physiologic or metabolic data (e.g., single photon emission computed tomography [SPECT]). Some modalities may actually be considered to provide both structural and functional information (e.g., magnetic resonance angiography [MRA]). This section presents some of the important technical and clinical aspects of current and advanced neuroimaging techniques used in the evaluation of the immature and developing central nervous system (CNS).

Structural Imaging

Ultrasonography

Ultrasonography (US) is a readily accessible, portable, fast, and multiplanar real-time modality.[3–7] It is less expensive than other cross-sectional modalities and relatively noninvasive (nonionizing radiation). It requires no contrast agent and infrequently requires patient sedation. The resolving power of US is based on variations in acoustic reflectance of tissues. Its diagnostic effectiveness, however, depends primarily on the skill and experience of the operator and interpreter. Also, for cranial and spinal imaging, US requires a window or path unimpeded by bone or air. This drawback limits its range of use in neuroimaging of the fetus (prenatal US), infant (open fontanelle and sutures), immature or dysplastic cranium or spine (e.g., dysraphism), orbit, and neck, or in surgical procedures (craniotomy and laminectomy).

The most common application of pediatric neurosonography is in the evaluation of intracranial abnormalities.[3–7] Other applications include fetal sonography, spinal US, sonography of neck masses, Doppler US, and interventional and intraoperative US. Probably the most important uses of US are (1) fetal and neonatal screening, (2) screening of the infant who cannot be examined in the radiology department (e.g., premature neonate with intracranial hemorrhage, extracorporeal membrane oxygenation [ECMO], intraoperatively), (3) when important adjunctive information is needed quickly (e.g., distinguishing cystic from solid masses; determining vascularity, vascular flow, or increased intracranial pressure), and (4) for real-time guidance and monitoring of invasive diagnostic or therapeutic surgical and interventional procedures.

In the last few years, advances in US techniques have continued to improve at a dramatic pace. The development of high-resolution transducers, improvements in color Doppler signal processing, and new scanning techniques have significantly improved our ability to visualize structural and vascular abnormalities in the neonatal brain.[10–20] Examples are the mastoid view to better visualize the posterior fossa,[11] the graded fontanelle compression Doppler technique to evaluate hydrocephalus,[18] and power Doppler.[19] Another advance in US technology is the development of vascular US contrast agents to amplify reflected sound waves.[20] Among these are a variety of microbubble-based preparations that currently are being developed. Potential applications include the detection of slow flow and the assessment of organ perfusion. Increased sensitivity and specificity also may soon be provided by advances in computerized analysis of textural features.[21] Specific applications of US in CP are covered in Chapter 3.

Computed Tomography

Although ionizing radiation is used in CT, current-generation scanners effectively collimate and restrict exposure to the immediate volume of interest.[3,4,6] Direct imaging usually is restricted to the axial or coronal plane. Reformatting from thin axial sections to other planes (e.g., coronal or sagittal) is the alternative. Projection scout images may provide information similar to plain films but with less spatial resolution. CT scanning of the pediatric CNS is usually accomplished using either the conventional or the helical-spiral technique.[22,23] CT requires sedation in infants and young children more often than does US but less often than does magnetic resonance imaging (MRI). The neonate or very young infant, however, may be examined while asleep after a feeding or during a nap. CT occasionally requires intravenous contrast enhancement and sometimes cerebrospinal fluid (CSF) contrast opacification. High-resolution bone and soft-tissue algorithms are important for demonstrating fine anatomy (e.g., skull base). Advances in computer display technology include image fusion (e.g., MRI/SPECT, CT/MRI), two-dimensional reformatting, three-dimensional volumetric and reconstruction methods, segmentation, and surface rendering techniques.[3] These high-resolution display techniques are used in the planning of stereotactic radiotherapy and radiosurgery, craniofacial reconstructive surgery, surgical stabilization of craniocervical anomalies and scoliosis, and real-time or stereotactic image guidance for interventional and neurosurgical procedures.

The role of CT has been redefined in the context of accessible and reliable US and MRI.[3–7] US is the procedure of choice for primary imaging or screening of the brain and spinal neuraxis in the neonate and young infant.[24] When US does not satisfy the clinical inquiry, or an acoustic window is not available, then CT becomes the primary modality for brain imaging in children, especially in acute or emergent presentations. CT is especially important for acute trauma, acute neurologic deficit, encephalopathy, increased intracranial pressure, macrocephaly, headache, unexplained or complicated acute episodic disorder (e.g., seizure, apnea), visual symptoms or signs, suspected CNS infection, shunted hydrocephalus with suspected shunt malfunction, and suspected postoperative complications. In these situations, CT is used primarily to screen for acute or subacute hemorrhage, edema, herniation, fractures, hypoxic-ischemic injury, focal infarction, hydrocephalus, tumor mass, or abnormal collection (e.g., pneumocephalus, abscess, empyema). Additional primary indications for CT include the evaluation of bony or air-space abnormalities of the skull base, cranial vault, orbit, paranasal sinuses, facial bones, and the temporal bone. Also, CT is the definitive procedure for detection and confirmation of calcification.[25] It is important too in the bony evaluation of a localized spinal column abnormality (e.g., trauma).

Secondary indications for CT are those that often are primary indications for MRI (see next section), in a setting in which MRI, though preferred to CT, is not readily available or feasible.[3–7]

Contraindications to CT in childhood are unusual, particularly with the proper application of radiation protection, the appropriate use of nonionic contrast agents, the proper administration of sedation or anesthesia, and the use of vital monitoring.

When CT is used, intravenous enhancement for blood-pooling effect (e.g., CT angiography) or blood-brain barrier disruption is recommended for the evaluation of suspected or known vascular malformation, infarction, neoplasm, abscess, or empyema.[3–7,26] Enhanced CT may help in the evaluation of a mass or hemorrhage of unknown etiology and might identify the membrane of a chronic subdural collection (e.g., in the case of child abuse).[27] By identifying the cortical veins, enhanced CT can distinguish between prominent low-density subarachnoid collections (benign extracerebral collections or benign external hydrocephalus of infancy) and low-density subdural collections (e.g., chronic subdural hematomas or hygromas). It also may help to differentiate infarction from neoplasm or abscess, serve as an indicator of disease activity (e.g., in degenerative or inflammatory disease and vasculitis), or provide a high-yield guide for stereotactic or open biopsy (e.g., tumor core). Ventricular or subarachnoid CSF contrast opacification might assist further in evaluating or confirming CSF compartment lesions or communication (e.g., arachnoid cyst or ventricular encystment). As a rule, and except for suppurative infection, MRI is the preferred alternative to contrast-enhanced CT in the circumstances just enumerated.

Magnetic Resonance Imaging

MRI is an established imaging technology based on the principle of nuclear magnetic resonance.[3–6] As one of the less invasive or relatively noninvasive imaging technologies, MRI neither is ionizing, as are CT and isotope scanning, nor requires a pathway unobstructed by bone or air, as does US. Furthermore, the MRI signal is exponentially derived from multiple parameters (e.g., T_1, T_2, proton density, T_2^*, proton flow, proton relaxation enhancement, and chemical shift). MRI also employs many more basic imaging techniques—spin echo, inversion recovery, gradient echo, and chemical shift—than do other modalities.

Advancing MRI capabilities promise to improve its sensitivity, specificity, and efficiency further.[28–76] These advances include the fluid attenuation inversion recovery technique (FLAIR), fat-suppression short T_1 inversion recovery imaging (STIR), and magnetization transfer imaging (MTI) for increased structural resolution.[28–34] Fast and ultrafast MRI techniques (fast spin echo, fast gradient echo, echo planar imaging) have also been developed to reduce imaging times, improve structural resolution, and provide functional resolution.[35–37] Important applications include vascular MRI, MRA, and perfusion MRI (PMRI)[38–43]; diffusion-weighted imaging (DWI)[44–51]; CSF flow and brain-cord motion imaging[52–56]; brain activation techniques[57–60]; and magnetic resonance spectroscopy (MRS).[61–69] Fast and ultrafast imaging techniques are also being used for morphometrics, treatment planning, and real-time MRI-guided surgical and interventional procedures.[70–76]

Although, in general, MRI is more expensive than US or CT, it is less expensive than the more invasive modalities such as angiography or myelography, which often require anesthesia. The role of MRI in studies of the pediatric CNS is defined by its superior sensitivity and specificity in a number of areas as compared to US and CT.[3–6] The availability of MRI has also redefined the roles of invasive procedures such as myelography, ventriculography, cisternography, and angiography.

MRI provides multiplanar imaging with equivalent resolution in all planes without the need to reposition the patient. Bone does not interfere with soft-tissue resolution, although metallic objects often produce signal void or field dis-

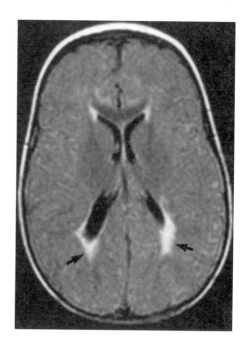

Figure 4.1   Fluid attenuation inversion recovery technique (FLAIR) magnetic resonance imaging of periventricular lesions. The axial FLAIR image vividly shows the high-intensity periventricular lesions (*arrows*) as contrasted against the low intensity of the fluid-attenuated cerebrospinal fluid off the lateral ventricles.

tortion artifacts. Some ferromagnetic or electronic devices (e.g., ferrous aneurysm clips and pacemakers) pose a hazard when MRI is employed, so these devices usually are contraindications to MRI use. MRI is not as rapid as US or CT, and patient sedation or anesthesia is required in most infants and younger children, because image quality is easily compromised by motion. MRI may not be as readily accessible to the pediatric patient as is US or CT and may not be feasible in emergencies or for intensive care cases unless magnet-compatible vital monitoring and support are available.

MRI demonstrates superior sensitivity and specificity in a number of circumstances, particularly with the addition of new techniques such as FLAIR, STIR, MTI, and DWI. The FLAIR sequence attenuates the signal from flowing water (i.e., CSF) and increases the conspicuity of nonfluid, water-containing lesions lying in close approximation to the CSF-filled subarachnoid and ventricular spaces (Figure 4.1).[28–30] The STIR technique suppresses fat signal to provide improved conspicuity of water-containing lesions in regions in which fat dominates (e.g., orbit, head and neck, spine).[6] The MTI method suppresses background tissues and increases conspicuity for vascular flow enhancement (e.g., MRA) and gadolinium enhancement (e.g., tumor seeding).[31–34] DWI is discussed later.

MRI is the imaging modality of choice in numerous clinical situations,[3–7] including developmental delay (e.g., static encephalopathy versus neurodegenerative disease); unexplained seizures (especially focal), unexplained neuroendocrine disorder, or unexplained hydrocephalus; the pretreatment evaluation of neoplastic processes and follow-up of tumor response and treatment effects; suspected infectious, postinfectious, and other inflammatory or noninflammatory encephalitides (e.g., encephalitis, postinfectious demyelination, vasculitis); migration and other submacroscopic dysplasias (e.g., cortical dysplasia); neurocutaneous syndromes (e.g., neurofibromatosis type 1, tuberous sclerosis); intractable or refractory epilepsy; vascular diseases, hemorrhage, and the sequelae of trauma.

MRI frequently offers greater diagnostic specificity than does CT or US for delineating vascular and hemorrhagic processes.[3-7] It affords clear depiction of vascular structures and abnormalities on the basis of proton flow parameters and software enhancements that do not require the injection of contrast agents (e.g., MRA). MRI with MRA can be used to differentiate arterial from venous occlusive disease. Using magnetic susceptibility sequences, MRI also provides more specific identification and staging of hemorrhage and clot formation according to the evolution of hemoglobin breakdown. MRI often is reserved for more definitive evaluation of hemorrhage and as an indicator or guide for angiography in a number of special situations. MRI may be used to evaluate an atypical or unexplained intracranial hemorrhage by distinguishing hemorrhagic infarction from hematoma and by distinguishing among the types of vascular malformations (e.g., cavernous malformation versus arteriovenous malformation [AVM]). In some cases of vascular malformation, MRA might obviate the need for conventional angiography in the follow-up of surgical therapy, interventional treatment, or radiosurgery.[40]

In the evaluation of intracranial vascular anomalies (e.g., vascular malformation, aneurysm), MRI may identify otherwise unsuspected prior hemorrhage (i.e., hemosiderin). When CT demonstrates a nonspecific, focal, high-density lesion (calcification versus hemorrhage), MRI may provide further specificity, for example, by distinguishing an occult vascular malformation (e.g., cavernous malformation) from a neoplasm (e.g., glioma). Used in conjunction with US or CT, MRI may provide additional information for differentiating benign infantile collections (i.e., external hydrocephalus) from subdural hematomas (e.g., in child abuse). MRI often also provides definitive evaluation of muscular and cutaneous vascular anomalies (i.e., hemangiomas, vascular malformations) that arise in parameningeal locations (e.g., head and neck, paraspinal) and either extend to involve the CNS directly or are associated with other CNS vascular or nonvascular abnormalities.

Functional Imaging

Nuclear Medicine

Whereas positron emission tomography (PET) has the unique ability to provide specific metabolic tracers (e.g., oxygen utilization and glucose metabolism), the wider availability, relative simplicity, and rapid technical advancement of SPECT allows more practical functional assessment of the pediatric CNS.[3,8,77-97] Current clinical and investigative applications of these technologies include the assessment of brain development and maturation,[79-81] focus localization in refractory childhood epilepsy (e.g., ictal perfusion SPECT, interictal

PET),[82–88] assessment of tumor progression versus treatment effects in childhood CNS neoplasia (perfusion and thallium SPECT, 18-fluorodeoxyglucose-PET),[89–94] the evaluation of occlusive cerebrovascular disease for surgical revascularization (e.g., perfusion SPECT),[9] the diagnosis of brain death (perfusion SPECT),[8,95] the use of brain activation techniques (e.g., perfusion SPECT, PET) in the elucidation of childhood cognitive disorders,[96,97] the assessment of CSF kinetics (e.g., in hydrocephalus, CSF leaks),[8] and spinal column screening (skeletal SPECT).[8]

Magnetic Resonance

As mentioned earlier, fast and ultrafast magnetic resonance techniques have been developed not only to provide more efficient and improved structural imaging but also to furnish functional and metabolic information.[28–76] Such techniques are MRS, PMRI, DWI, MRA, CSF flow and brain-cord motion imaging, and brain activation MRI.

Spectroscopy MRS offers a noninvasive in vivo approach to biochemical analysis.[61–69] Furthermore, MRS provides additional quantitative information regarding cellular metabolites, as signal intensity is linearly related to steady-state metabolite concentration. MRS can detect cellular biochemical changes before the detection of morphologic changes by MRI or other imaging modalities. MRS may therefore provide further insight into both follow-up assessment and prognosis.

With advances in instrumentation and methodology, and using the high inherent sensitivity of hydrogen-1, single voxel and multivoxel proton MRS now is carried out with relatively short acquisition times to detect low-concentration metabolites in healthy and diseased tissues. P-31 spectroscopy has also been developed for pediatric use. Currently, MRS is used primarily in the assessment of brain development and maturation, perinatal brain injury, childhood CNS neoplasia, and metabolic and neurodegenerative disorders.

Perfusion Imaging PMRI currently is being used to evaluate cerebral perfusion dynamics through the application of a dynamic contrast-enhanced T_2*-weighted MRI technique.[43] This new technique is undergoing further development to qualify and quantify normal and abnormal cerebrovascular dynamics of the developing brain by analyzing hemodynamic parameters, including relative cerebral blood volume, relative cerebral blood flow, and mean transit time, all as complements to conventional MRI.

Current applications of this and non–contrast-enhanced methods of PMRI include the evaluation of ischemic cerebrovascular disease (e.g., hypoxic-ischemic encephalopathy, moyamoya, sickle-cell disease), the differentiation of tumor progression from treatment effects, and brain activation imaging. One of the most active areas of research is the localization of brain activity, an area previously dominated by PET. *Functional MRI* is the terminology often applied to brain activation imaging, in which local or regional changes in cerebral blood flow are displayed that accompany stimulation or activation of sensory (e.g., visual), motor, or cognitive centers.[57–60] Brain activation MRI may eventually provide important information regarding cognitive and behavioral disorders. Also, it may ultimately serve as a guide for safe and effective tumor resection, AVM resection, and seizure ablation.

Diffusion-Weighted Imaging DWI provides information based on differences in the rate of diffusion of water molecules and is especially sensitive to intracellular changes.[44–51] The rate of diffusion, or the apparent diffusion coefficient (ADC), is higher for free or pure water (e.g., extracellular) than for macromolecular bound water (e.g., intracellular). The ADC varies according to the microstructural or physiologic state of a tissue.

Current clinical applications include the assessment of brain maturation, the evaluation of ischemia, and the characterization of tumors. A particularly important application of DWI is in the early detection of diffuse and focal hypoxic-ischemic injury. The ADC of water is reduced within minutes of an ischemic insult and is progressive within the first hour. Bright signal is demonstrated on DWI at a time when conventional imaging is negative and likely reflects intracellular (cytotoxic) edema. Further investigation is under way regarding the roles of DWI, PMRI, and MRS in the early diagnosis and treatment of potentially reversible ischemic injury.

Flow and Motion Imaging Motion-sensitive MRI techniques are used not only to evaluate vascular flow (e.g., MRA) and perfusion but also to demonstrate the effect of pulsatile cardiovascular flow on other fluid tissues (e.g., CSF) and on nonfluid tissues such as the brain and spinal cord.[52–56] Using cardiac or pulse gating, these MRI techniques may be used to evaluate, preoperatively and postoperatively, abnormalities of CSF dynamics (e.g., hydrocephalus, hydrosyringomyelia), as well as abnormalities of brain motion (e.g., Chiari malformation) and spinal cord motion (e.g., tethered cord syndrome).

SPECIFIC APPLICATIONS

Congenital and Developmental Abnormalities

Congenital and developmental abnormalities of the CNS may result from defective formation, postformational destruction, or disordered maturation. These anomalies probably are best classified according to gestational timing (Table 4.1) and include disorders of dorsal and ventral neural tube development; disorders of neural, glial, and mesenchymal development; encephaloclastic processes; and disorders of myelination and cortical maturation.[5,6,98]

Developmental anomalies readily identified by (prenatal or postnatal) US or CT are the *gross* formational defects of categories I–IV and the *gross* encephaloclastic lesions of category V (see Table 4.1). This is especially true for those abnormalities involving the ventricular system or containing CSF.[5,6]

Table 4.1 Classification of Central Nervous System Malformations by Gestational Timing

I. Disorders of dorsal neural tube development (3–4 wks)
 Anencephaly
 Cephaloceles
 Chiari malformations
 Spinal dysraphism*
 Hydrosyringomyelia

II. Disorders of ventral neural tube development (5–10 wks)
 Holoprosencephaly
 Agenesis septum pellucidum
 Optic and olfactory hypoplasia or aplasia*
 Pituitary-hypothalamic hypoplasia or aplasia*
 Cerebellar hypoplasia or aplasia
 Dandy-Walker-Blake spectrum
 Craniosynostosis

III. Disorders of neural and glial migration and cortical organization (2–5 mos)
 Schizencephaly*
 Neuronal heterotopia*
 Agyria or pachygyria*
 Lissencephaly
 Polymicrogyria (cortical dysplasias)*
 Agenesis corpus callosum

IV. Disorders of neural, glial, and mesenchymal proliferation, differentiation,
  and histogenesis (2–6 mos)
 Micrencephaly
 Megalencephaly
 Hemimegalencephaly
 Aqueductal anomalies*
 Colpocephaly
 Neurocutaneous syndromes*
 Vascular anomalies
 Malformational tumors
 Arachnoid cysts

V. Encephaloclastic processes (>5–6 mos)
 Hydranencephaly
 Porencephaly
 Multicystic encephalopathy
 Encephalomalacia
 Leukomalacia
 Hemiatrophy
 Hydrocephalus
 Hemorrhage
 Infarction

VI. Disorders of myelination (7 mos–2 yrs)
 Hypomyelination*
 Delayed myelination*
 Dysmyelination*
 Demyelination*

*MRI often or usually is needed for detection.
Sources: Modified from M van der Knaap, J Valk. Congenital abnormalities of the CNS. AJNR Am J Neuroradiol 1988;9:315; and SM Wolpert, P Barnes. MRI in Pediatric Neuroradiology. St. Louis: Mosby–Year Book, 1992;41–82.

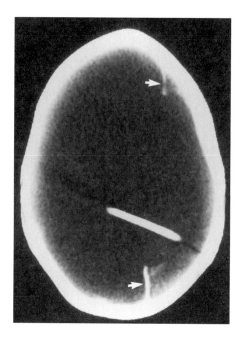

Figure 4.2 Hydranencephaly. Axial computed tomography shows extensive supratentorial cerebrospinal fluid low densities, no cerebral cortex (the isodense band beneath the calvaria represents beam-hardening artifact), a ventricular shunt catheter, and remnants of the falx cerebri (*arrows*).

Among such abnormalities are hydrocephalus, hydranencephaly (Figure 4.2), holoprosencephaly (Figure 4.3), absent septum pellucidum, agenesis of the corpus callosum, porencephaly, open schizencephaly, the Dandy-Walker-Blake spectrum, arachnoid cysts, and cephaloceles.[99-106] US may not clearly distinguish between hydranencephaly (absent cerebral mantle) and severe hydrocephalus (attenuated cerebral mantle). Other anomalies often delineated by US or CT include Chiari II malformation, lissencephaly, and vascular malformations such as the Galenic malformation.[5,6] In fact, any lesion detected by US, particularly a cystic one, should be examined with Doppler US to determine whether it is vascular in nature.[7]

Encephaloclastic processes are those destructive lesions of the already formed brain and may result from a variety of prenatal or perinatal insults including hypoxia-ischemia and infection (see Table 4.1). MRI occasionally may demonstrate subtle abnormalities not revealed by US or CT (e.g., periventricular leukomalacia; see Figure 4.1).

MRI is important when US or CT fails to satisfy the clinical investigation. MRI often provides a more complete delineation of complex CNS anomalies for diagnosis, treatment, prognosis, and genetic counseling.[5,6] In fact, ultrafast MRI techniques are increasingly being used prenatally to evaluate for fetal CNS abnormalities in at-risk pregnancies or as detected by obstetric US (Figure 4.4).[107] Furthermore, MRI often is indicated if more specific treatment is planned beyond simple shunting of hydrocephalus. Examples include manage-

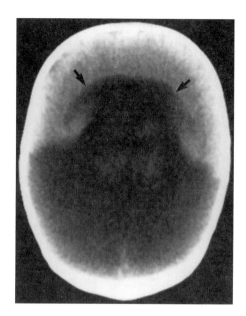

Figure 4.3 Alobar holoprosencephaly. Axial computed tomography shows a monoventricular chamber (*arrows*) with a large dorsal cyst, continuity of the frontal cerebrum across the midline, absence of the corpus callosum and septum pellucidum, no interhemispheric fissure, and no falx.

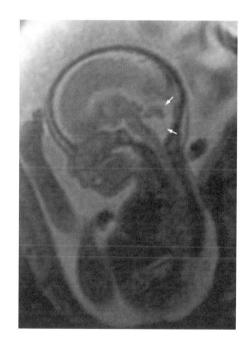

Figure 4.4 Fetal magnetic resonance imaging (MRI) at 20 weeks' gestation. Sagittal ultrafast MRI shows a Dandy-Walker-Blake spectrum anomaly of the hindbrain (*arrows*) and partial agenesis of the corpus callosum. (Courtesy of Dr. Debra Levine, Beth Israel Hospital, Boston, MA.)

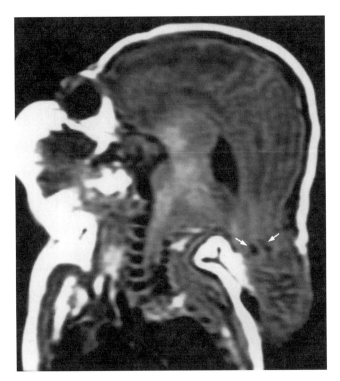

Figure 4.5 Occipital cephalocele. Sagittal T_1-weighted magnetic resonance imaging shows dysplastic occipital lobe tissue and anomalous venous structures (*arrows*) within the cephalocele, microcephaly, Chiari III hindbrain malformation, agenesis of the corpus callosum, and colpocephaly.

ment of the sequelae of the Chiari II malformation after closure of a myelomeningocele (e.g., hydrosyringomyelia), reduction or closure of a cephalocele (i.e., vascular and neural anatomy; Figure 4.5), and the decision, in the Dandy-Walker-Blake spectrum, of whether cyst shunting or combined cyst-and-ventricular shunting should be performed (presence or absence of a widely patent aqueduct; Figure 4.6).[101–103] Preoperative arterial and venous mapping may be done noninvasively using Doppler US, MRA, or computed tomographic angiography (CTA). Intraoperative guidance may be provided by real-time and Doppler US. Patients with craniosynostosis initially are evaluated with plain films.[6] Those with multiple suture involvement, especially when associated with craniofacial syndromes, often require more extensive evaluation, including three-dimensional CT and, occasionally, MRI.

Sonography is useful for screening of dysraphic myelodysplasia in the fetus (e.g., myelomeningocele, Chiari II malformation) and in the neonate and young infant.[5–7] It can also detect a variety of skin-covered dysraphic abnormalities, including lipomyelomeningocele, diastematomyelia, dermal sinuses, and the caudal dysplasias. Spinal US may be most effective for screening to rule out tethered cord in small infants with low-yield presentations (e.g., sacral dimple only) or with ambiguous findings on lumbosacral spine films and to evaluate other organ systems for anomalies (e.g., hydronephrosis or solitary kidney).

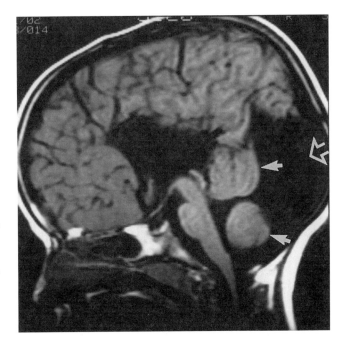

Figure 4.6 Dandy-Walker-Blake cyst. Sagittal T_1-weighted magnetic resonance imaging shows partial vermian agenesis (*upper arrow*), a large retro-cerebellar cyst (*open arrow*), interposed cerebellar tonsil (*lower arrow*), agenesis of the corpus callosum, and hydrocephalus.

MRI is the definitive modality for diagnosis, surgical planning, and follow-up.[5,6] Myelography or myelographic CT occasionally is needed in patients who have metallic spinal instrumentation, as artifacts often compromise MRI scan quality.

Nonenhanced spinal CT, however, often is used for evaluating the dysraphic bony anatomy. Myelographic CT may seldom be needed to better delineate nerve roots, septation in diastematomyelia, or tethering bands in meningocele manque. Occasionally, sonography may be used for postoperative follow-up to detect cord retethering (diminished cord pulsation), although operative scarring often makes assessment difficult. CSF motion and spinal cord motion MRI sequences are also being developed to assist in this difficult evaluation.

MRI is often required to delineate structurally the more subtle anomalies arising as disorders of migration and cortical organization (category III; Figures 4.7–4.10) or as disorders of proliferation, differentiation, and histogenesis (category IV; Figure 4.11; see Table 4.1).[104,105] The perfusional and metabolic characteristics of these anomalies (e.g., cortical dysplasias, hemimegalencephaly) may be investigated with SPECT and PET, respectively, in children with medically refractory partial epilepsy who are candidates for focal surgical ablation.[8,82–88] For added precision, the SPECT or PET data may be fused with the MRI data to provide a higher-resolution spatial display of the functional infor-

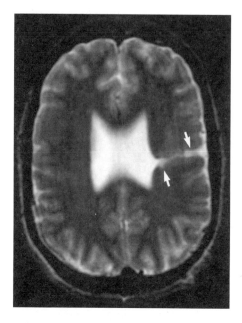

Figure 4.7 Schizencephaly and absent septum pellucidum. Axial T_2-weighted magnetic resonance imaging shows a left frontal complete cerebral cleft (*arrows*) lined by dysplastic gray matter and mild ventriculomegaly with no identifiable septal leaflets.

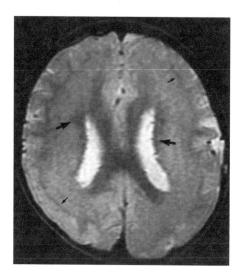

Figure 4.8 Laminar heterotopias. Axial T_2-weighted magnetic resonance imaging shows that the subcortical cerebral white matter has been largely replaced by gray matter isointensities. Some periventricular and cortical myelinated white matter remnant intensities are seen (*arrows*) along with a pachygyric cortex.

mation.[91] MRS and PMRI with brain activation eventually might contribute to the evaluation and treatment of these patients.[84]

MRI is now the preferred modality for the screening and definitive evaluation of the dysplastic, neoplastic, and vascular manifestations of the neurocutaneous syndromes.[5,6,108] After initial screening with US or CT, MRI also is considered the primary technology for treatment planning and follow-up of vas-

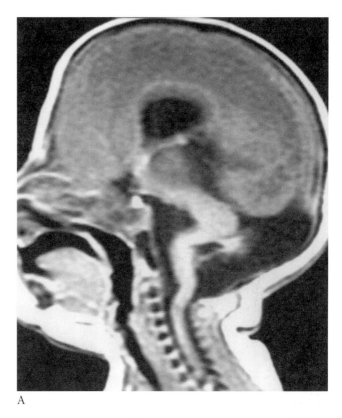

A

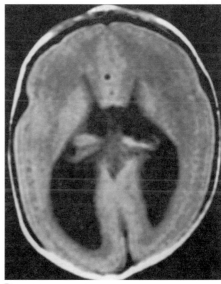

Figure 4.9 Walker-Warburg syndrome, lissencephaly, and cerebrocerebellar malformation. Sagittal (A) and axial (B) T$_1$-weighted magnetic resonance imaging shows an agyric cerebral cortex, a monoventricular chamber, hydrocephalus, and a Dandy-Walker-Blake hindbrain malformation.

B

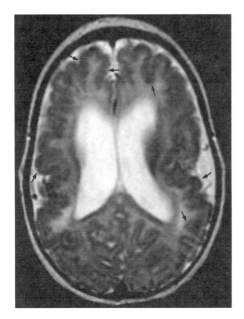

Figure 4.10 Diffuse polymicrogyria and cytomegalovirus infection. Axial T_2-weighted magnetic resonance imaging shows ventriculomegaly, white matter high-intensity abnormalities, and a serrated appearance of the cerebral cortex (*arrows*).

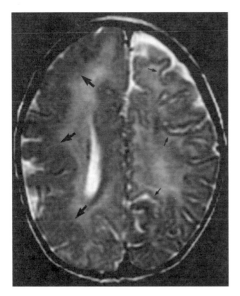

Figure 4.11 Hemimegalencephaly. Axial T_2-weighted magnetic resonance imaging shows a pachygyric right cerebral cortex (*large arrows*), abnormal white matter high intensities, and a dilated right lateral ventricle. A normal cerebral cortical ribbon is shown on the left (*small arrows*).

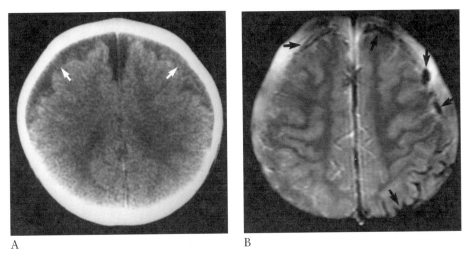

A   B

Figure 4.12 Subdural hematomas resulting from child abuse. (A) Axial nonenhanced computed tomography shows nonspecific extracerebral low densities (*arrows*). (B) Axial T$_2$-weighted magnetic resonance imaging shows that the collections are subdurally located and that the intensities represent hemorrhages of varying age (*arrows*).

cular malformations and developmental tumors.[6] Although arachnoid cysts often are readily delineated by US or CT, MRI may be necessary for confirmation (i.e., to exclude solid tumor) and for surgical planning.[6] FLAIR or diffusion MRI may easily distinguish an arachnoid cyst from a dermoid or epidermoid cyst. Myelination and disorders of myelination can be precisely assessed only by MRI, as discussed later.[5,6,109] The MRI findings, however, are often nonspecific regarding causation, particularly in the first year of life, because of the watery character of the immature brain. MRS may add specificity to the diagnostic evaluation of these infants.[62,63,66,67]

Hydrocephalus

In infants with macrocephaly, the differential diagnosis of exclusion commonly includes subdural collections and hydrocephalus. When nonspecific extracerebral collections first are demonstrated by US or nonenhanced CT, further imaging usually is indicated for clarification (Figure 4.12). The critical point is to differentiate between benign infantile extracerebral collections (i.e., transient external hydrocephalus due to immaturity of the arachnoid villi) and subdural hematomas (e.g., in child abuse).[5,6,13] In the former, Doppler US may confirm the subarachnoid location of the collections (deep to the cortical veins) and obviate the need for enhanced CT or MRI. In the latter, Doppler US shows that the collections occupy the subdural space (superficial to the cortical veins) or occupy both spaces. If CT does not show findings characteristic of hemorrhage, then MRI is required to confirm the hemorrhagic nature of the collection (see Figure

4.12). Hemorrhages or other injuries of varying age suggest repetitive episodes and are highly suspicious for nonaccidental trauma, or child abuse, particularly when the findings are out of proportion to the history and other existing conditions (e.g., vascular, hematologic, or metabolic disease) are ruled out.[6,27,110,111]

The vast majority of childhood hydrocephalus occurs in infancy, and the most common cause is acquired adhesive ependymitis or arachnoiditis after hemorrhage or infection.[6,99] Hydrocephalus is a well-known sequela of neonatal intracranial hemorrhage, especially in premature infants (germinal matrix or intraventricular hemorrhage). Prenatal infection (e.g., TORCH [toxoplasmosis, rubella, cytomegalovirus, and herpes simplex]) or postnatal infection (e.g., meningitis) may also lead to hydrocephalus. By far the most common developmental source of hydrocephalus is the Chiari II malformation associated with myelocele or myelomeningocele, which often develops after repair of the spinal defect.[6,101] Other common developmental causes are aqueductal anomalies (forking, stenosis, septation, gliosis) and the Dandy-Walker-Blake spectrum of retrocerebellar cysts (see Figure 4.6).[6] Less common or rare causes of hydrocephalus include atresia of the foramen of Monro, skull base anomaly (e.g., achondroplasia), intracranial cyst, craniosynostosis, encephalocele, holoprosencephaly (see Figure 4.3), hydranencephaly (see Figure 4.2), and lissencephaly (see Figure 4.9).[6]

Neoplasm as an expanding mass or an obstructive lesion is a rare cause of elevated pressure or hydrocephalus in infancy. Most masses of infancy are cystic or cystlike and include the Dandy-Walker-Blake spectrum (see Figure 4.6), arachnoid or glioependymal cysts (retrocerebellar, suprasellar, intraventricular, quadrigeminal plate cistern), porencephaly (Figure 4.13), encephalocele (see Figure 4.5), and the vein of Galen malformation (varix) as a blood-filled cyst.[6] The rare neoplasms occurring in the first 2 years of life are astrocytomas, choroid plexus tumors, germ cell tumors, embryonal tumors (e.g., permeative neuroectodermal tumor [PNET], medulloblastoma), and mesenchymal neoplasms (e.g., rhabdoid tumor).[5,6] Tumors have a predilection for the midline and along the ventricular pathways, including the posterior fossa about the fourth ventricle and aqueduct (e.g., medulloblastoma, ependymoma, ependymoblastoma, rhabdoid tumor, medulloepithelioma), and the supratentorial compartment about the third ventricle (astrocytoma, germ cell tumors) and lateral ventricles (choroid plexus papilloma and carcinoma).

Hydrocephalus in the fetus and infant, especially when of a developmental or acquired non-neoplastic origin, is diagnosed easily with US or CT before shunting.[3-7] Doppler US using the graded fontanelle compression technique may be employed to identify infants with ventriculomegaly and increased intracranial pressure and to help determine the need for and timing of shunting.[18]

MRI may be indicated to delineate hydrocephalus further when surgery is more specifically directed beyond simple shunting (e.g., in the case of a retrocerebellar cyst, isolation of the fourth ventricle, porencephaly, postventriculitis encystment, or a ventricular tumor).[5,6] Proper catheter placement for management of hydrocephalus related to a cyst in the Dandy-Walker-Blake spectrum prevents upward or downward herniation due to unbalanced decompression of one compartment relative to the other.[6] Endoscopic third-ventricle ventricu-

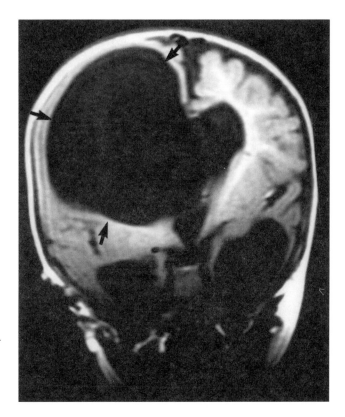

Figure 4.13 Porencephaly and hydrocephalus. Coronal T_1-weighted magnetic resonance imaging shows a large right cerebral cystic cavity (*arrows*) that communicates with an enlarged ventricular system.

loscopy is a relatively new neurosurgical procedure that is usually employed beyond infancy. It is indicated for decompression of hydrocephalus due to aqueductal stenosis in the absence of communicating hydrocephalus or immaturity of the arachnoid villa CSF absorption mechanism.[99]

Although CT may be a practical screening examination after infancy, MRI is preferred because neoplasm becomes the leading consideration.[6] The multiplanar and multiparametric capability of MRI makes it the procedure of choice for delineating anatomy and the extent of tumor for planning surgical therapy, radiotherapy, and chemotherapy, as well as for follow-up of tumor response and treatment effects.

MRI readily confirms CSF-containing compartments and lesions (e.g., arachnoid cysts) without requiring cisternography or ventriculography. The proton flow characteristics of CSF make CSF contrast opacification unnecessary in these circumstances, although occasionally intravenous gadolinium enhancement is needed.[6] MRI may offer more supportive or causative information when the CT or US demonstrates nonspecific ventriculomegaly. Supportive information that may confirm hydrocephalus includes MRI demonstration of accentuated CSF flow voids, other abnormalities of CSF dynamics, and periventricular edema. Unexplained hydrocephalus requires a thorough investigation for an occult neoplastic or inflammatory process.[6] MRI may demonstrate a periaqueductal tumor in "presumed" aqueductal stenosis, or leptomeningeal enhancement in inflammatory or neoplastic infiltration (e.g., granulomatous infection, tumor seeding).

The follow-up imaging of shunted, non-neoplastic hydrocephalus may be adequately accomplished with US or CT.[6] US is also an ideal guide for shunt placement intraoperatively and for shunt placement evaluation on follow-up. After the acoustic window is lost in older infants and children, CT becomes the procedure of choice for routine follow-up and for evaluation of shunt complications, including malfunction and subdural fluid collections.[6] MRI might provide multiplanar anatomic and multiparametric delineation, including CSF flow dynamics, especially for complex, compartmentalized, or encysted hydrocephalus.[6]

Along with CT (and a comparison with previous CT studies), imaging often also includes shunt series radiographs (head and neck, thorax, abdomen, and pelvis) or US to evaluate for ventriculoperitoneal shunt system discontinuity and abdominal complications.[6] Ventricular shunt tap is occasionally necessary, whereas contrast shuntogram is rarely needed. Occasionally, CT with CSF contrast enhancement may be necessary for evaluation of the complex, encysted, or compartmentalized system, to assist in proper drainage or shunt catheter placement. Isolation of the fourth ventricle may occur after lateral ventricular shunting, owing to secondary aqueductal closure in the presence of an existing outlet fourth ventricular obstruction.[6] Expansion of the fourth ventricle results from continued choroid plexus CSF production, and progressive compression of the brain stem might be present. Isolation of the fourth ventricle can occur after shunting of hydrocephalus for Chiari II malformation or shunting of outlet foraminal adhesive occlusion from infection or hemorrhage. Again, multiplanar MRI or CSF contrast-enhanced CT may assist in preoperative planning, whereas stereotactic techniques or intraoperative US are used to facilitate catheter placement.

Neurovascular Disease

Neurovascular disease characteristically presents as an acute neurologic event (e.g., paresis, seizure). A recently discovered but fixed deficit (e.g., hemiplegia) may be the first indication of a remote prenatal or perinatal neurovascular injury. Imaging assists in the clinical evaluation and differentiation of hypoxia-ischemia, hemorrhage, and occlusive vascular disease.[5,6,112–114]

Diffuse Hypoxic-Ischemic Injury Prenatal or perinatal partial, prolonged hypoxic-ischemic encephalopathy (HIE) may be associated with periventricular injury to the preterm fetus or neonate (see Figures 4.1, 4.14) or cortical and subcortical border zone cerebral injury during term gestation (Table 4.2 and Figure 4.15).[5,6,9,112] More extensive fetal or neonatal brain

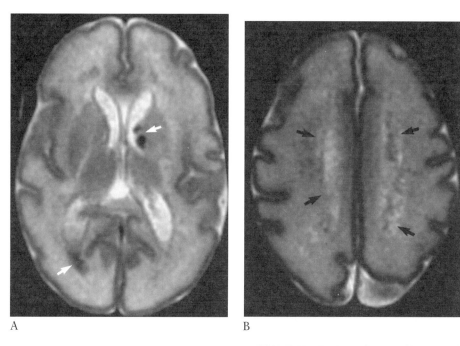

A   B

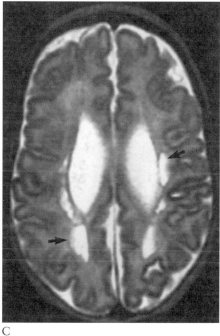

Figure 4.14 Preterm partial hypoxic-ischemic encephalopathy. (A,B) Axial T$_2$-weighted magnetic resonance imaging (MRI) in the acute to subacute stage at 30 weeks' gestation shows hypointense germinal matrix and intraventricular hemorrhage (*white arrows*) and periventricular high-intensity injury (*black arrows*). (C) Axial T$_2$-weighted MRI in the chronic stage at 40 weeks' gestation shows high-intensity periventricular cysts and gliosis (*arrows*) plus ventriculomegaly. Note the progress in myelination and cortical development comparing images A and B to image C. (Courtesy of Dr. Petra Huppi, Brigham and Women's Hospital, Boston, MA.)

C

Table 4.2 Imaging Patterns of Diffuse Hypoxic-Ischemic Encephalopathy (HIE)*

Hemorrhage
Germinal matrix-intraventricular hemorrhage
Choroid plexus-intraventricular hemorrhage
Subarachnoid hemorrhage
Partial HIE
Preterm: periventricular leukomalacia
Full-term and post-term: cortical or subcortical injury (border-zone, watershed, parasagittal)
Intermediate: combined or transitional pattern
Profound HIE
Thalamic and basal ganglia injury
Brain stem injury
Hippocampal injury
Cerebral white matter injury
Paracentral injury
Global injury (prolonged profound)
Combined partial and prolonged HIE

*Depend on gestational and chronologic age, duration, and severity of the insult.
Sources: Modified from AJ Barkovich. Pediatric Neuroimaging. New York: Raven, 1995; and JJ Volpe. Neurology of the Newborn. Philadelphia: Saunders, 1995.

injury may occur with more profound insults and involve the thalami, basal ganglia, brain stem, hippocampi, and perirolandic cortex (Figure 4.16).[5,6,9,112] Imaging may demonstrate early edema, necrosis, or hemorrhagic infarction. The long-term result is a static encephalopathy (i.e., CP), and imaging might demonstrate porencephaly, hydranencephaly, atrophy, periventricular leukomalacia, cystic encephalomalacia (Figure 4.17), or mineralization (Figure 4.18). The more subtle ischemic periventricular white matter lesions occasionally are better delineated by US than by CT or MRI, in which the density and intensity character of immature white matter often obscures the injury. However, CT and MRI often show gray matter injury better than does US. Advances in the development of PMRI, DWI, and MRS have the potential to add diagnostic sensitivity and specificity for the early institution of neuroprotective measures to treat potentially reversible HIE.[43,45,61,62,64,69]

Intracranial Hemorrhage Intracranial hemorrhage may result from parturient trauma, hypoxia-ischemia, a coagulopathy (e.g., thrombocytopenia, disseminated intravascular coagulation, ECMO), or vaso-occlusive disease (e.g., venous thrombosis).[5,6,9,112–114] Hemorrhage may occasionally be associated with infection (e.g., herpes simplex virus type 2). Vascular malformations that produce intracranial hemorrhage (e.g., AVM, cavernous malformations, developmental venous anomalies, and telangiectasias) are rare in the neonate and young

Figure 4.15 Full-term partial hypoxic-ischemic encephalopathy. Sagittal T₁-weighted (A) and axial T₂-weighted (B) magnetic resonance imaging (MRI) in the acute to subacute phase show bilateral parasagittal cerebral cortical and subcortical high-intensity abnormalities (*arrows*) in a watershed or border-zone distribution at 40 weeks' gestation. Axial T₂-weighted MRI (C) during the chronic phase shows atrophic and gliotic high-intensity abnormalities (*arrows*) in a similar distribution plus ventriculomegaly.

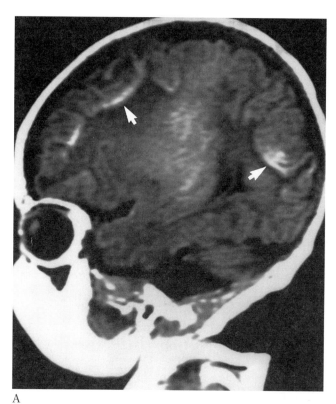

A

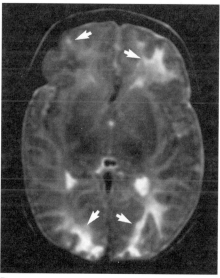

B

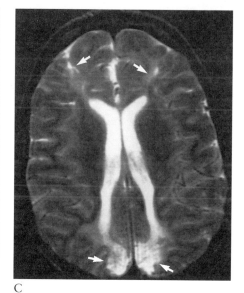

C

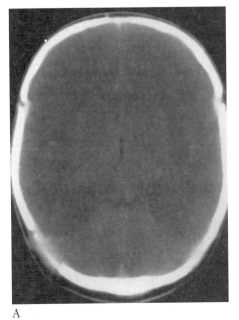

A

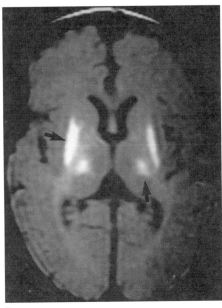

B

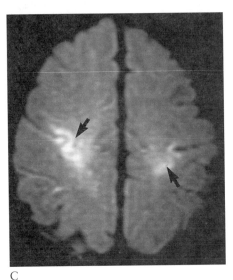

C

Figure 4.16 Full-term profound hypoxic-ischemic encephalopathy. (A) Axial nonenhanced computed tomography in the acute phase shows extensive low-density abnormality with loss of gray and white matter differentiation involving the cortical and subcortical cerebrum as well as the basal ganglia, thalami, and deep capsular tracts. The "spared" cerebellum appears to be of relatively higher density. (B,C) Axial proton density magnetic resonance imaging in the subacute to chronic phase shows bilateral high-intensity abnormalities (*arrows*) in the putamina, ventrolateral thalami, centrum semiovale, and paracentral (perirolandic) cortex.

infant and usually are not encountered until later in childhood.[114] Aneurysms are exceedingly rare in children but may be developmental, associated with a syndrome (e.g., Turner's syndrome), or related to trauma or infection (mycotic aneurysm). The vein of Galen malformations are subclassified as choroidal, mural, and AVM types. They rarely hemorrhage and more commonly present in infancy with congestive heart failure, cerebral ischemia, or hydrocephalus.[114]

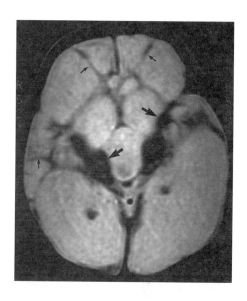

Figure 4.17 Cystic encephalomalacia. Axial T_2-weighted magnetic resonance imaging in the chronic phase of a prolonged, profound hypoxic-ischemic encephalopathy at term shows extensive bilateral high-intensity cerebral cavitation and ventriculomegaly with hypointense septation (*small arrows*) and hypointense mineralization of the basal ganglia and thalami (*larger arrows*).

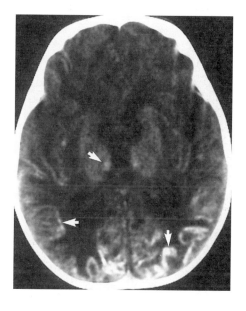

Figure 4.18 Mineralizing encephalomalacia. Axial nonenhanced computed tomography after extracorporeal membrane oxygenation in the chronic phase of a combined partial prolonged and profound hypoxic-ischemic encephalopathy at term shows extensive low densities throughout the cerebrum plus high-density calcification (*arrows*) of the cerebral cortex, basal ganglia, and thalamus.

US or CT remains the primary imaging choice in acute situations.[5–7,9] Acute intracranial hemorrhage, particularly subarachnoid, is diagnosed most specifically by CT (Figure 4.19), though MRI may provide better specificity beyond the acute phases (see Figures 4.12, 4.14). Hemorrhagic manifestations of HIE in the premature infant that are readily detected by US include germinal matrix hemorrhage, intraventricular hemorrhage, and periventricular hemorrhagic infarction.[115] Choroid plexus hemorrhage and hemorrhagic infarction in the full-term

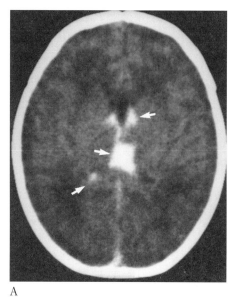

A

Figure 4.19 Venous thrombosis with hemorrhagic infarction. (A) Axial nonenhanced computed tomography shows high-density thalamic, subependymal, and intraventricular hemorrhages (*arrows*). (B) Sagittal T_1-weighted magnetic resonance imaging shows high-intensity methemoglobin (*arrows*) within the thrombosed straight and superior sagittal dural venous sinuses.

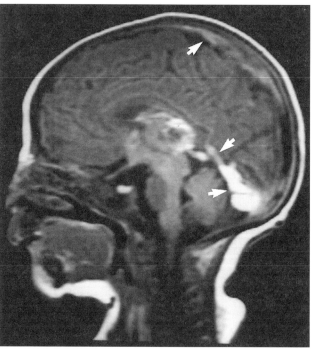

B

infant are also easily demonstrated. Portable US may effectively delineate the potential hemorrhagic or ischemic sequelae of ECMO.[7] Although CT has been more reliable, high-resolution US using transfontanelle and transcranial approaches, including the mastoid view, can now accurately detect extracerebral hemorrhage (subdural and subarachnoid) and posterior fossa collections (cerebellar or subdural).[11] Color Doppler US, MRA, and CTA are all able to identify and distinguish the types of Galenic malformations and provide follow-up. Angiography is more specifically directed to the definitive interventional or surgical management of these and other vascular anomalies.[114] Real-time Doppler US provides intraprocedural guidance and monitoring.

Occlusive Neurovascular Disease Occlusive neurovascular disease in the neonate and young infant may be arterial or venous in origin and typically results in focal or multifocal lesions within the distribution of the occluded vessel or vessels.[5,6,113,114] Arterial occlusive disease may be partial or complete and due to stenosis, thrombosis, or embolization.[6,9,113,114] The result may be ischemia edema, ischemic infarction (Figure 4.20), hemorrhagic infarction (see Figure 4.19), and then atrophy. Arterial occlusive disease may occur as a prenatal or perinatal event (emboli of placental origin or from involuting fetal vessels), as a complication of infection (e.g., meningitis), with congenital heart disease, or from a hypercoagulopathy. Other very rare causes include trauma, vascular dysplasia, and metabolic disorders (e.g., mitochondrial cytopathies) (Table 4.3).

Conditions commonly associated with cortical or dural venous sinus occlusive disease include infection, dehydration, perinatal encephalopathy, cyanotic congenital heart disease, polycythemia, other hypercoagulable states (see Figure 4.19), disseminated intravascular coagulation, and trauma (Table 4.4).[6,113] Color Doppler US can be used as a noninvasive tool for initial identification and monitoring of these infants.[113] MRI may be more sensitive and specific than US or CT for ischemic infarction, hemorrhagic infarction, and venous thrombosis.[6,113]

MRA or CTA may also contribute to the diagnosis of arterial or venous occlusion and clarify the need for cerebral angiography, particularly when anticoagulation or thrombolysis is being considered.[114] As mentioned earlier, PMRI, DWI, and MRS have the potential to contribute to the early diagnosis and timely treatment of ischemic insults.

Acute myelopathy due to hypoxia-ischemia, spontaneous vascular occlusion, or spontaneous hemorrhage is extremely rare in childhood.[6] Spinal MRI is the primary and often the definitive procedure to evaluate spinal cord infarction or hemorrhage. Spinal angiography is necessary to evaluate fully the vascular abnormality in anticipation of surgery or interventional therapy. The muscular and cutaneous vascular anomalies of childhood include hemangiomas and the vascular malformations (e.g., AVM, lymphatic malformations, venous malformations). These often involve the head and neck region or the paraspinal region and are evaluated definitively by a combination of Doppler US and MRI.

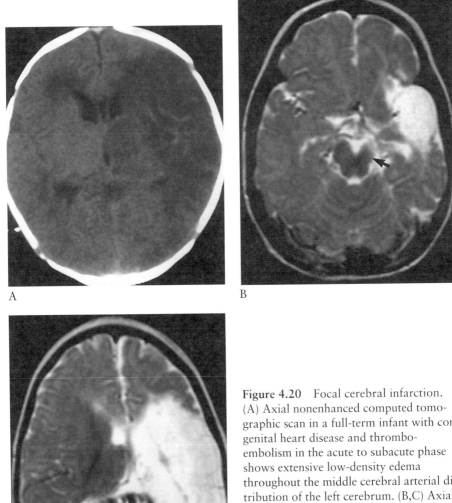

A

B

C

Figure 4.20 Focal cerebral infarction. (A) Axial nonenhanced computed tomographic scan in a full-term infant with congenital heart disease and thromboembolism in the acute to subacute phase shows extensive low-density edema throughout the middle cerebral arterial distribution of the left cerebrum. (B,C) Axial T_2-weighted magnetic resonance imaging in the chronic phase shows extensive high-intensity cavitation, gliosis, and atrophy in the involved distribution, with dilatation of the left lateral ventricle plus findings of wallerian degeneration (*arrow*). Also, crossed cerebellar diaschisis may occasionally be seen in such cases.

Table 4.3 Occlusive Neurovascular Disease in the Fetus, Neonate, and Infant

Idiopathic
    Vascular maldevelopment
       Atresia
       Hypoplasia
    Vasculopathy
       Familial proliferative
       Isoimmune thrombocytopenia
    Vasospasm
       Maternal cocaine use
    Vascular distortion
       Extreme head and neck motion
    Extracorporeal membrane oxygenation
    Emboli
       Involuting fetal vessels
       Congenital heart disease
       Catheterized vessels

Thrombosis
    Meningitis
    Hypoxic-ischemic encephalopathy (HIE) or disseminated intravascular coagulation (DIC)
    Dehydration or hypernatremia
    Sepsis or DIC
    Polycythemia or hyperviscosity
    Protein S or C deficiency
    Antithrombin III deficiency
    Antiphospholipid antibodies

Thromboembolic
    Placental vascular anastomoses
    Cotwin fetal death
    Fetofetal transfusion

HIE or thromboembolism

Source: Modified from JJ Volpe. Neurology of the Newborn. Philadelphia: Saunders, 1995.

Trauma

With improvements in resolution and the use of additional views (e.g., mastoid view), US may be used as the primary modality for evaluating the newborn with intrapartum trauma.[7,11,112,115] CT, however, is usually the modality of choice for delineating extracerebral hemorrhage and posterior fossa hemorrhage (Figure 4.21).[6,111] CT is sufficiently sensitive and specific for acute hemorrhage and the complications or sequelae of fractures.

Occasionally, skull films will demonstrate a skull fracture not shown by CT. MRI often is reserved for circumstances in which neurologic deficits persist and the CT scan is negative or nonspecific. In this situation, MRI may reveal

Table 4.4 Occlusive Neurovascular Disease in the Older Child

Cardiac disease
    Congenital heart disease
    Mitral valve prolapse
    Cardiomyopathies
    Endocarditis
    Cardiac tumors

Dissection

Arteriopathy
    Fibromuscular dysplasia
    Marfan syndrome
    Takayasu arteritis
    Kawasaki disease
    Moyamoya
    Vasculitis
    Polyarteritis nodosa
    Lupus erythematosus

Hypercoagulable state
    Protein S or C deficiency
    Antithrombin III deficiency
    Antiphospholipid antibodies
    Heparin cofactor II deficiency
    Dehydration
    Nephrotic syndrome
    Oncologic disease

Infection

Hemolytic uremic syndrome

Hemoglobinopathies
    Sickle-cell disease

Treatment of oncologic disease
    Radiotherapy
    Chemotherapy

Metabolic disease
    Mitochondrial disorders
    Homocystinuria
    Dyslipoproteinemia
    Fabry disease

Sources: Adapted from JJ Volpe. Neurology of the Newborn. Philadelphia: Saunders, 1995; and WS Ball. Cerebrovascular occlusive disease in childhood. Neuroimaging Clin North Am 1994;4:393–422.

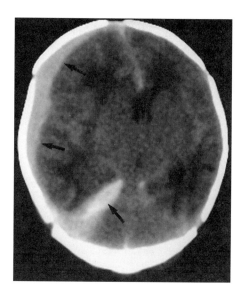

Figure 4.21 Parturient trauma. Axial nonenhanced computed tomographic scan in a full-term neonate shows high-density acute subdural hemorrhagic collections (*arrows*) along the tentorium and about the frontotemporal cerebral convexity on the right.

lesions such as brain stem infarction, axonal shear injury, and cortical contusion, or sequelae such as gliosis, microcystic encephalomalacia, and hemosiderin deposition.[5,6,111] MRI often is more specific than CT for hemorrhage beyond the acute or subacute stage (see Figure 4.12).

Color Doppler US, contrast-enhanced CT, or MRI may distinguish external hydrocephalus (dilated subarachnoid spaces) from chronic subdural hematomas (e.g., in child abuse) when nonenhanced CT demonstrates nonspecific extracerebral collections.[5,6,13] Furthermore, hemosiderin as demonstrated by MRI is confirmation of a previous hemorrhage. In children with atypical intracranial hemorrhage (hemorrhage out of proportion to the history of trauma), MRI may detect an existing vascular malformation, show a hemorrhagic neoplasm, or suggest child abuse (e.g., interhemispheric subdural hematoma [Figure 4.22], hemorrhages of varying ages).[6,27,110,111]

Traumatic spinal column or neuraxis injury in the neonate and young infant may be intrapartum or postnatal and accidental or nonaccidental.[6] Initial evaluation should include plain films of the spine or a skeletal survey if child abuse is suspected. Radionuclide bone scanning (e.g., skeletal SPECT imaging) may demonstrate traumatic bone abnormalities not revealed on radiography.[8] The initial bone survey or bone scan may be negative in the acute phase of child abuse. A follow-up survey or scan a few weeks later may demonstrate fractures in the healing phase. CT is used to evaluate spinal column injury, and US may be used to screen for intraspinal injury.[6] Radiologic abnormality or changing clinical signs may provide the indication for MRI. Neurologic symptoms and signs out of proportion to the history of trauma should suggest the possibility of an existing spinal anomaly (e.g., craniocervical anomaly), a pathologic fracture, or

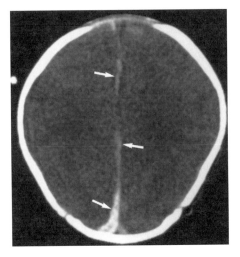

Figure 4.22 Interhemispheric subdural hematoma as a result of child abuse. Axial nonenhanced computed tomographic scan in a young infant shows parasagittal and convexity high-density acute hemorrhagic collections (*arrows*) plus extensive cerebral low densities with loss of cerebral gray and white matter differentiation. The latter finding often is consistent with associated hypoxic-ischemic encephalopathy (e.g., strangulation, suffocation, apnea) or extensive shear injury.

child abuse. Injuries of varying ages should also be a warning sign of repeated inflicted trauma.

MRI obviates the need for myelography in acute trauma patients with progressive myelopathy or radiculopathy (e.g., intraspinal hemorrhage, cord contusion, cord transection, or brachial plexus injury). MRI is also the procedure of choice for evaluating the sequelae of spinal cord trauma (e.g., syrinx, myelomalacia).

Neonatal and Congenital Infections

US or CT is often used to delineate CNS infection (Table 4.5) and the sequelae or complications that may accompany TORCH infections and infantile meningitis, such as cisternal exudate, ventriculitis, hydrocephalus, effusion, empyema, abscess, cystic encephalomalacia, edema, cerebritis, infarction, and calcification (Figures 4.23, 4.24).[5-7,116,117] In the absence or nonspecificity of findings on US or CT, MRI may provide more definitive evaluation (e.g., cytomegalovirus [see Figure 4.10], herpesvirus, human immunodeficiency virus). CT or MRI with intravenous contrast enhancement may also be preferred for the diagnosis and follow-up of suppurative collections.

Infectious or postinfectious encephalitis beyond the neonatal stage is usually viral or postviral in origin.[116,117] The former includes herpes simplex virus type 1 and human immunodeficiency virus infections. The latter includes acute disseminated encephalomyelitis. MRI is often more sensitive than CT in demonstrating encephalitis and acute disseminated encephalomyelitis. Much less common are the granulomatous infections (tuberculosis, fungal and parasitic infections).[116,117] Tuberculous CNS infection tends to occur in infancy and classically produces a basilar meningitis with basal ganglia infarction. Tuberculomas are another manifestation. Cysticercosis is a common cause of focal encephalitis, and seizures occur later in childhood. Calcification might not be present on CT at initial presentation.

Table 4.5   Congenital and Infantile Central Nervous System Infections

TORCH
   Toxoplasmosis
   Other (e.g., syphilis)
   Rubella
   Cytomegalovirus
   Herpes simplex virus type 2
   Human immunodeficiency virus

Meningitis
   Group B streptococcal
   Listeria monocytogenes
   Gram-negative (*Escherichia coli; Proteus, Pseudomonas, Citrobacter* spp.)
   Staphylococcal
   Pneumococcal
   Haemophilus influenzae B
   Neisseria meningitidis
   Other (e.g., viral)

Cerebritis, abscess, and empyema

Encephalitides
   Viral (e.g., herpes simplex virus type 1)
   Acute disseminated encephalomyelitis
   Other (e.g., Rasmussen, subacute sclerosing panencephalitis, progressive multifocal
      leukoencephalopathy)

Granulomatous and parasitic infections
   Tuberculosis
   Fungal
   Cysticercosis
   Lyme disease
   Other

Source: Adapted from PD Barnes, TY Poussaint, PE Burrows. Imaging of pediatric central nervous system infections. Neuroimaging Clin North Am 1994;4:367–392.

Recurrent CNS infection may require investigation for a parameningeal focus (e.g., sinus or mastoid infection, dermal sinus, primitive neurenteric connection, CSF leak after trauma, dermoid or epidermoid cyst).[6,116] Brain abscess or empyema may be associated with gram-negative meningitis (e.g., *Citrobacter*) in the neonate.[116] Suppurative collections related to sinus infection, trauma, surgery, sepsis, the immunocompromised state, or uncorrected cyanotic congenital heart disease primarily occur in older children.[6] Contrast-enhanced CT usually suffices for diagnosis and follow-up. Occasionally, multiplanar T_2-weighted MRI or gadolinium-enhanced T_1-weighted MRI is needed to delineate subtle collections for drainage. Contrast-enhanced stereotactic CT or intraoperative US may provide direct guidance.

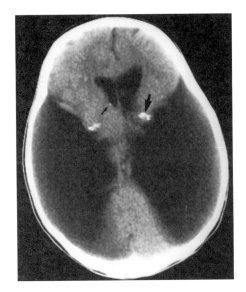

Figure 4.23 Toxoplasmosis. Axial nonenhanced computed tomographic scan in a newborn in the chronic phase shows bilateral low-density porencephaly, hydrocephalus, and high-density calcifications (*arrows*).

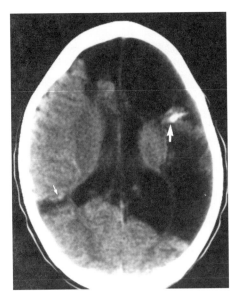

Figure 4.24 Herpes simplex virus type 2 viral encephalitis. Axial nonenhanced computed tomographic scan in a young infant in the chronic phase shows asymmetric cystic encephalomalacia with calcifications (*arrows*) and ventriculomegaly.

Plain films or SPECT are recommended for the screening of suspected spinal column infection.[6] CT or MRI often is needed for definitive diagnosis and for treatment follow-up. MRI is the procedure of choice for evaluating spinal neuraxis infections (e.g., dermal sinus with abscessed dermoid cyst). Gadolinium enhancement is an important finding.

Metabolic and Neurodegenerative Disorders

In the evaluation of developmental delay (e.g., static encephalopathy versus neurodegenerative disease), MRI is the only modality that can provide an accurate assessment of brain maturation based on myelination and cortical development.[5,6,118,119] The clinical hallmark of a neurodegenerative disorder is progressive neurologic impairment in the absence of a CNS tumor or another readily identifiable process (e.g., infection). These are rare disorders that often are untreatable. Many are heredofamilial and metabolic, such that genetic counseling and prenatal screening are important when possible. Metabolic and degenerative disorders may be classified in a number of ways, including anatomic predilection (e.g., gray matter, white matter, both) and metabolic defect. Diagnosis is primarily a clinical one and involves metabolic testing (e.g., enzymatic assays) or biopsy of CNS or extra-CNS tissues.

MRI is superior to CT in evaluating disease extent and anatomic distribution. Occasionally, MRI may demonstrate characteristic imaging findings (e.g., Zellweger syndrome). Proton MRS has the potential to contribute specific metabolic characterization of these disorders. Stereotactic CT or MRI may serve as a guide for biopsy.

Neoplastic Diseases

The classification of CNS tumors is based primarily on pathologic criteria.[5,6,120,121] Anatomic predilection and corresponding clinical signs provide another basis for classifying intracranial tumors in childhood, as follows: cerebral hemispheric tumors, tumors about the third ventricle, posterior fossa tumors, and parameningeal tumors.[6] The rare intracranial neoplasms occurring in infancy are optic or hypothalamic astrocytomas, choroid plexus tumors, the desmoplastic ganglioglioma, germ cell tumors (e.g., teratoma), embryonal tumors (e.g., PNET, medulloblastoma, ependymoblastoma, medulloepithelioma), and mesenchymal neoplasms (e.g., rhabdoid tumor, meningeal sarcoma).[5,6] Parameningeal tumors are those that arise extradurally and often directly invade the CNS. Common parameningeal tumors of infancy include neuroblastoma, histiocytosis, hemangioma, rhabdomyosarcoma, other sarcomas, PNET, and melanotic progonoma.

Although US or CT might detect the vast majority of intracranial masses in childhood, MRI is the procedure of choice for definitive evaluation, including treatment planning and the follow-up of tumor response and treatment effects.[6,120–122] Furthermore, the superior sensitivity of MRI makes it the definitive procedure for the detection of tumors that are often occult to CT or US, particularly in unexplained focal seizure disorders, unexplained hydrocephalus, unexplained neuroendocrine disorders (e.g., diencephalic syndrome), and for cervicomedullary junction tumors and leptomeningeal neoplastic processes. MRI is an important adjunct to CT in evaluating parameningeal or extradural tumors that encroach on or invade the CNS. Craniospinal MRI with gadolinium enhancement is important for assessing tumor seeding, especially in medulloblastoma, germ cell tumors, and malignant glial tumors. Doppler can characterize the degree of intratumoral vascularity, identify its vascular supply, and determine obstruction of adjacent venous sinuses. Although MRI is sensitive to treatment effects (e.g., ischemic or hemorrhagic vasculopathy), functional or metabolic imaging (e.g., SPECT, PET, PMRI, MRS) may add specificity in differentiating between necrosis and tumor progression or recurrence.[6,8,69,122]

Neoplastic diseases of the spine and spinal neuraxis occur primarily in older children and are classified anatomically as extradural, intradural, or intramedullary.[6] Extradural tumors may be relatively benign (e.g., congenital hemangioma) or relatively malignant and invasive (e.g., neuroblastoma, PNET, sarcoma, histiocytosis). SPECT imaging may provide superior sensitivity in detecting multiple lesions.[8] Common intradural extramedullary neoplasms of childhood include schwannoma, neurofibroma, and seeding. Astrocytoma, ependymoma, and ganglioglioma make up the majority of intramedullary tumors in children and often are associated with cysts or hydrosyringomyelia. Although CT may be indicated for single-level lesions, MRI is recommended for the definitive evaluation of all spinal column and spinal neuraxis tumors.[6] Spinal MRI is indicated particularly in children with atypical scoliosis when hydrosyringomyelia is demonstrated and a developmental cause (e.g., Chiari I malformation) must be distinguished from a neoplastic cause (e.g., astrocytoma).

REFERENCES

1. Much L, Alberman E, Hagberg B, et al. Cerebral palsy epidemiology. Dev Med Child Neurol 1992;34:547–551.
2. Kuban KCK, Leviton A. Cerebral palsy. N Engl J Med 1994;330:188–195.
3. Barnes PD, O'Tuama L, Tzika AA. Investigating the pediatric central nervous system. Curr Opin Pediatr 1993;5:643–652.
4. Barnes PD. Imaging of the central nervous system in pediatrics and adolescence. Pediatr Clin North Am 1992;39:743–776.
5. Barkovich AJ. Pediatric Neuroimaging. New York: Raven, 1995.
6. Wolpert SM, Barnes P. MRI in Pediatric Neuroradiology. St. Louis: Mosby–Year Book, 1992;41–82.
7. Teele R, Share J. Ultrasonography of Infants and Children. Philadelphia: Saunders, 1991.
8. Treves ST (ed). Pediatric Nuclear Medicine (2nd ed). New York: Springer-Verlag, 1995.
9. Volpe JJ. Neurology of the Newborn. Philadelphia: Saunders, 1995.
10. Anderson N, Allan R, Darlow B, et al. Diagnosis of intraventricular hemorrhage in the newborn: value of sonography via the posterior fontanelle. AJR Am J Roentgenol 1994;63:893.
11. Buckley KM, Taylor GA, Estroff JA, et al. Use of the mastoid fontanelle for improved sonographic visualization of the neonatal midbrain and posterior fossa. AJR Am J Roentgenol 1997;168:1021–1025.
12. Dean LM, Taylor GA. The intracranial venous system in infants: normal and abnormal findings on duplex and color Doppler sonography. AJR Am J Roentgenol 1995;164:151.
13. Chen C-Y, Chou T-Y, Zimmerman RA, et al. Pericerebral fluid collection: differentiation of enlarged subarachnoid spaces from subdural collections with color Doppler US. Radiology 1996;201:389.

14. Goh D, Minns RA, Hendry GMA, et al. Cerebrovascular resistive index assessed by duplex Doppler sonography and its relationship to intracranial pressure in infantile hydrocephalus. Pediatr Radiol 1992;22:246.
15. Seibert JJ, McCowan TC, Chadduck WM, et al. Duplex pulsed Doppler US versus intracranial pressure in the neonate: clinical and experimental studies. Radiology 1989;171:155.
16. Taylor GA, Short LB, Walker LK, et al. Intracranial blood flow: quantification with duplex Doppler and color Doppler flow US. Radiology 1990;176:231.
17. Westra SJ, Curran JG, Duckwiler GR, et al. Pediatric intracranial vascular malformations: evaluation of treatment results with color Doppler US. Radiology 1991; 186:775.
18. Taylor GA, Madsen JR. Hemodynamic response to fontanelle compression in neonatal hydrocephalus: correlation with intracranial pressure and need for shunt placement. Radiology 1996;201:685.
19. Rubin JM, Bude RO, Carson PL, et al. Power Doppler: a potentially useful alternative to mean-frequency based color Doppler sonography. Radiology 1994;190:853.
20. Goldberg BB, Liu JB, Forsberg G. Ultrasound contrast agents: a review. US Med Biol 1994;20:319.
21. Barr LL, McCullough PJ, Ball WS Jr, et al. Quantitative sonographic feature analysis of clinical infant hypoxia. AJNR Am J Neuroradiol 1996;17:1025.
22. Coleman LT, Zimmerman RA. Pediatric craniospinal spiral CT: current applications and future potential. Semin Ultrasound CT MR 1994;15:148.
23. White KS. Helical/spiral CT scanning: a pediatric radiology perspective. Pediatr Radiol 1996;26:5–14.
24. Blankenberg FG, Norbash AM, Lane B, et al. Neonatal intracranial ischemia and hemorrhage: diagnosis with US, CT, and MR imaging. Radiology 1996;199: 253–259.
25. Legido A, Zimmerman R, Packer R, et al. Significance of basal ganglia calcification on CT in children. Pediatr Neurosci 1988;14:64.
26. Zeman RK, Silverman PM, Vieco PT, Costello P. CT angiography. AJR Am J Roentgenol 1995;165:1079–1088.
27. Kleinman P. Diagnostic Imaging of Child Abuse. Baltimore: Williams & Wilkins, 1987.
28. DeCoene B, Hajnal JV, Gatehouse P, et al. MR of the brain using fluid-attenuated inversion recovery (FLAIR) pulse sequences. AJNR Am J Neuroradiol 1992;13: 1555–1564.
29. Rydberg JN, et al. Initial clinical experience in MR imaging of the brain with a fast fluid-attenuated inversion-recovery pulse sequence. Radiology 1994;193:173–180.
30. Simonson TM, et al. Echo-planar FLAIR imaging in evaluation of intracranial lesions. Radiographics 1996;16:575–584.
31. Finelli DA, et al. Cerebral white matter: technical development and clinical applications of effective magnetization transfer (MT) power concepts for high-power, thin-section, quantitative MT examinations. Radiology 1996;199:219–226.
32. Grossman RI, et al. Magnetization transfer: theory and clinical applications in neuroradiology. Radiographics 1994;14:279–290.
33. Santry GE, Mulkern RV. Magnetization transfer in MR imaging: a report from the relaxometry and biophysics committee of the SMRI. J Magn Reson Imaging 1995; 5:121–124.
34. Wolff SD, Balaban RS. Magnetization transfer imaging: practical aspects and clinical applications. Radiology 1994;192:593–599.
35. Engelbrecht V, Malms J, Kahn T, et al. Fast spin echo MR imaging of the pediatric brain. Pediatr Radiol 1996;26:259–264.
36. Edelman RR, Wielopolski P, Schmitt F. Echo-planar MR imaging. Radiology 1994;192:600–612.

37. DeLaPaz RL. Echo-planar imaging. Radiographics 1994;14:1045–1058.
38. Robertson RL, Blaustein PA, Gonzalez RG. Intracranial MRA. In KE Yucel (ed), Magnetic Resonance Angiography: A Practical Approach. New York: McGraw-Hill, 1995.
39. Siebert JE, Pernicone JR, Potchen EJ. Physical principles and application of MRA. Semin Ultrasound CT MR 1992;13:227.
40. Maas K, Barkovich AJ, Dong L, et al. Selected indications for and applications of magnetic resonance angiography in children. Pediatr Neurosurg 1994;20:113–125.
41. Edelman RR, Mattle HP, Atkinson DJ, et al. Cerebral blood flow: assessment with dynamic contrast-enhanced $T_2{}^*$-weighted MR imaging at 1.5 T. Radiology 1990; 176:211–220.
42. Kucharczyk J, Vexler ZS, Roberts TP, et al. Echo-planar perfusion-sensitive MR imaging of acute cerebral ischemia. Radiology 1993;188:711–717.
43. Tzika A, Massoth R, Ball W Jr, et al. Cerebral perfusion in children: detection with dynamic contrast-enhanced T_2-weighted images. Radiology 1993;87:449–458.
44. Chien D, Kwong KK, Gress DR, et al. MR diffusion imaging of cerebral infarction in humans. AJNR Am J Neuroradiol 1992;13:1097–1102.
45. Cowan FM, Pennock JM, Hanrahan JD, et al. Early detection of cerebral infarction and hypoxic ischemic encephalopathy in neonates using diffusion-weighted magnetic resonance imaging. Neuropediatrics 1994;25:172–175.
46. Harada K, Fujita N, Sakurai K, et al. Diffusion imaging of the human brain: a new pulse sequence application for a 1.5-T standard MR system. AJNR Am J Neuroradiol 1991;12:1143–1148.
47. Le Bihan D, Turner R, Douek P, Patronas N. Diffusion MR imaging: clinical applications. AJR Am J Roentgenol 1992;159:591–599.
48. Le Bihan D. Diffusion/perfusion MR imaging of the brain: from structure to function. Radiology 1990;177:328–329.
49. Sakuma H, Nomura Y, Takeda K, et al. Adult and neonatal human brain: diffusional anisotropy and myelination with diffusion-weighted MR imaging. Radiology 1991;180:229–233.
50. Sevick RJ, Kanda F, Mintorovitch J, et al. Cytotoxic brain edema: assessment with diffusion-weighted MR imaging. Radiology 1992;185:687–690.
51. Sorensen AG, Buonanno FS, Gonzalez RG, et al. Hyperacute stroke: evaluation with combined multisection diffusion-weighted and hemodynamically weighted echo-planar MR imaging. Radiology 1996;199:391–401.
52. Bhadelia RA, Bogdan AR, Wolpert SM, et al. Cerebrospinal fluid flow waveforms: analysis in patients with Chiari I malformation by means of gated phase-contrast MR imaging velocity measurements. Radiology 1995;196:195–202.
53. Feinberg DA. Modern concepts of brain motion and cerebrospinal fluid flow. Radiology 1992;185:630-632.
54. Maier SE, Hardy CJ, Jolesz FA. Brain and cerebrospinal fluid motion. Radiology 1994;193:477–483.
55. Poncelet BP, Wedeen VJ, Weisskoff RM, Cohen MS. Brain parenchyma motion: measurement with cine echo-planar MR imaging. Radiology 1992;185:645–651.
56. Wolpert SM, Bhadelia RA, Bogdan AR, Cohen AR. Chiari I malformations: assessment with phase-contrast velocity MR. AJNR Am J Neuroradiol 1994;15:1299–1308.
57. Connelly A, Jackson GD, Frackowiak RS, et al. Functional mapping of activated human primary cortex with a clinical MR imaging system. Radiology 1993;188:125–130.
58. Li A, Yetkin FZ, Cox R, Haughton VM. Ipsilateral hemisphere activation during motor and sensory tasks. AJNR Am J Neuroradiol 1996;17:651–656.
59. Rosen BR, Aronen HJ, Kwong KK, et al. Advances in clinical neuroimaging: functional MR imaging techniques. Radiographics 1993;13:889–896.

60. Sorensen AG, Rosen BR. Functional MRI of the Brain. In SW Atlas (ed), Magnetic Resonance Imaging of the Brain and Spine (2nd ed). Philadelphia: Lippincott–Raven, 1996.

61. Boesch C, Martin E. Combined application of MR imaging and spectroscopy in neonates and children: installation and operation of a 2.35-T system in a clinical setting. Radiology 1988;168:481.

62. Grodd W, Krageloh-Mann I, Klose U, et al. Metabolic and destructive brain disorders in children: findings with localized proton MR spectroscopy. Radiology 1991;181:173–181.

63. Kimura H, Fujii Y, Itoh S, et al. Metabolic alterations in the neonate and infant brain during development: evaluation with proton MR spectroscopy. Radiology 1995;194:483–489.

64. Moorcraft J, Bolas NM, Ives NK, et al. Spatially localized magnetic resonance spectroscopy of the brains of normal and asphyxiated newborns. Pediatrics 1991; 87:273–282.

65. Sutton LN, Wang Z, Duhaime AC, et al. Tissue lactate in pediatric head trauma: a clinical study using 1H NMR spectroscopy. Pediatr Neurosurg 1995;22:81–87.

66. Tzika AA, Vigneron D, Ball W, et al. Localized proton MR spectroscopy of the brain in children. J Magn Reson Imaging 1993;3:719–729.

67. Tzika AA, Ball WS Jr, Vigneron DB, et al. Clinical proton MR spectroscopy of neurodegenerative disease in childhood. AJNR Am J Neuroradiol 1993;14: 1267–1281.

68. van der Knaap MS, van der Grond J, van Rijen PC, et al. Age-dependent changes in localized proton and phosphorus MR spectroscopy of the brain. Radiology 1990;176:509–515.

69. Wang Z, Zimmerman RA, Sauter R. Proton MR spectroscopy of the brain: clinically useful information obtained in assessing CNS diseases in children. AJNR Am J Neuroradiol 1996;167:191–199.

70. Alexander E 3rd, Kooy HM, van Herk M, et al. Magnetic resonance image-directed stereotactic neurosurgery: use of image fusion with computerized tomography to enhance spatial accuracy. J Neurosurg 1995;83:271–276.

71. Anzai Y, Desalles AA, Black KL, et al. Interventional MR imaging. Radiographics 1993;13:897–904.

72. Jackson GD. New techniques in magnetic resonance and epilepsy. Epilepsia 1994;35(suppl 6):S2–S13.

73. Jolesz FA, Silverman SG. Interventional magnetic resonance therapy. Semin Intervention Radiol 1995;12:20–27.

74. Kikinis R, Gleason PL, Moriarty TM, et al. Computer-assisted interactive three-dimensional planning for neurosurgical procedures. Neurosurgery 1996;38:640–649.

75. Schaefer GB, Thompson JN Jr, Bodensteiner JB, et al. Quantitative morphometric analysis of brain growth using magnetic resonance imaging. J Child Neurol 1990; 5:127–130.

76. Schenck JF, Jolesz FA, Roemer PB, et al. Superconducting open-configuration MR imaging system for image-guided therapy. Radiology 1995;195:805–814.

77. Chugani HT. Functional brain imaging in pediatrics. Pediatr Clin North Am 1992;39:777–799.

78. Legido A, Price ML, Wolfson B, et al. Technetium ^{99m}Tc-HMPAO SPECT in children and adolescents with neurologic disorders. J Child Neurol 1993;8:227–234.

79. Chiron C, Raynaud C, Maziere B, et al. Changes in regional cerebral blood flow during brain maturation in children and adolescents. J Nucl Med 1992;33:696–703.

80. Chugani HT, Phelps ME, Mazziotta JC. Positron emission tomography study of human brain functional development. Ann Neurol 1987;22:487–497.

81. Chugani HT, Phelps ME. Maturational changes in cerebral function in infants determined by 18-FDG positron emission tomography. Science 1986;231:840–843.

82. Chugani HT. The role of PET in childhood epilepsy. J Child Neurol 1994;9: S82–S88.

83. Harvey AS, Berkovic SF. Functional neuroimaging with SPECT in children with partial epilepsy. J Child Neurol 1994;9:S71–S81.

84. Jack CR Jr. Epilepsy: surgery and imaging. Radiology 1993;189:635–646.

85. Janicek MJ, O'Tuama LA, Treves ST. Quantitative evaluation of ^{99m}Tc-hexamethylpropyleneamineoxime brain SPECT in childhood-onset epilepsy. J Nucl Biol Med 1992;36:319–323.

86. Mastin ST, Drane WE, Gilmore RL, et al. Prospective localization of epileptogenic foci: comparison of PET and SPECT with site of surgery and clinical outcome. Radiology 1996;199:375–380.

87. Packard AB, Roach PJ, Davis RT, et al. Ictal and interictal technetium-99m-bicisate brain SPECT in children with refractory epilepsy. J Nucl Med 1996;37:1101–1106.

88. Ryvlin P, Philippon B, Cinotti L, et al. Functional neuroimaging strategy in temporal lobe epilepsy: a comparative study of ^{18}FDG-PET and ^{99m}Tc-HMPAO-SPECT. Ann Neurol 1992;31:650–656.

89. Delbeke D, Meyerowitz C, Lapidus RL, et al. Optimal cutoff levels of F-18 fluorodeoxyglucose uptake in the differentiation of low-grade from high-grade brain tumors with PET. Radiology 1995;195:47–52.

90. Holman LB, Zimmerman RE, Johnson KA, et al. Computer-assisted superimposition of magnetic resonance and high-resolution technetium-99m-HMPAO and thallium-201 SPECT images of the brain. J Nucl Med 1991;32:1478–1484.

91. Habboush IH, Mitchell KD, Mulkern RV, et al. Registration and alignment of three-dimensional images: an interactive visual approach. Radiology 1996; 199:573–578.

92. Kahn D, Follett KA, Bushnell DL, et al. Diagnosis of recurrent brain tumor: value of ^{201}Tl SPECT vs ^{18}F-fluorodeoxyglucose PET. AJR Am J Roentgenol 1994; 163:1459–1465.

93. Levin DN, Hu XP, Tan KK, et al. The brain: integrated three-dimensional display of MR and PET images. Radiology 1989;172:783–789.

94. O'Tuama LA, Treves ST, Larar JN, et al. Thallium-201 versus technetium-99m-MIBI in evaluation of childhood brain tumors: a within-subject comparison. J Nucl Med 1993;34:1045–1051.

95. Laurin NR, Driedger AA, Hurwitz GA, et al. Cerebral perfusion imaging with technetium-99m HM-PAO in brain death and severe central nervous system injury. J Nucl Med 1989;30:1627–1635.

96. George MS, Ruig HA, Costa DC, et al. Neuroactivation and Neuroimaging with SPECT. London: Springer-Verlag, 1991.

97. O'Tuama LA, Treves ST. Brain SPECT for behavior disorders in children. Semin Nucl Med 1993;23:255–264.

98. van der Knaap M, Valk J. Congenital abnormalities of the CNS. AJNR Am J Neuroradiol 1988;9:315.

99. McComb JG. Cerebrospinal fluid physiology of the developing fetus. AJNR Am J Neuroradiol 1992;13:595–600.

100. Fitz CR. Holoprosencephaly and septo-optic dysplasia. Neuroimaging Clin North Am 1994;4:263–282.

101. McLone DG, Naidich TP. Developmental morphology of the subarachnoid space, brain vasculature and contiguous structures, and the cause of the Chiari II malformation. AJNR Am J Neuroradiol 1992;13:463–482.

102. Naidich TP, Altman NR, Braffman BH, et al. Cephaloceles and related malformations. AJNR Am J Neuroradiol 1992;13:655–690.

103. Altman NR, Naidich TP, Braffman BH. Posterior fossa malformations. AJNR Am J Neuroradiol 1992;13:691–724.

104. Barkovich AJ, Gressens P, Evrard P. Formation, maturation, and disorders of brain neocortex. AJNR Am J Neuroradiol 1992;13:423–446.
105. Barkovich AJ, Lyon G, Evrard P. Formation, maturation, and disorders of white matter. AJNR Am J Neuroradiol 1992;13:447–462.
106. Flodmark O. Neuroradiology of selected disorders of the meninges, calvarium, and venous sinuses. AJNR Am J Neuroradiol 1992;13:483–492.
107. Levine D, Hatabu H, Gaa J, et al. Fetal anatomy revealed with fast MR sequences. AJR Am J Roentgenol 1996;167:905–908.
108. Braffman B, Naidich TP. The phakomatoses. Neuroimaging Clin North Am 1994;4:299–348.
109. Bird C, Hedberg M, Drayer B, et al. MR assessment of myelination in infants and children: useful marker sites. AJNR Am J Neuroradiol 1989;10:731–740.
110. Harwood-Nash DC. Abuse to the pediatric central nervous system. AJNR Am J Neuroradiol 1992;13:569–576.
111. Zimmerman RA, Bilaniuk LT. Pediatric head trauma. Neuroimaging Clin North Am 1994;4:349–366.
112. Rorke LB, Zimmerman RA. Prematurity, postmaturity, and destructive lesions in utero. AJNR Am J Neuroradiol 1992;13:517–536.
113. Ball WS. Cerebrovascular occlusive disease in childhood. Neuroimaging Clin North Am 1994;4:393–422.
114. Burrows PE, Robertson RL, Barnes PD. Angiography and the evaluation of cerebrovascular disease in childhood. Neuroimaging Clin North Am 1996;3:561–588.
115. Boyer RS. Neuroimaging of premature infants. Neuroimaging Clin North Am 1994;4:241–262.
116. Barnes PD, Poussaint TY, Burrows PE. Imaging of pediatric central nervous system infections. Neuroimaging Clin North Am 1994;4:367–392.
117. Fitz CR. Inflammatory diseases of the brain in childhood. AJNR Am J Neuroradiol 1992;13:551–568.
118. Naidich TP, Grant JL, Altman N, et al. The developing cerebral surface: anatomy, US, and MRI. Neuroimaging Clin North Am 1994;4:201–240.
119. Kendall BE. Disorders of lysosomes, peroxisomes, and mitochondria. AJNR Am J Neuroradiol 1992;13:621–654.
120. Edwards-Brown MK. Supratentorial brain tumors. Neuroimaging Clin North Am 1994;4:437–457.
121. Vezina LG, Packer RJ. Infratentorial brain tumors of childhood. Neuroimaging Clin North Am 1994;4:423–436.
122. Ball WS, Prenger EC, et al. Neurotoxicity of radio/chemotherapy in children: pathologic and MR correlation. AJNR Am J Neuroradiol 1992;13:761–776.

5

Perinatal Aspects of Cerebral Palsy

Jan Goddard-Finegold

Cerebral palsy is a consequence of damage to the developing brain and can result from a number of different causes. Hypoxic-ischemic injury to the brain is the perinatal insult most frequently associated with both neonatal encephalopathy and subsequent neurologic sequelae, including cerebral palsy, in survivors. However, toxic, metabolic, infectious, genetic, and traumatic insults and congenital malformations also can cause antenatal or perinatal brain defects sufficient to produce cerebral palsy. Notably, preterm infants without demonstrable signs of encephalopathy or evidence of intrapartum hypoxic-ischemic injury can later show signs of cerebral palsy.[1] A proportion of both preterm and full-term infants may have antenatal brain injury that is not symptomatic at birth, and some infants, most often preterm infants, will suffer neurologic sequelae as a consequence of postnatal disease and adverse postnatal events. In this chapter, the statistics and epidemiology, concepts of pathophysiology, and clinical aspects of perinatal brain injury are discussed.

CURRENT STATISTICS AND EPIDEMIOLOGY OF PERINATAL BRAIN INJURY

Perinatal hypoxia-ischemia sufficient to cause neurologic signs and symptoms in the newborn period is thought to occur in 2–6 per 1,000 full-term infants and in considerably more preterm infants.[2] In a study conducted in the 1980s, preterm infants of less than 1,500-g birth weight were believed to have signs of birth asphyxia in 60% of cases.[3] Early intervention strategies in the current care of very low–birth-weight infants have contributed to a decrease in this number today.

Because the outcome of both preterm and full-term patients is related both to the duration and degree of the insult and to the duration and degree of the resulting encephalopathy (among other factors), the number of infants who survive hypoxic-ischemic insult with neurologic sequelae evidenced as cerebral palsy is a fraction of those who sustain the varying degrees of insult.[4–7] The mortality from hypoxia-ischemia currently ranges from 9% to 35%.[4–7] Small-for-gestational-age infants and twins are at greater risk for cerebral palsy than are appropriate-for-gestational-age singleton infants.[8–10] Preterm infants are up to 10–20 times more likely to have cerebral palsy than are full-term infants, and preterm infants are more likely than full-term infants to sustain and suffer consequences from adverse postnatal insults.[8,11]

Survivors of neonatal encephalopathy believed to be due to hypoxia-ischemia have varying degrees of neurologic sequelae that are related to the duration and degree of the injury and the encephalopathy.[12,13] Almost all full-term infants with mild encephalopathy in the neonatal period are neurologically normal at later follow-up, whereas those with moderate encephalopathy have a 20–35% risk of later neurologic sequelae. Those with severe encephalopathy have a 75% risk of dying in the newborn period, and survivors have a virtually universal risk of neurologic sequelae.[7,12,13]

As previously stated, the predominant cause of neonatal encephalopathy is hypoxia-ischemia, and cerebral palsy consists of neurologic signs and symptoms that occur frequently as a result of significant hypoxic-ischemic brain injury. However, hypoxia-ischemia is not the only cause of neonatal encephalopathy and, in some cases, despite the presence of clear-cut signs of encephalopathy, determining whether significant hypoxia-ischemia actually has occurred is difficult. Clearly, toxic, metabolic, infectious, genetic, traumatic, and other causes must be considered.

Viewed from another perspective, intrapartum hypoxia-ischemia is not the only, or even a frequent, cause of cerebral palsy. Surveys in the 1980s of members of the population who have cerebral palsy showed that perinatal hypoxic-ischemic brain injury accounts for a relatively small proportion of cases in that group (8–22%).[3,14] Currently, for most patients with cerebral palsy, a history of intrapartum abnormalities or neonatal encephalopathy is not found, suggesting that their cerebral palsy is a result of remote antepartum brain injury, genetic abnormalities, malformation syndromes, undiagnosed intrauterine infections, or other, undefined causes. The prevalence of cerebral palsy reported in a survey in California was 1.1 per 1,000 singleton births and 12 per 1,000 twin pregnancies.[9] A compilation of figures from many studies showed rates of 1.3 per 1,000 in survivors of more than 2,500-g birth weight and 8.5 per 1,000 in the 1,500- to 2,499-g birth weight category, with an overall prevalence for all neonatal survivors of 2.3 per 1,000.[15–17] However, a study published in 1996 by Hack and colleagues[11] reported a 43% survival and 10% incidence of cerebral palsy in surviving infants of birth weights less than 750 g, suggesting that the extremely low–birth-weight population is adding a considerable number of infants to the population with cerebral palsy.

In fact, data compiled by Bhushan and colleagues[17] indicate that the numbers of both very low–birth-weight survivors without cerebral palsy and those with cerebral palsy have increased over the past decade. Most of the data for these studies were compiled in the late 1980s and early 1990s. Because larger numbers of extremely low–birth-weight infants currently are surviving, the percentage of people in the population with cerebral palsy secondary to problems of prematurity might increase over the next decade.

Hypoxic-ischemic brain insult severe enough to cause encephalopathy has been estimated to occur before labor in 20% of cases, during delivery in 35% of cases, both before and during delivery in 35% of cases, and in the early postnatal period in 10% of cases.[18] These numbers vary in different series, but they all indicate that a significant prenatal component is involved in a large proportion of infants with hypoxic-ischemic injury.[19-21] Though preterm infants are at increased risk of both intrapartum and postpartum hypoxia-ischemia, preterm labor and preterm delivery might occur after such infants have sustained significant antenatal brain injury.[22-26] We are learning that fetuses with preexisting brain injury may be prone to preterm labor. Some infants with significant antepartum brain injury might not exhibit abnormal neurologic signs at birth and yet will begin to show signs of cerebral palsy early in life. This seems to be especially true for antenatally acquired cystic periventricular leukomalacia (PVL). As Bejar and associates[25] and Grafe[26] have shown, a significant proportion of preterm infants who are evaluated with ultrasound examinations of the brain shortly after birth, as well as infants who are stillborn, have easily identified, already established central nervous system (CNS) lesions. Thus, documentation of lesions that are present at birth, when possible, is important for providing a clearer understanding of the most likely causes of cerebral palsy and other neurologic deficits in both individual patients and in the population at large.

HYPOXIC-ISCHEMIC BRAIN INJURY

Basic Premises

Hypoxia-ischemia, by definition, is a state characterized by lack of oxygen and lack of sufficient blood flow to an organ. Brain infarction occurs in adult primates when cerebral blood flow is less than 8–12 ml/min/100 g tissue, depending on the duration of the ischemia.[27-29] The level of blood flow that is sufficient in newborns is likely to be less than this, as resting cerebral blood flow in newborns (approximately 20 ml/min/100 g) is less than that of adults.[30] Altman and colleagues[31] have shown that some preterm newborns can survive intact after sustaining cerebral blood flows of less than 5 ml/min/100 g for relatively long periods of time.

Hypoxia can occur without ischemia under circumstances of inadequate inspired oxygen and inadequate oxygen-carrying capacity (severe anemia, blood loss, carbon monoxide poisoning) or if ventilation is transiently curtailed but cardiac function is maintained, at least temporarily. Hypoxia leads to anaerobic cellular metabolism and metabolic acidosis.

That ischemia, and ischemia plus hypoxia, are clear antecedents to brain injury has long been known, whereas hypoxia alone is less likely to produce irreversible brain damage,[32] although hypoxia and systemic acidosis can lead to cardiovascular compromise and hypotension (with resulting brain ischemia and brain injury). Questions of graded neuropathologic effects of hypoxia, especially for the pathogenesis of epilepsy, have been raised, however. At least one study has shown loss of a specific neuronal population in a primate model after asphyxia without marked hypotension.[33]

Injury to the brain after hypoxia-ischemia can be due to the effects of reperfusion. In fact, reperfusion injury is, in some cases, more deleterious than the injury caused by ischemia alone. Reperfusion injury results from a number of proposed physiologic processes, including the release of oxygen free radicals and subsequent free radical–induced oxidation membrane injury.[34]

Respiratory failure is a common cause of asphyxia, with consequent decreased oxygen intake and decreased removal of carbon dioxide. Respiratory acidosis occurs as carbon dioxide builds up, and a mixed acidosis occurs as cellular metabolism becomes anaerobic and lactate is produced.

Mechanisms of Cellular Injury After Hypoxia-Ischemia and Reperfusion

Experimental studies of hypoxia-ischemia show that the earliest cellular responses to hypoxia include the release of adenosine and the opening of potassium channels, which cause the cell membrane to hyperpolarize.[35] This hyperpolarization reduces the neuron's ability to produce action potentials and is coupled with depression of calcium currents and decreased release of synaptic neurotransmitters. During these events, intracellular calcium increases, activating calcium-dependent potassium channels and further increasing membrane hyperpolarization. As adenosine triphosphate concentrations decrease, the excitability of the neuron is limited further. These events likely serve to spare energy during periods when oxygen is not available; they are reversed when perfusion and oxygenation return to normal. In addition, studies have shown that hypoxia-ischemia alters the binding characteristics of hexokinase, an enzyme that is vital for glucose metabolism, making this enzyme less available for any glucose that is present.[36] Apparently, this effect is not immediately reversible, persisting for several hours into oxygenation and reperfusion.[36]

When tissue oxygen lack continues, other mechanisms become important for cellular injury, including release of glutamate, production of neuronal and vascular nitric oxide, and the release of oxygen free radicals.[35,37,38] The role of glutamate as a neurotransmitter and as a major factor in excitotoxic neuronal injury after hypoxia-ischemia is supported by a plethora of data.[35,39] Of the four receptor types for glutamate, the most avid is the N-methyl-D-aspartate (NMDA) receptor. NMDA is the most physiologically active of the receptors, and the channels that are activated by it are voltage dependent and calcium permeable and cause depolarization of neurons.[35,40,41] When NMDA channels open, therefore, further depolarization of neurons occurs, and the neurons accumulate intracellular calcium.

Under normal physiologic conditions, glutamate is intracellular and is not accessible to NMDA receptors, and synaptically released glutamate, when present extracellularly, is rapidly pumped back across the cell membrane. During hypoxia-ischemia, however, these mechanisms fail, and glutamate is not transported out of the extracellular space. Toxic levels of glutamate can accumulate during ongoing hypoxia-ischemia, leading to eventual cell death, which is hypothesized to occur owing to lethal accumulation of intracellular calcium. Areas that are the most sensitive to hypoxic-ischemic injury have been shown to be those with the highest densities of NMDA receptors. In addition, the NMDA receptor densities in the brain change with development, providing a possible mechanism for age-related changes in "selective vulnerabilities" to hypoxic-ischemic injuries.[42,43]

Possible preventive agents against hypoxic-ischemic brain injury include the NMDA-receptor antagonists and drugs that block endogenous glutamate release (adenosine). However, these agents have considerable clinical toxicities, and finding preventive agents with acceptable levels of clinical toxicity will be a major accomplishment.[44,45]

Other agents thought to play a role in hypoxic-ischemic brain injury include nitric oxide (NO) and oxygen free radicals. NO is a vasodilating agent that is produced by some neurons, glia, and endothelial cells.[37] NO synthase converts L-arginine to NO and citrulline and, when L-arginine is present, NO is preferentially made by NO synthase. When L-arginine is not present, NO synthase in the brain generates superoxide and hydrogen peroxide.[46,47] Interestingly, when NO combines with superoxide, a toxic compound, peroxynitrite is formed. This toxin can contribute to neuronal damage, and so NO can be helpful in stimulating vasodilation and increasing blood flow during hypoxia-ischemia. However, it can also be deleterious, as excessive NO can excite NMDA receptors and increase the production of free radicals (peroxynitrite).[37,48]

Despite the frequent occurrence of hypoxia-ischemia and its noteworthy impact on brain injury, other types of injury *do* occur in the brain, and other metabolic factors can aggravate hypoxic-ischemic injury. As has been stressed previously, brain injury also occurs after prolonged hypoglycemia, with significant and prolonged hyperammonemia, with the buildup or absence of other metabolic products, and in the face of severe hyperbilirubinemia.[49] Bacterial, viral, fungal, and parasitic infections of the newborn brain can cause single or multifocal lesions and, though traumatic brain injury occurs infrequently at birth, such trauma can result in cerebral contusion, axonal tearing, and hemorrhage. Hemorrhage is believed to exacerbate hypoxic-ischemic and reperfusion injuries by providing excess ferrous iron to react with hydrogen peroxide that is generated during reperfusion. The reaction of hydrogen peroxide with ferrous iron results in the production of toxic hydroxy radicals, which can, if unchecked by antioxidant mechanisms, initiate lipid peroxidation and disruption of cellular membranes.[49,50]

Intrauterine Asphyxia

Intrauterine asphyxia is a term used to denote the failure of normal gas exchange in the fetus when the fetus still is dependent on the placenta. Intrauterine asphyxia can occur secondary to numerous causes, including interruption of the umbilical circulation, inadequate perfusion of the maternal side of the placenta, or impaired maternal oxygenation. Postnatal asphyxia can occur when there is failure of neonatal lung function or failure of transition from the fetal to the neonatal circulation (among other causes).[51]

Asphyxia is one cause of abnormal fetal movement or abnormal heart tones before labor. Asphyxia may also be suspected if a fetus responds abnormally to testing using an intrauterine biophysical profile or if a fetus shows abnormal or autonomic responses during labor.[52] Infants who are depressed at birth, are acidotic, and require ventilatory assistance may also have suffered intrauterine asphyxia. However, the great majority of infants who are depressed at birth have had transient, late, depressive events with a low likelihood of sequelae, and a low Apgar score alone is a poor indicator of neurologic outcome.[53,54] When resuscitated quickly, most affected infants will not have neonatal encephalopathy.

A number of causes of neonatal depression are not synonymous with intrauterine asphyxia. Among these are CNS congenital anomalies, effects of drugs, vagal responses to head compression or suctioning, or preexisting neurologic damage.[43,55,56]

In an infant who exhibits a mixed acidosis, the likelihood of having had inadequate respiratory gas exchange is likely. If an infant has very low Apgar scores that persist (0–3 for >5 minutes), severe acidosis (pH <7.0), neonatal encephalopathy and, in many cases, some degree of systemic organ injury, then asphyxia significant enough to cause neurologic sequelae is a likely etiology.[57]

Neonatal Encephalopathy Due to Asphyxia or Hypoxia-Ischemia

Neonatal encephalopathy is a term most frequently used to describe the abnormal neurologic status of the newborn with significant asphyxial or hypoxic-ischemic insult. However, a cause for neonatal encephalopathy should only be ascribed after the appropriate history, physical examination, and diagnostic tests have been evaluated. Encephalopathy in the newborn can be attributed to a number of causes, including head trauma or cerebral hemorrhage, CNS infection, metabolic disorders, toxic effects of drugs, and disorders that may cause secondary asphyxia (congenital anomalies, congenital muscular dystrophies or myopathies).

The degrees of severity of neonatal encephalopathy have been described by Sarnat and Sarnat,[12] Volpe,[58] and Novotny,[59] among others. Mild encephalopathy is characterized by alterations in consciousness, including lethargy, irritability, and hyperalertness for varying periods of time. The infants frequently are jittery, feed poorly, and have abnormal sleep cycles, although findings on neurologic examination are not marked. The cranial nerve examination is normal, whereas muscle tone and deep tendon reflexes may be increased. Pupillary dilation and tachycardia (autonomic signs) might be seen. The Moro reflex may be exaggerated, but most of the primitive reflexes are normal. The infant with mild encephalopathy, by definition, does not have seizures.

The moderately encephalopathic infant is hypotonic and lethargic and feeds poorly. Autonomic findings include constricted pupils and bradycardia in some cases and possibly abnormal movements, such as spontaneous myoclonus or extrapyramidal dysfunction. Reflexes are usually increased, clonus is usually present, and the gag reflex may be depressed. Frequently, seizures occur within the first 24 hours.

The infant with severe encephalopathy is usually comatose and flaccid, and reflexes are absent. Often, the infant must be mechanically ventilated due to apnea, and the infant may be bradycardic and hypotensive. The pupils are often fixed or slowly reactive, and the dolls' eye reflex is absent. Seizures may occur, or these infants may have severely depressed electroencephalograms or electroencephalograms with burst-suppression patterns.

The neurologic sequelae in babies with encephalopathy secondary to hypoxia-ischemia are related to the degree of encephalopathy. Infants who have neonatal depression (low Apgar scores, delayed respirations, meconium staining, or problems of fetal heart rate or pattern) but who do not have neonatal encephalopathy are not likely to have neurologic sequelae unless previous brain damage has occurred earlier in utero.[60] Furthermore, infants who recover quickly from neonatal encephalopathy and in whom a normal neurologic examination is obtained by the end of the first postnatal week have a high likelihood of normal outcome.[7]

Neonatal Encephalopathy Due to Other Causes

Other encephalopathies in the newborn can be metabolic, toxic, infectious, or bilirubin-induced.[49] All these etiologies must be considered in the assessment of the encephalopathic newborn, as treatment often is etiology-specific and, in some cases, life- or disability-sparing. This is especially true for some of the metabolic encephalopathies.

Metabolic Encephalopathy

A metabolic encephalopathy occurs when there is lack of a vital substrate (such as glucose) or an accumulation of a metabolic product that is toxic when present in above-normal concentrations. A number of metabolic disorders has been identified in which the buildup of toxic products is the key feature of the condition. Well-known disorders are those in which ammonia, branched-chain amino acids, or ketoacids are in excess. Others include disorders of propionate and methylmalonate metabolism; pyruvate and mitochondrial metabolism; defects of medium-chain acyl–coenzyme A dehydrogenase; glutaric acidemia; glutathione synthetase deficiency; molybdenum cofactor deficiency; and problems of carbohydrate metabolism (e.g., galactosemia, glycogen storage disease type 1; fructose-1,6-diphosphatase deficiency, and phosphoenolpyruvate carboxykinase deficiency).[49]

Correction of hypoglycemia is extremely important, as glucose is the primary source of fuel for the brain. Produced primarily in the liver and transported to the brain by the blood, its transport into the brain depends on transporter proteins that carry glucose molecules across the blood-brain barrier.

Glucose transporter protein deficiency disorders have been described and are characterized by seizures, microcephaly, and mental retardation in affected infants.[61] In addition to the clinical status, the laboratory hallmark of glucose transporter deficiency is a low cerebrospinal fluid glucose with normal serum glucose values. Some patients with this disorder respond to a ketogenic diet.

For brain energy, normal newborn infants can metabolize ketones in addition to or other than glucose. Ketones reach the brain easily by carrier-mediated transport. Nevertheless, in hypoglycemic infants, ketones are not available in adequate supply, and ketone levels do not increase (as they would in older infants and children) during hypoglycemia or fasting.[62] This shortage may be attributable to lack of substrate for ketone synthesis by the liver in the newborn period and puts the severely hypoglycemic newborn at risk for hypoglycemic brain injury. Clinically, hypoglycemia is defined as a plasma glucose level of less than 40 mg/dl in an infant of any gestational age.[63] This plasma glucose level is a reasonable level at which to initiate glucose therapy, although it does not necessarily correlate with symptomatology. The mechanisms for hypoglycemic brain injury are not known completely, although some data suggest that hypoglycemia-induced brain injury is not likely a result of depletion of adenosine triphosphate and may be due to release of excitotoxins.[64,65]

Documentation of hyperammonemia early in the course of metabolic encephalopathy is also extremely important. Hyperammonemia and encephalopathy are associated with hepatic dysfunction and with inborn errors of urea cycle metabolism. Infants with these disorders usually become symptomatic when protein enters the diet via milk. Symptoms of irritability, lethargy, poor feeding, seizures, and coma usually become apparent quickly and lead to death if the infant is untreated. The enzyme deficiencies most often encountered include carbamoyl-phosphate synthetase deficiency, ornithine transcarbamylase deficiency, argininosuccinate deficiency, argininosuccinase deficiency, and arginase deficiency.[66] Ammonia affects cellular membrane pumps, other membrane properties, and synaptic mechanisms and has pathologic effects on glial cells.[66]

Drug-Related Encephalopathy
Neurologic depression in the newborn can be secondary to toxic effects of drugs, including general anesthetic in the mother, transferal of local anesthetic to a fetus, or accidental injection of local anesthetic directly into the fetus.[67,68] Neonates can also exhibit withdrawal symptoms when they have been exposed to addictive agents in utero, and infants who are severely affected can demonstrate an encephalopathic picture with seizures. Narcotic addiction causes an abstinence syndrome of persistent wakefulness, irritability, jitteriness, crying, hyperactivity, hyperreflexia, hyperthermia and sweating, excessive but inefficient sucking, diarrhea and vomiting, rhinorrhea, tachypnea, hiccups, poor weight gain, and seizures (infrequently).[69] Cocaine is known to be a nervous system stimulant and a potent vasoconstrictor, and its use during pregnancy has been associated with placental abruption as well as with cerebral infarcts in newborns.[69,70] In addition, cocaine-exposed babies can have a number of symptoms

in the newborn period, including poor feeding, sleeplessness, tremors and irritability, and decreased birth weight, length, and head circumference.[71]

Infection-Induced Encephalopathy

CNS infection should be high on the list of differential diagnoses for any infant with encephalopathy in the newborn period. Encephalopathy is an especially prominent feature of viral infections of the CNS, because viral infections very quickly can cause cell death, impaired synaptic transmission, abnormal metabolism of neurotransmitters, cell membrane fusion, and other neurochemical abnormalities and cellular dysfunctions in the brain.[72] Brain necrosis and hemorrhage occur frequently during viral encephalitides, especially when due to herpesviruses. Intracellular inclusions can also be found in some viral infections of the nervous system (e.g., herpesvirus, cytomegalovirus).[73] Viral infections in newborns usually cause alterations in consciousness, abnormal neurologic signs, hypothermia or hyperthermia, and seizures. Herpesvirus type 2 is often found in such situations.

Bacterial, spirochetal, fungal, and parasitic (*Toxoplasma gondii*) infections of the nervous system also occur in the newborn infant. Suspicion should always be high for these infections, especially in preterm infants and in infants who have had complications during the neonatal period.

Since the late 1970s, we have learned that effects of maternal infections, other than direct infection of the fetus, may cause brain injury in the fetus.[74] Some hypothesize that cytokines produced by a fetus as a response to maternal infection can produce brain lesions.[74] A number of studies in animals support this hypothesis and, in human infants, Perlman and colleagues[75] have shown a relationship between the presence of maternal chorioamnionitis and the presence of cystic PVL in the preterm neonate.

Encephalopathy Related to Bilirubin Toxicity

Another form of metabolic and toxic encephalopathy is bilirubin toxicity in the neonate.[49] For many years, we have known that bilirubin, when dissociated from albumin and present in sufficient quantity in cerebrospinal fluid, can cause staining of brain nuclei.[76,77] It has also been shown that the distance between susceptible neurons and capillary ultrafiltrate is smaller in the neonatal brain and that clearance of bilirubin from cerebrospinal fluid is slower in the neonate than in adults.[78,79] These data, among others, provide some explanations for the enhanced vulnerability of the newborn nervous system to bilirubin toxicity.

Bilirubin has several avenues by which it can induce toxicity. In brain slices, bilirubin is seen to depress oxygen utilization and, at high concentrations, it uncouples oxidative phosphorylation.[80,81] It has been shown to affect water, potassium, and sodium transport across membranes.[82,83] Bilirubin affects neuronal transport and enzyme systems, and neuronal swelling is found in kernicteric brains.[84] Physiologic studies have shown that bilirubin decreases nerve conduction.[84] The electroencephalographic tracing can be abolished in adult brains by unconjugated bilirubin.[85] Other known adverse effects of bilirubin all can contribute to bilirubin encephalopathy.

The clinical condition of bilirubin encephalopathy is called *kernicterus*.[86,87] A neonate with kernicterus shows lethargy in the first 48 postnatal hours, an incomplete Moro response, and opisthotonic posturing after abrupt postural changes.[87] Other abnormal findings include an ineffective suck and a cerebral (high-pitched) cry. Abnormal eye movements frequently consist of persistent downward gaze and rotary nystagmus. Other findings include periods of hypothermia and hyperthermia. Terminally, decerebrate posturing occurs.

The neuropathology of kernicterus includes (in descending order of frequency) involvement of the basal ganglia (caudate nucleus, lentiform nucleus, globus pallidus), cerebellum, hippocampus, medulla, subthalamic nuclei, thalamus, fourth ventricle, dentate nucleus, olivary nuclei, nuclei in the floor of the fourth ventricle, midbrain, spinal cord, ependyma, pons, mamillary bodies, and cerebral cortex.[88] Bilirubin pigment is found in these regions along with swelling and vacuolization of neurons.[89,90]

The American Academy of Pediatrics[91] has published guidelines for the treatment of hyperbilirubinemia in the newborn. When jaundice occurs in an infant before 24 postnatal hours, it is considered pathologic, and the infant requires further workup and possible early therapy. When jaundice occurs after 24 hours in otherwise healthy infants, the infants are treated with phototherapy when the bilirubin is greater than 15 mg/dl (μmol/liter) in the first 25–48 hours and with exchange transfusion if the bilirubin is 20 mg/dl or greater in the first 25–48 hours (though intensive phototherapy may be tried first). The reader should refer to the guidelines from the American Academy of Pediatrics for further details.

BRAIN LESIONS AND CEREBRAL PALSY

Cerebral palsy encompasses an entire spectrum of neurologic deficits. The hallmark of cerebral palsy is a lesion that is basically static, usually having been incurred at one point in the brain's developmental history. Unfortunately, even static lesions can interfere with further developmental processes and, likewise, the effects of static lesions may not be apparent until a number of years after the insult.

The newborn brain is believed to have more equipotentiality than do older brains, to be less susceptible to hypoxia, and to have a greater degree of plasticity. However, each of these concepts is limited. *Equipotentiality* refers to the ability of one part of the developing brain to assume the functions of another part of the brain. For instance, in the case of damage to the speech area of an individual's brain, often the patient can develop speech on the other side of the brain, but this is not without cost. Research in this field has shown that when the function of one area is taken over by another area of the brain, that substitute area then loses at least some ability to perform its primary function.[92] In addition, when areas of the brain die because of hypoxia-ischemia, infection, trauma, hemorrhage, or metabolic disease, they cannot be rebuilt and, thus, become areas of permanent injury.

Nonetheless, some infants with apparently extensive lesions show only minimal deficit.[93] This finding may be attributable to the fact that the infant brain has some capacity to alter ongoing developmental processes to accommodate for injury. For instance, neuronal and synaptic pruning are normal parts of the developmental sequences. After brain injury, pruning in some areas can be curtailed to allow survival of more neurons or synapses. This type of homeostatic adjustment is termed *plasticity* and becomes increasingly limited as the course of normal developmental processes continues.

At any time during development, components of the nervous system appear to be selectively vulnerable to injury. Cellular susceptibilities depend on maturation, metabolic factors, metabolic rate, and presence and density of certain receptor types. Ferriero and colleagues[94] have shown that NADPH (reduced nicotinamide adenine dinucleotide phosphate)-diaphorase–containing neurons are less susceptible to hypoxic-ischemic injury. Oka and associates[95] have shown that oligodendroglia are very susceptible to excitotoxic injury and that, surprisingly, in these cells the mechanism of injury involves depletion of cystine via a transmembrane glutamate-cystine exchange. This depletion leads to decreased levels of glutathione (a product of cystine) and resulting free radical injury (as glutathione provides defense against free radical injury).

In addition, receptor-mediated glutamate injury occurs in neurons. Greenamyre and colleagues[96] have shown that glutamate receptors seem to be highly concentrated in the basal ganglia in the perinatal period, whereas McDonald and associates[97] have shown that the glutamate receptor subtype most clearly related to neuronal death in the striatum is the subtype of greatest density in that region in the perinatal period.

Vascular distributions during development also affect patterns of ischemic injury in preterm and full-term brains and seem to play a role in the vulnerability of certain areas to injury.[49]

Thus, many interacting processes contribute to the pathologic outcome when the fetal or newborn brain has been injured, and a number of potential causes exist for fetal or neonatal brain injury that subsequently will manifest as cerebral palsy.

Sites and Types of Brain Lesions

As mentioned earlier in this chapter, severe hypoxia-ischemia frequently results in brain lesions, and their location and extent differ in full-term and preterm brains. In the full-term newborn, injury is more likely to occur in the cerebral cortex, the CA1 region of the hippocampus, Purkinje cells of the cerebellum, and anterior horn cells in the spinal cord.[98] Full-term and preterm infants seem to have an equal predisposition to injury of the basal ganglia, thalamus, and cranial nerve nuclei of the brain stem, whereas preterm infants are at particular risk for neuronal injury in the subiculum of the hippocampus, the ventral pons, the inferior olivary nuclei, the internal granule cells of the cerebellum, and diffusely in the spinal cord.[98]

The differences in neuronal susceptibilities to injury are believed to depend on variations in neuronal differentiation and in vascular distributions between the full-term and the preterm infant. The preterm infant brain has more cortical vascular anastomoses, whereas the full-term infant brain has more areas in which anastomoses are less prominent, giving rise to so-called watershed or border-zone regions between major arterial territories. Involvement of a watershed region is exemplified by parasagittal injury in the full-term infant, which involves gray and white matter and is greatest in the posterior cerebrum, where the border-zone region for all three major cerebral vessels is present.[99] PVL (white matter injury) occurs in both full-term and preterm infants but is particularly prevalent in the preterm infant.[100,101] Perlman and associates[75] reported an incidence of cystic PVL of 3.2% in infants weighing less than 1,500 g at birth. The most frequent sites of occurrence for this lesion are at the level of the occipital radiation at the trigone of the lateral ventricles and at the level of the cerebral white matter around the foramen of Monro.[102,103] These two regions are particularly prominent border zones between penetrating branches of major arteries in the preterm brain.

The pathologic process involved in PVL includes necrosis of cells and processes, resulting in positive periodic acid–Schiff staining of cells and axonal swellings. Macrophages infiltrate the affected areas, and astrocytes become activated. Oligodendroglial cells are particularly susceptible to injury in these regions. The final outcome commonly is cyst formation or cavitary lesions, and hemorrhage occurs into areas of necrosis approximately 25% of the time.[101] Cystic lesions usually are apparent within 7 days to 3 weeks after acute injury, and sometimes gliosis occurs, causing cysts or cavities to shrink over time. Loss of normal white matter may cause secondary enlargement of the ventricles. Cavitation is a feature of the immature brain and probably is related to the high water content in the immature brain, the low myelin content, and the relatively limited glial response. The association between PVL, especially cystic PVL, and cerebral palsy is high.[104–107] If cystic lesions are apparent on neuroimaging in the first postnatal days, then the injury occurred before labor and birth.

PVL probably is the consequence of more than one type of injury. For some time, PVL has been hypothesized to be due to loss of blood supply when perfusion pressure falls, at the places where the vessels do not fully penetrate (border zones). In these areas, perfusion may fail when systemic blood pressure falls, especially if the range of autoregulation (the range of blood pressures over which cerebral blood flow remains constant) is impaired or extremely narrow. Impaired autoregulation may be common in the preterm infant. Ranges of autoregulation seem to vary between species and with development, can be impaired at all stages by hypoxia, and can be affected by various pharmacologic agents.[108,109]

Early studies in animals suggested that endotoxemia could result in lesions that resembled PVL, and epidemiologic studies have shown that preterm infants born to mothers with premature rupture of membranes or chorioamnionitis are at increased risk for PVL.[75,110] Cytokine production by fetal lymphocytes in response to maternal infection may cause injury to the developing fetal white matter; prenatal infection, too, might cause dissolution of white matter.[74] In addition, myelination glia may have selective susceptibilities to various types of insults, including hypoxia, acidosis, hypoglycemia, and ischemia and reperfusion injury.[49]

Fetal brains can incur ischemic infarctions that may lead to cavitation or loss of brain tissue as a result of focal or multifocal vascular occlusions, hemorrhage, or loss of blood flow that leads to necrosis in vascular territories. In the second trimester, these events usually result in porencephaly or hydranencephaly, whereas in the third trimester, they more often cause cystic encephalomalacia.[111–114]

The pathology of injured neurons includes nuclear abnormalities (pyknosis and chromatolysis) and neuronal loss.[115] Ulegyria are lesions of the cortical sulcus, including loss of neurons and gliosis at the depths of the sulci. Cortical layer III is particularly susceptible to neuronal loss. Abnormal myelinated fibers called *plaques fibromyeliniques* may infiltrate the lesions; these can be seen also after injury to the basal ganglia and thalamus (status marmoratus).[115]

Intraventricular hemorrhage is a lesion found mainly, but not exclusively, in preterm infants, with highest incidences in the lowest-birth-weight infants.[113,116–119] In the past, the highest grades of intraventricular hemorrhage were associated with greater degrees of neurologic sequelae in survivors.[120–124] However, infants with severe neurologic sequelae and intraventricular hemorrhage usually have additional brain lesions, including PVL and pontosubicular necrosis.[125,126]

The worst prognosis appears to be that for the infant with intraventricular hemorrhage and periventricular hemorrhagic infarction. This infarction is usually unilateral and occurs when there is substantial intraventricular hemorrhage on the same side. Current theory holds that the large intraventricular clot impairs venous return in the white matter around the ventricle, causing extensive venous infarction, necrosis, and hemorrhage.[127]

Brain Lesions and Neurologic Outcome

Varying degrees of neuronal loss can occur in the cortex, hippocampus, thalamus, basal ganglia, brain stem, cerebellum, and spinal cord after hypoxic-ischemic, infectious, toxic, traumatic, or metabolic injuries. As mentioned earlier, periventricular white matter injury and combinations of gray and white matter injury (especially parasagittal injury) can occur under various circumstances. Neurologic sequelae can be directly related to the location and extent of injury in the brain, with cognitive defects, vision loss, or seizure disorders associated with cortical neuronal necrosis, as well as to injury in association areas. Thalamic injury can cause intellectual deficit as well as spastic quadriparesis, and injury to the basal ganglia causes movement disorders (dystonia, choreoathetosis).[128] Spastic pareses, the most common of which is spastic diplegia, are associated with PVL, and hypotonia often is a consequence of cerebral injury or spinal cord injury (loss of anterior horn cells). Cerebral parasagittal injury results in proximal limb weakness, usually greater in the upper than in the lower extremities, whereas spastic diplegia secondary to PVL usually results in lower-extremity weakness that is greater than upper-extremity weakness.

Difficulties with sucking, swallowing, and facial movement can be related to brain stem injury or to cerebral injury (pseudobulbar palsy). If damage occurs to brain stem dorsal cochlear nuclei or to the cochlea itself, hearing will be lost. Hypothalamic damage can result in precocious puberty. Hemiparesis usually is present in infants with middle cerebral artery territory unilateral cerebral infarction.

Imaging of Perinatal Brain Injury

Imaging of the brain in the first postnatal days is usually accomplished by ultrasonography. This assessment provides information regarding ventricular size and the presence of periventricular or intraventricular hemorrhage, periventricular echodensities or cystic lesions, hyperechoic lesions of the deep gray nuclei, and gross malformations of the brain.[129] Ultrasound examination usually is followed by computed tomography or magnetic resonance imaging, when possible, to define lesions better and to determine whether more subtle pathologic processes are present.

Several studies of preterm infants have been completed to determine the relationship of ultrasonographically defined lesions and outcome. Pidcock and colleagues[105] studied 288 infants of less than 33 weeks' gestational age. Of the 288 infants, 127 survived, and 26 developed spastic cerebral palsy. All 26 infants had moderate or severe periventricular echodensities on ultrasound examination, and all 26 developed cysts in the periventricular region. Mild or moderate periventricular echodensities were present in the other 101 infants, none of whom developed cerebral palsy. In this study, the presence of moderate or severe periventricular echodensities with large cyst formation was the most predictive finding for cerebral palsy (efficiency of 92%).[105]

A more recent study assessed the relationship of neonatal cranial ultrasound abnormalities to cognitive outcomes at 6 years of age.[130] Parenchymal lesions with ventricular enlargement were associated significantly with mental retardation and with borderline intelligence in this population; approximately one-half of the cases of mental retardation were related to parenchymal lesions and ventricular enlargement in the absence of other lesions. Both parenchymal lesions and ventricular enlargement reflect white matter damage and, thus, the conclusion of this study was that prevention of white matter damage would considerably enhance cognitive outcomes for very low-birth-weight infants.[130]

Fazzi and associates[107] evaluated children at 5–7 years of age who had had PVL from infancy. The 37 children with PVL were divided into three groups based on the ultrasound scans. Group 1 consisted of infants with cystic PVL in whom the cysts were unilateral or bilateral and measured greater than 5 mm in diameter (14 cases). Group 2 consisted of infants with small focal cystic PVL

(<5 mm; 11 cases). Group 3 consisted of infants with periventricular echodensities (prolonged flare) without cysts (12 cases).

All children in group 1 (14 of 14) developed cerebral palsy, whereas only two of 11 in group 2 developed cerebral palsy. In group 3, cerebral palsy was seen in six and mild neurologic signs in four (10 of 12). In this study, the location of the lesions also was important, with small frontal lesions having a more favorable prognosis than parieto-occipital or fronto-parieto-occipital lesions. This study showed that although large cystic lesions clearly are prognostic for cerebral palsy, persisting echodensities without cysts are also associated with cerebral palsy and milder neurologic sequelae in a number of cases.[107]

NEW AVENUES FOR PREVENTION OF INTRAUTERINE AND NEONATAL BRAIN INJURY

Knowledge of some of the underlying mechanisms of neuronal and glial injury has led to studies of pharmacologic agents that might be protective against hypoxia-ischemia. Current problems revolve around the safety of various agents and the consequences of the side effects they engender. Specific interest has been directed toward NMDA receptor antagonists, modulators of nitric oxide, antioxidant compounds, iron chelators, and modest hypothermia, all of which have ameliorated brain injury to varying extents after hypoxia-ischemia in animals or in tissue culture models.[131,132] Some of these agents may hold great promise as prophylactic agents in the future but, at present, the risk-benefit ratios are not clearly defined.

Other agents have been used with varying degrees of success for preventing intraventricular hemorrhage. The best known are phenobarbital and indomethacin, which have been given to preterm neonates postnatally to reduce surges in cerebral blood flow or to extend the range of cerebral autoregulation.[107,108,133–135] These agents are not used in every nursery, and whether the decrease seen nationwide in the incidence of intraventricular hemorrhage is attributable to use of these drugs or to better respiratory therapy and surfactant use, increasing use of prenatal steroids, or minimal stimulation protocols is not yet clear. A review of the evidence suggests that prenatal steroids not only prevent respiratory distress syndrome in small preterm infants but are highly effective for prevention of intraventricular hemorrhage.[135]

Although a majority of individuals with cerebral palsy do not have perinatal etiologies for their brain injury, it is nevertheless important to determine for which infants acquired perinatal or postnatal brain injury can be predicted, and possibly prevented. Ideally, this determination should be possible before delivery but, regardless of when the determination is made, the information would still be beneficial to protect the newborn brain from secondary forms of damage. New methods for assessing brain oxygenation and blood flow, such as near-infrared spectroscopy, nuclear magnetic resonance spectroscopy, and various forms of functional brain imaging, may help us to achieve this goal.

REFERENCES

1. Low JA, Froese AB, Galbraith RS, et al. The association between preterm newborn hypotension and hypoxemia and outcome during the first year. Acta Paediatr 1993;82:433–437.
2. Levene HL, Kornberg J, Williams THC. The incidence and severity of post-asphyxial encephalopathy in full-term infants. Early Hum Dev 1985;11:21–26.
3. Blair E, Stanley FJ. Intrapartum asphyxia: a rare cause of cerebral palsy. J Pediatr 1988;112:515–519.
4. Robertson C, Finer N. Term infants with hypoxic-ischemic encephalopathy: outcome at 3–5 years. Dev Med Child Neurol 1985;27:473–484.
5. Minchom P, Niswander K, Chalmers I, et al. Antecedents and outcome of very early neonatal seizures in infants born at or after term. Br J Obstet Gynaecol 1987; 94:431–439.
6. Holden KR, Mellits ED, Freeman JM. Neonatal seizures: 1. Correlation of prenatal and perinatal events with outcomes. Pediatrics 1982;70:165–176.
7. Finer NN, Robertson CM, Richards RT, et al. Hypoxic ischemic encephalopathy in term neonates: perinatal factors and outcome. J Pediatr 1981;98:112–117.
8. Ellenberg J, Nelson KB. Birthweight and gestational age in children with cerebral palsy or seizure disorders. Am J Dis Child 1979;133:1044–1048.
9. Grether JK, Nelson KB, Cummins SK. Twinning and cerebral palsy: experience in four northern California counties, births 1983 through 1985. Pediatrics 1993; 92:854–858.
10. McCarton CM, Wallace IF, Divon M, Vaughan HG Jr. Cognitive and neurologic development of the premature, small for gestational age infant through age 6: comparison by birth weight and gestational age. Pediatrics 1996;98:1167–1178.
11. Hack M, Friedman H, Fanaroff AA. Outcomes of extremely low birth weight infants. Pediatrics 1996;98:931–937.
12. Sarnat HB, Sarnat MS. Neonatal encephalopathy following fetal distress—a clinical and electroencephalographic study. Arch Neurol 1976;33:696–705.
13. Robertson CMT, Finer NN, Grace MGA. School performance of survivors of neonatal encephalopathy associated with birth asphyxia at term. J Pediatr 1989; 114:753–760.
14. Torfs CP, van den Berg BJ, Oechsli FW, et al. Prenatal and perinatal factors in the etiology of cerebral palsy. J Pediatr 1990;116:615–619.
15. Stanley FJ, Watson L. The cerebral palsies in Western Australia: trends, 1968–1981. Am J Obstet Gynecol 1988;158:89–93.
16. Pharoah POD, Cooke T, Cooke RWI, Rosenbloom I. Birthweight specific trends in cerebral palsy. Arch Dis Child 1990;65:602–606.
17. Bhushan V, Paneth N, Kiely JL. Impact of improved survival of very low birth weight infants on recent secular trends in the prevalence of cerebral palsy. Pediatrics 1993;91:1094–1100.
18. Volpe JJ. Neurology of the Newborn (3rd ed). Philadelphia: Saunders, 1995;314–372.
19. Holm VA. The causes of cerebral palsy: a contemporary perspective. JAMA 1982; 247:1473–1477.
20. O'Reilly DE, Walentynowicz JE. Etiological factors in cerebral palsy: an historical review. Dev Med Child Neurol 1981;23:633–642.
21. Hagberg B, Hagberg G, Olow I, et al. The changing panorama of cerebral palsy in Sweden: V. The birth year period 1979–1982. Acta Paediatr Scand 1989;78:283–290.
22. Ellis WG, Goetzmann BW, Lindenberg JA. Neuropathologic documentation of prenatal brain damage. Am J Dis Child 1988;142:858–866.
23. Sinha SK, D'Souza SW, Rivlin E, Chiswick ML. Ischemic brain lesions diagnosed at birth in preterm infants: clinical events and developmental outcome. Arch Dis Child 1990;65:1017–1020.

24. Skolnick A. New ultrasound evidence appears to link prenatal brain damage, cerebral palsy. JAMA 1991;265:948–949.
25. Bejar R, Wozniak P, Allard M, et al. Antenatal origin of neurologic damage in newborn infants: I. Preterm infants. Am J Obstet Gynecol 1988;159:357–363.
26. Grafe MR. The correlation of prenatal brain damage with placental pathology. J Neuropathol Exp Neurol 1994;53:407–415.
27. Garcia JH, Mitchem HC, Briggs L, et al. Transient focal ischemia in subhuman primates. J Neuropathol Exp Neurol 1983;42:44–60.
28. Morawetz RB, Crowell RH, DeGirolami U, et al. Regional cerebral blood flow thresholds during cerebral ischemia. Fed Proc 1979;48:2493–2494.
29. Morawetz RB, DeGirolami U, Ojemann RG, et al. Cerebral blood flow determined by hydrogen clearance during middle cerebral artery occlusion in unanesthetized monkeys. Stroke 1978;9:143–149.
30. Edwards AD, McCormick DC, Roth SC, et al. Cerebral hemodynamic effects of treatment with modified natural surfactant investigated by near infrared spectroscopy. Pediatr Res 1992;32:532–536.
31. Altman DI, Powers WJ, Perlman JM, et al. Cerebral blood flow requirement for brain viability in newborn infants is lower than in adults. Ann Neurol 1988;24:218–226.
32. Vannucci RC. Heterogeneity of Hypoxic-Ischemic Thresholds in Experimental Animals. In HC Lou, JF Larsen, JH Thaysen (eds), Brain Lesions in the Newborn: Hypoxic and Haemodynamic Pathogenesis. Copenhagen: Munksgaard, 1994; 192–208.
33. Sloper JJ, Johnson P, Powell TPS. Selective degeneration of interneurons in the motor cortex of infant monkeys following controlled hypoxia: a possible cause of epilepsy. Brain Res 1980;198:204–209.
34. Chan PH. Role of oxidants in ischemic brain damage. Stroke 1996;27:1124–1129.
35. Rothman SM. Biochemistry of Hypoxic-Ischemic Brain Injury. In RA Polin, WW Fox (eds), Fetal and Neonatal Physiology. Philadelphia: Saunders, 1992;1608–1613.
36. Gray SM, Adams V, Yamashita Y, et al. Hexokinase binding in ischemic and reperfused piglet brain. Biochem Med Metabol Biol 1994;53:145–148.
37. Faraci FM, Brian JE. Nitric oxide and the cerebral circulation. Stroke 1994; 25:692–703.
38. Vannucci RC. Perinatal hypoxic-ischemic encephalopathy. Neurologist 1995;1: 35–52.
39. Monaghan DT, Holets VR, Toy DW, et al. Anatomical distribution of four pharmacologically distinct 3H-L glutamate binding sites. Nature 1983;306:176–179.
40. Mayer ML, Westbrook GL, Guthrie PB. Voltage-dependent block by Mg^{2+} of NMDA responses in spinal cord neurons. Nature 1984;309:261–263.
41. Mayer ML, MacDermott AB, Westbrook GL, et al. Agonist- and voltage-gated calcium entry in cultured mouse spinal cord neurons under voltage clamp measured using arsenazo III. J Neurosci 1987;7:3230–3244.
42. McDonald JW, Johnston MV. Non-ketotic hyperglycinemia: pathophysiological role of the N-methyl-D-aspartate type amino acid receptors [letter]. Ann Neurol 1990; 27:449.
43. Goddard-Finegold J. The Intrauterine Nervous System. In HW Taeusch, RA Ballard (eds), Diseases of the Newborn (7th ed). Philadelphia: Saunders (in press).
44. Goldberg MP, Monyer H, Weiss JH, et al. Adenosine reduces cortical neuronal injury induced by oxygen or glucose deprivation in vitro. Neurosci Lett 1988; 89:323–327.
45. Swan JH, Evans MC, Meldrum BS. Ischaemic brain damage: protection by 2-chloroadenosine, a modulator of excitatory neurotransmission. J Cereb Blood Flow Metab 1987;7:S145.
46. Pou S, Pou WS, Bredt DS, et al. Generation of superoxide by purified brain nitric oxide synthase. J Biol Chem 1992;267:24173–24176.

47. Manzoni O, Prezeau L, Marin P, et al. Nitric oxide–induced blockade of NMDA receptors. Neuron 1992;8:653–662.
48. Iadecola C. Bright and dark sides of nitric oxide in ischemic brain injury. Trends Neurosci 1997;20:132–139.
49. Goddard-Finegold J, Mizrahi EM, Lee RT. The Postnatal Nervous System. In HW Taeusch, RA Ballard (eds), Diseases of the Newborn (7th ed). Philadelphia: Saunders (in press).
50. Halliwell B, Gutteridge JMC. Oxygen toxicity, oxygen radicals, transition metals, and disease. J Biochem 1984;219:1–14.
51. Sunshine P. Epidemiology of Perinatal Asphyxia. In DK Stevenson, P Sunshine (eds), Fetal and Neonatal Brain Injury: Mechanisms, Management, and the Risks of Practice. Philadelphia: BC Decker, 1989;2–11.
52. Carmichael L, Campbell K, Patrick J. Fetal breathing, gross fetal body movements, and maternal and fetal heart rates before spontaneous labor at term. Am J Obstet Gynecol 1984;148:675–679.
53. Sykes GS, Molloy PM, Johnson P, et al. Do Apgar scores indicate asphyxia? Lancet 1982;1:494–496.
54. Silverman F, Surdan J, Wasserman J, et al. The Apgar score: is it enough? Obstet Gynecol 1985;66:331–336.
55. O'Brien WF, Davis SE, Grissom MP, et al. Effect of cephalic pressure on fetal cerebral blood flow. Am J Perinatol 1984;1:223–226.
56. Badawi N, Kurinszuk J, Blair E, et al. Early prediction of the development of microcephaly after hypoxic-ischemic encephalopathy in the newborn [letter to the editor]. Pediatrics 1996;97:151–152.
57. American College of Obstetricians and Gynecologists. Fetal and neonatal neurologic injury [ACOG Tech Bull No. 163]. Int J Gynecol Obstet 1993;41:97–101.
58. Volpe JJ. Hypoxic-Ischemic Encephalopathy: Clinical Aspects. In Neurology of the Newborn (3rd ed). Philadelphia: Saunders, 1995;314–372.
59. Novotny EJ. Hypoxic-Ischemic Encephalopathy. In DK Stevenson, P Sunshine (eds), Fetal and Neonatal Brain Injury: Mechanisms, Management, and the Risks of Practice. Philadelphia: BC Decker, 1989;113–122.
60. Nelson KB, Ellenberg JH. The asymptomatic newborn and risk of cerebral palsy. Am J Dis Child 1987;141:1333–1335.
61. DeVivo D, Trifiletti RR, Jacobson RI, et al. Defective glucose transport across the blood-brain barrier as a cause of persistent hypoglycorrhachia, seizures, and developmental delay. N Engl J Med 1991;325:703–709.
62. Stanley CA, Anday EK, Baker L, et al. Metabolic fuel and hormone responses to fasting in newborn infants. Pediatrics 1979;64:613–619.
63. Ogata ES. Carbohydrate Homeostasis. In GB Avery, MA Fletcher, MG MacDonald (eds), Neonatology: Pathophysiology and Management of the Newborn (4th ed). Philadelphia: Lippincott, 1994;568–584.
64. Auer RN. Progress review: hypoglycemic brain damage. Stroke 1986;17:699–708.
65. Wieloch T. Hypoglycemia-induced neuronal damage prevented by an N-methyl-D-aspartate antagonist. Science 1985;230:681–683.
66. Lockwood AH. Ammonia-Induced Encephalopathy. In DW McCandless (ed), Cerebral Energy Metabolism and Metabolic Encephalopathy. New York: Plenum, 1985;203–222.
67. Morishima HO, Heymann MA, Rudolph AM, et al. Toxicity of lidocaine in the fetal and newborn lamb and its relationship to asphyxia. Am J Obstet Gynecol 1972;112:72–79.
68. Sinclair JC, Fox HJ, Lentz JF. Intoxication of the fetus by a local anesthetic: a newly recognized complication of maternal and caudal anesthesia. N Engl J Med 1965;273:1173–1177.

69. Cohen RS, Benitz WE, Stevenson DK. Fetal Injury from Drug Abuse in Pregnancy: Alcohol, Narcotic, Cocaine, and Phencyclidine. In DK Stevenson, P Sunshine (eds), Fetal and Neonatal Brain Injury: Mechanisms, Management, and the Risks of Practice. Philadelphia: BC Decker, 1989;57–64.

70. Chasnoff IF, Bussey ME, Savich R, et al. Perinatal cerebral infarction and maternal cocaine use. J Pediatr 1986;108:456–459.

71. Oro AS, Dixon SD. Perinatal cocaine and methamphetamine exposure: maternal and neonatal correlates. J Pediatr 1987;111:571–578.

72. Rammohan KW, Farooqui AA, Horrocks LA. Neurochemical Effects of Viral Infections in the Central Nervous System. In DW McCandless (ed), Cerebral Energy Metabolism and Metabolic Encephalopathy. New York: Plenum, 1985;433–445.

73. Fishman MA. Infectious Diseases. In RB David (ed), Pediatric Neurology for the Clinician. Norwalk, CT: Appleton & Lange, 1992;249–268.

74. Adinolfi M. Infectious diseases in pregnancy, cytokines, and neurological impairment; an hypothesis. Dev Med Child Neurol 1993;35:549–553.

75. Perlman JM, Risser R, Broyles RS. Bilateral cystic periventricular leukomalacia in the premature infant: associated risk factors. Pediatrics 1996;97:822–827.

76. Diamond I, Schmid R. Experimental bilirubin encephalopathy. The mode of entry of bilirubin ^{14}C into the central nervous system. J Clin Invest 1966;45:678–689.

77. Ernster L, Herlin L, Zetterstrom R. Experimental studies on the pathogenesis of kernicterus. Pediatrics 1957;20:647–652.

78. Bass NH, Lundborg P. Postnatal development of bulk flow in the cerebrospinal fluid system of the albino rat: clearance of carboxyl (^{14}C) insulin after intrathecal infusion. Brain Res 1973;52:323–332.

79. Davson H, Kleeman CR, Levin E. Quantitative studies of the passage of different substances out of the cerebrospinal fluid. J Physiol 1962;161:126–142.

80. Day R. Inhibition of brain respiration in vitro by bilirubin. Reversal of inhibition by various means. Proc Soc Exp Biol 1954;85:261–264.

81. Mustafa MG, Cowger ML, King TE. Effects of bilirubin on mitochondrial reactions. J Biol Chem 1969;244:6403–6414.

82. Corchs JL, Serrani RE, Palchick M. Effects of bilirubin on potassium (86Rb+) influx and ionic content in Ehrlich ascites cells. Biochim Biophys Acta 1979;555:512–518.

83. Brem AS, Cashore WJ, Pacholski M. Effects of bilirubin on transepithelial transport of sodium, water, and urea. Kidney Int 1985;27:51–57.

84. Hansen TWR, Paulsen O, Gjerstad L, et al. Short-term exposure to bilirubin reduces synaptic activation in rat transverse hippocampal slices. Pediatr Res 1988;23:453–456.

85. Wennberg RP, Hance AJ. Experimental bilirubin encephalopathy: importance of total protein, protein binding, and blood brain barrier. Pediatr Res 1986;20:789–792.

86. Schmorl G. Zur Kenntnis des Ikterus neonatorum, insbesondere der dabei auf tretenden Gehirnveraenderungen. Verh Dtsch Pathol Ges 1903;6:109–115.

87. Odell GB, Schutta HS. Bilirubin Encephalopathy. In DW McCandless (ed), Cerebral Energy Metabolism and Metabolic Encephalopathy. New York: Plenum, 1985;229–261.

88. Claireaux AE, Cole PG, Lathe GH. Icterus of the brain in the newborn. Lancet 1953;2:1226–1230.

89. Vaughn VC III, Allen FH Jr, Diamond LK. Erythroblastosis fetalis: IV. Further observations on kernicterus. Pediatrics 1950;6:706–716.

90. Schutta HS, Johnson L, Neville HE. Mitochondrial abnormalities in bilirubin encephalopathy. J Neuropathol Neurol 1970;29:296–305.

91. American Academy of Pediatrics, Provisional Committee for Quality Improvement and Subcommittee on Hyperbilirubinemia. Practice parameter: management of hyperbilirubinemia in the healthy term newborn. Pediatrics 1994;94:558–565.

92. Vargha-Khadem F, Isaacs E, Muter V. A review of cognitive outcome after unilateral lesions sustained during childhood. J Child Neurol 1994;9(suppl 2):67–73.

93. Fawer CL, Levene MI, Dubowitz LMS. Intraventricular hemorrhage in a preterm neonate: discordance between clinical course and ultrasound scan. Neuropediatrics 1983;14:242–244.

94. Ferriero DM, Arcavi LJ, Sagar SM, et al. Selective sparing of NADPH-diaphorase neurons in neonatal hypoxia-ischemia. Ann Neurol 1988;24:670–676.

95. Oka A, Belliveau MJ, Rosenberg PA, et al. Vulnerability of oligodendroglia to glutamate: pharmacology, mechanisms, and prevention. J Neurosci 1993;13:1441–1453.

96. Greenamyre T, Penney JB, Young AB, et al. Evidence for transient perinatal glutamatergic innervation of globus pallidus. J Neurosci 1987;7:1022–1030.

97. McDonald JW, Johnston MV, Young AB. Differential ontogenic development of three receptors comprising the NMDA receptor/channel complex in the rat hippocampus. Exp Neurol 1990;110:237–247.

98. Armstrong DD. Neonatal Encephalopathies. In S Duckett (ed), Pediatric Neuropathology. Baltimore: Williams & Wilkins, 1995;334–352.

99. Brierley JB, Excell BJ. The effects of profound systemic hypotension upon the brain of M. rhesus: physiological and pathological observations. Brain 1966;89:269–298.

100. Banker BQ, Larroche JC. Periventricular leukomalacia of infancy. A form of neonatal anoxic encephalopathy. Arch Neurol 1962;7:386–410.

101. Armstrong D, Norman MG. Periventricular leucomalacia in neonates. Complications and sequelae. Arch Dis Child 1974;49:367–375.

102. Volpe JJ. Hypoxic-Ischemic Encephalopathy: Neuropathology and Pathogenesis. In Neurology of the Newborn (3rd ed). Philadelphia: Saunders, 1995;279–313.

103. Shuman RM, Selednik LJ. Periventricular leukomalacia: a one-year autopsy study. Arch Neurol 1980;37:231–235.

104. Jongmans M, Henderson S, deVries L, et al. Duration of periventricular densities in preterm infants and neurological outcome at 6 years of age. Arch Dis Child 1993;69:9–13.

105. Pidcock FS, Graziani LJ, Stanley C, et al. Neurosonographic features of periventricular echodensities associated with cerebral palsy in preterm infants. J Pediatr 1990;116:417–422.

106. Fazzi E, Lanzi G, Gerardo A, et al. Neurodevelopmental outcome in very-low-birth-weight infants with or without periventricular haemorrhage and/or leukomalacia. Acta Paediatr 1992;81:808–811.

107. Fazzi E, Orcesi S, Caffi L, et al. Neurodevelopmental outcome at 5–7 years in preterm infants with periventricular leukomalacia. Neuropediatrics 1994;25:134–139.

108. Yamashita Y, Goddard-Finegold J, Contant CF, et al. Phenobarbital and cerebral blood flow during hypotension in newborn pigs. Pediatr Res 1993;33:598–602.

109. Louis PT, Yamashita Y, Del Toro J, et al. Brain blood flow responses to indomethacin during hemorrhagic hypotension in newborn piglets. Biol Neonate 1994;66:359–366.

110. Gilles FH, Leviton A, Kerr CS. Endotoxin leucoencephalopathy in the telencephalon of the newborn kitten. J Neurol Sci 1976;27:183–191.

111. Larroche JC. Fetal encephalopathies of circulatory origin. Biol Neonate 1986;50:61–74.

112. Scher MS, Belfar H, Martin J, et al. Destructive brain lesions of presumed fetal onset: antepartum causes of cerebral palsy. Pediatrics 1991;88:898–906.

113. Amato M, Huppi P, Herschkowitz N, et al. Prenatal stroke suggested by intrauterine ultrasound and confirmed by magnetic resonance imaging. Neuropediatrics 1991;22:100–102.

114. Fernandez F, Perez-Higueras A, Hernandez R, et al. Hydranencephaly after maternal butane gas intoxication during pregnancy. Dev Med Child Neurol 1986;28:361–363.

115. Friede RL. Developmental Neuropathology (2nd ed). New York: Springer-Verlag, 1989;82–98.
116. Goddard-Finegold J, Mizrahi EM. Understanding and preventing perinatal, intracerebral, peri- and intraventricular hemorrhage. J Child Neurol 1987;2:170–185.
117. Papile LA, Burstein J, Burstein R, et al. Incidence and evolution of subependymal and intraventricular hemorrhage: a study of infants with birth weights less than 1,500 gm. J Pediatr 1978;92:529–534.
118. Ahmann PA, Lazzara A, Dykes FD, et al. Intraventricular hemorrhage in the high-risk preterm infant: incidence and outcome. Ann Neurol 1980;7:118–124.
119. Shinnar S, Molteni RA, Gammon K, et al. Intraventricular hemorrhage in the preterm infant: a changing outlook. N Engl J Med 1982;306:1464–1468.
120. Williamson WD, Desmond MM, Wilson GW, et al. Early neurodevelopmental outcome of low birth weight infants surviving neonatal intraventricular hemorrhage. J Perinat Med 1982;10:34–41.
121. Papile LA, Munsick-Bruno G, Schaefer A. The relationship of cerebral intraventricular hemorrhage and early childhood neurologic handicaps. J Pediatr 1983; 103:273–277.
122. Kitchen WH, Rickards AL, Ryan MM, et al. Improved outcome to two years of very low-birthweight infants: fact or artifact? Dev Med Child Neurol 1986;28: 579–588.
123. Yu VYH, Downe L, Astbury J, et al. Perinatal factors and adverse outcome in extremely low birthweight infants. Arch Dis Child 1986;61:554–558.
124. Skouteli HN, Dubowitz LMS, Levene MI, et al. Predictors for survival and normal neurodevelopmental outcome of infants weighing less than 1,001 grams at birth. Dev Med Child Neurol 1985;27:588–595.
125. Armstrong DL, Sauls CD, Goddard-Finegold J. Neuropathologic findings in short-term survivors of intraventricular hemorrhage. Am J Dis Child 1987;141: 617–621.
126. Skullerud K, Westre B. Frequency and prognostic significance of germinal matrix hemorrhage, periventricular leukomalacia, and pontosubicular necrosis in preterm infants. Acta Neuropathol 1986;70:257–261.
127. Volpe JJ. Intracranial Hemorrhage: Germinal Matrix–Intraventricular Hemorrhage of the Premature Infant. In Neurology of the Newborn (3rd ed). Philadelphia: Saunders, 1995;373–402.
128. Malamud N. Status marmoratus: a form of cerebral palsy following either birth injury or inflammation of the central nervous system. J Pediatr 1950;37:610–619.
129. Latchaw RE, Truwit CE. Imaging of perinatal hypoxic-ischemic brain injury. Semin Pediatr Neurol 1995;2:72–89.
130. Whitaker AH, Feldman JF, Van Rossem R, et al. Neonatal cranial ultrasound abnormalities in low birth weight infants: relation to cognitive outcomes at six years of age. Pediatrics 1996;98:719–729.
131. Miller VS. Pharmacologic management of neonatal cerebral ischemia and hemorrhage: old and new directions. J Child Neurol 1993;8:7–18.
132. Vannucci RC. Current and potentially new management strategies for perinatal hypoxic-ischemic encephalopathy. Pediatrics 1990;85:961–968.
133. Donn SM, Roloff DW, Goldstein GW. Prevention of intraventricular haemorrhage in preterm infants by phenobarbitone—a controlled trial. Lancet 1981;2: 215–217.
134. Goddard-Finegold J. Pharmacologic Prevention of IVH. In TN Hansen, N McIntosh (eds), Current Topics in Neonatology. London: Saunders (in press).
135. National Institutes of Health. Consensus Statement: Effect of Corticosteroids for Fetal Maturation on Perinatal Outcomes. Bethesda, MD: National Institutes of Health, 1994;12.

6

Genetic Evaluation of Cerebral Palsy

Stuart K. Shapira

The genetic approach to a child or adult with cerebral palsy relies on the fact that the cerebral palsy phenotype is not attributable to a single entity. Typical cerebral palsy generally is attributable to prenatal or birth-related events. When patients with cerebral palsy are evaluated for risk factors, only 6–14% of patients can be identified as having had intrapartum asphyxia.[1–5] In most cases, evidence for asphyxial damage is not present. Central nervous system damage due to infections in the first year of life account for another 6% of affected patients.[5] In addition, prenatal risk factors, such as viral infections, some toxin or drug exposures, and maternal iodine deficiency, account for an even smaller percentage of cerebral palsy patients.[6,7] Therefore, in most cerebral palsy patients, other causes explain the phenotype. Identifying those patients in whom there is an underlying genetic condition as the basis for their phenotype often is diagnostically challenging but must be undertaken to provide optimal medical management for the patient and appropriate future reproductive counseling for the family.

FEATURES OF CEREBRAL PALSY

Cerebral palsy connotes motor impairment resulting from a significant disorder in the pyramidal or extrapyramidal system or both; however, when the brain injury is more severe, visual, auditory, and cognitive impairment and epilepsy may accompany the motor impairment. Cerebral palsy is a chronic, nonprogressive encephalopathy, although the neurologic manifestations might evolve over time. In addition, the features of cerebral palsy can be highly variable and have been subdivided into the following types: spastic diplegic, quadriplegic (tetraplegic and double hemiplegic), and hemiplegic; dyskinetic (athetoid and dystonic); ataxic and atonic. Thus, the variable nature of cerebral palsy must be considered in the context of evaluating for a genetic etiology of the phenotype.

The diagnosis of cerebral palsy generally presumes that genetic disorders have been considered, as genetic and neurodevelopmental conditions can cause the features of cerebral palsy. Various static pathologic conditions that result in motor dysfunction may result from genetic factors, and differentiating between these and nongenetic causes is essential because each might carry different

173

implications for prognosis, treatment, and recurrence risk of cerebral palsy in future pregnancies. Genetic and neurodevelopmental conditions are best considered according to the types of cerebral palsy that can result.

Spastic Diplegic Cerebral Palsy

Spastic diplegia may be associated with periventricular leukomalacia, which has been shown in some circumstances to be caused by hypoperfusion of periventricular structures at a vulnerable time during brain development.[8,9] Therefore, diplegia may result from vascular anomalies of the central nervous system, structural brain anomalies that affect vascular flow, and ischemic events from congenital infection, toxins and drugs (such as cocaine), hemorrhage, and factors affecting cardiac output (e.g., arrhythmias, cardiomyopathy).

Spastic diplegia primarily involves the lower extremities, resulting in gait disturbances, with scissoring and tightness of the adductors of the thighs and, often, ankle clonus. Genetic syndromes that manifest primarily with lower-extremity motor dysfunction in infancy and childhood should be considered in the evaluation of spastic diplegia (Table 6.1). A typical example is argininemia, a metabolic disorder of ureagenesis in which spasticity affects the lower extremities more than the upper extremities and seizures, growth failure, and progressive psychomotor retardation are seen.[10] This condition has been mistaken for diplegic cerebral palsy in several patients.[11]

Thorough evaluation of the brain and the spinal cord, comprehensive neurologic assessment for a neuropathy, chromosome analysis, and metabolic testing are indicated in the workup of diplegia (Table 6.2).

Spastic Quadriplegic Cerebral Palsy

Spastic quadriplegia results from cortical and subcortical insults that manifest as severe dysfunction, usually with bulbar palsies, visual disturbances, epilepsy, severe cognitive impairment, microcephaly, and growth failure. Often, cerebral atrophy and gliosis are seen also. The causes vary but include congenital infections, fetal toxin or drug exposure (such as methylmercury or alcohol), neonatal and infantile infectious encephalitides, structural brain anomalies, intraventricular hemorrhage, perinatal hypoxic-ischemic encephalopathy, chromosomal abnormalities, various genetic syndromes, infantile lysosomal storage disorders and leukodystrophies, and several disorders of amino acid metabolism.

Genetic conditions with global neurodevelopmental features resulting from severe cortical dysfunction require consideration in the workup of spastic quadriplegia (see Table 6.1). The distinguishing feature of many genetic causes of the quadriplegia phenotype, particularly the neurometabolic disorders, is the progressive nature of the encephalopathy. An example is Tay-Sachs syndrome, a lysosomal storage disorder manifesting as progressive motor weakness, spasticity, loss of developmental milestones, seizures, and blindness.[12] Progressive deterioration and encephalopathy would necessitate the search for a neurode-

Table 6.1   Genetic and Neurodevelopmental Conditions with Features of Cerebral Palsy

Diplegia
   Brain dysgenesis
   Chromosomal anomalies
   Argininemia
   Hereditary sensory and motor neuropathies
   Club feet
   Spina bifida
   Tethered cord
   Familial spastic diplegia

Quadriplegia
   Brain dysgenesis
   Chromosomal anomalies
   Leukodystrophies
   Lysosomal storage disorders
   Organic acidopathies
   Nonketotic hyperglycemia
   Urea cycle disorders
   Phenylketonuria (untreated)
   MCAD deficiency
   Peroxisomal disorders
   Walker-Warburg syndrome
   Menke's syndrome
   Cockayne's syndrome
   Rett syndrome
   Hyperexplexia
   Thanatophoric congenital stiffness

Hemiplegia
   Brain dysgenesis
   Neurocutaneous syndromes
   Mitochondrial disorders (MELAS, etc.)
   Tourette's syndrome

Dyskinesia
   Mitochondrial disorders
   Glutaric acidemia type 1
   Juvenile Huntington's disease
   Lesch-Nyhan syndrome
   Wilson's disease
   Salla disease
   Dystonia musculorum deformans
   Nonketotic hyperglycinemia
   Sarcosinemia
   Hypoparathyroidism, hypocalcemic syndromes
   Ceroid lipofuscinosis
   Neuraxonal dystrophy
   Segawa syndrome
   Rett syndrome
   Tourette's syndrome

Table 6.1 (continued)

Ataxia
Spinocerebellar ataxia
Friedreich ataxia
Ataxia telangiectasia
Carbohydrate-deficient glycoprotein syndrome
Joubert syndrome
Pelizeus-Merzbacher disease
Neuraxonal dystrophy
Hartnup disease
Refsum disease
Behr syndrome
Marinesco-Sjögren's syndrome
Gillespie syndrome
Mitochondrial disorders (NARP, etc.)
Salla disease
Nucleoside phosphorylase deficiency
Rett syndrome
Familial ataxia syndromes

MCAD = medium-chain acyl–coenzyme A dehydrogenase; MELAS = mitochrondrial encephalopathy, lactic acidosis, and strokelike episodes; NARP = neuropathy, ataxia, retinitis pigmentosa.

generative cause of such a child's problems, even though some features akin to cerebral palsy might be present.

Thorough evaluation of the brain, comprehensive neurologic assessment for a neuropathy, chromosome analysis, and metabolic testing should be considered in the workup of quadriplegia (see Table 6.2).

Hemiplegic Cerebral Palsy

The most common cerebral palsy phenotype among full-term infants and the second most common among premature infants is hemiplegia.[13] Hemiplegia among full-term infants generally occurs from events in the third trimester that result in hypoperfusion, though congenital brain malformations and infarction events within the distribution of the middle cerebral artery also can be the cause.[14,15] The condition may be difficult to diagnose in the first 3 months of life; asymmetry of deep tendon reflexes and fisting may be the earliest signs. In some cases, hemiplegia may be so mild as to remain undetected until walking is achieved; there may be toe walking, and the affected leg often is dragged. Other accompanying features can include learning disabilities, focal seizures, visual field defects, and scoliosis. In particular, hemiplegia due to an insult in the postnatal period (e.g., tumor, meningitis, trauma) will more likely be accompanied by epilepsy. Other nongenetic causes of hemiplegia include fetal exposure to alcohol and postnatal lead intoxication.[16]

Table 6.2 Testing for Genetic and Neurodevelopmental Conditions with Features of Cerebral Palsy

---

Brain MRI scan
    Cerebral malformation
    Cerebellar anomaly
    Porencephalic cyst
    Hydrocephalus
    Arnold-Chiari malformation
    Basal ganglia anomaly
    Leukodystrophy
    Walker-Warburg syndrome
    Sturge-Weber syndrome
    Joubert syndrome
    Ataxia telangiectasia

Spinal MRI scan
    Spina bifida
    Tethered cord

Chromosome analysis
    Chromosomal abnormality

Plasma amino acid analysis
    Argininemia
    Urea cycle disorders
    Phenylketonuria
    Nonketotic hyperglycinemia
    Sarcosinemia

Cerebrospinal fluid amino acid analysis
    Nonketotic hyperglycinemia

Urine amino acid analysis
    Hartnup disease

Urine organic acid analysis
    Organic acidopathies
    Glutaric acidemia type 1
    MCAD deficiency

Very-long-chain fatty acids
    Peroxisomal disorders

Phytanic acid
    Refsum disease

White blood cell enzyme assay
    Leukodystrophy
    Lysosomal storage disorder
    Neuraxonal dystrophy

Red blood cell enzyme assay
    Lesch-Nyhan syndrome
    Argininemia
    Nucleoside phosphorylase deficiency

Table 6.2 (continued)

Serum copper, urine copper
Serum ceruloplasmin
  Menke's syndrome
  Wilson's disease

Transferrin isoelectric focusing
  Carbohydrate-deficient glycoprotein syndrome

Ophthalmologic evaluation
  Lysosomal storage disorder
  Wilson's disease
  Ceroid lipofuscinosis
  Mitochondrial disorder
  Ataxia telangiectasia
  Refsum disease
  Marinesco-Sjögren's syndrome
  Joubert syndrome
  Behr syndrome
  Gillespie syndrome

Nerve conduction studies
  Hereditary sensory and motor neuropathy

Nerve biopsy
  Neuraxonal dystrophy
  Hereditary sensory and motor neuropathy

Muscle biopsy
  Mitochondrial disorder

Mitochondrial enzyme studies (preferably on muscle)
  Mitochondrial disorder

DNA mutation analysis
  Mitochondrial disorder
  MCAD deficiency
  Spinocerebellar ataxia
  Friedreich's ataxia
  Huntington's disease
  Hereditary sensory and motor neuropathy (Charcot-Marie-Tooth disease)

MRI = magnetic resonance imaging; MCAD = medium-chain acyl–coenzyme A dehydrogenase.

Very few genetic or neurodevelopmental anomalies present with features of spastic hemiplegia. Rare familial cases of hemiparesis with schizencephaly have been reported, suggesting the possible involvement of genetic factors in this phenotype.[17]

Several neurocutaneous syndromes (e.g., incontinentia pigmenti, Sturge-Weber syndrome, phacomatosis pigmentovascularis, hypomelanosis of Ito) should not be mistaken for hemiplegic cerebral palsy because of their classic cutaneous manifestations. Mitochondrial disorders that predispose to strokelike episodes (e.g., mitochondrial encephalomyopathy, lactic acidosis, and strokelike episodes [MELAS]) may mimic spastic hemiplegia, though clinically they are different, being progressive neurodegenerative disorders, often accompanied by other motor and cognitive abnormalities.[18]

Thorough brain imaging for central nervous system abnormalities and a skin examination should be part of the evaluation of hemiplegia. Additional metabolic and DNA mutation studies for a mitochondrial disorder should be considered if the clinical course is progressive (see Table 6.2).

Dyskinetic Cerebral Palsy

Full-term infants who suffer an insult to the basal ganglia, most often due to obvious perinatal insults, will manifest features of dyskinetic cerebral palsy. Signs generally include dystonia with severe motor disability and preservation of primitive neonatal reflexes, though more severe ischemic damage to cortical and subcortical regions can result in other cerebral palsy phenotypes, particularly quadriplegia.[15,19] Choreoathetoid cerebral palsy is much less common today as a result of treatment to avoid kernicterus, although hypoxic-ischemic insults to the basal ganglia can result in choreoathetosis and spasticity. In severe cases, opisthotonos occurs, in addition to dyskinetic movements of the tongue, palate, and facial muscles.

Genetic conditions in which a movement disorder (dystonia, athetosis) is a component will have to be considered in patients with dyskinetic cerebral palsy (see Table 6.1). In the differential diagnosis, genetic disorders that cause progressive damage to the basal ganglia (e.g., certain mitochondrial conditions, glutaric acidemia type 1, juvenile Huntington's disease, Lesch-Nyhan syndrome, Wilson's disease) should be high on the list of conditions mimicking dyskinetic cerebral palsy.

Brain imaging for basal ganglia anomalies and specialized metabolic and DNA mutation studies ultimately will be necessary to test for these conditions (see Table 6.2).

Ataxic Cerebral Palsy

Ataxic cerebral palsy is relatively rare and frequently progresses from initial hypotonia. The earliest signs are truncal ataxia and head titubation; subsequently, intention tremor may become prominent. Congenital ataxic cerebral palsy generally results from prenatal dysgenetic supratentorial or infratentorial abnormalities in brain development, although it can occur from cerebellar lesions (vascular malformations, tumors, Arnold-Chiari malformation, colloid cysts) and with hydrocephalus. Other nongenetic causes of cerebellar dysfunction include fetal exposure to alcohol.

Most childhood ataxias have a genetic basis and will follow a progressive, degenerative course, in contrast to the static course of ataxic cerebral palsy (see Table 6.1). The well-described ataxic syndromes (e.g., juvenile spinocerebellar ataxia, ataxia-telangiectasia) generally present in older children, although the age at which ataxia develops varies significantly. In addition, numerous rare familial ataxic syndromes have been described.[20–26]

Brain imaging for cerebellar abnormalities and metabolic and DNA mutation studies for inherited ataxic syndromes should be part of the workup of ataxic cerebral palsy (see Table 6.2).

GENETIC AND METABOLIC WORKUP OF CEREBRAL PALSY

The diagnostic testing for genetic or neurodevelopmental etiologies of a cerebral palsy phenotype will depend on the presenting symptoms and signs and the results of a good clinical and neurologic evaluation. Various tests to assist in the diagnostic evaluation of cerebral palsy for specific conditions are listed in Table 6.2. A brain magnetic resonance imaging (MRI) scan may prove useful in detecting cerebral malformations and dysgenesis (atrophy, hydrocephalus, agenesis of the corpus callosum, porencephalic cyst, Walker-Warburg lissencephaly) and cerebellar anomalies, Arnold-Chiari malformation, and hypoplasia (Joubert syndrome, ataxia-telangiectasia, and carbohydrate-deficient glycoprotein syndrome). A diagnosis of ataxia-telangiectasia can be further supported by telangiectasias on ophthalmologic examination, an elevated blood alpha-fetoprotein level, low IgA level, and abnormal chromosomal breakage and translocations. Carbohydrate-deficient glycoprotein syndrome is diagnosed by an abnormal transferrin isoelectric focusing. White matter abnormalities may suggest a leukodystrophy, which often is accompanied by an elevated cerebrospinal fluid (CSF) protein level, but should be confirmed by white blood cell enzyme assay in Krabbe's disease and metachromatic leukodystrophy. Adrenoleukodystrophy is diagnosed by very-long-chain fatty acid levels, and Canavan's disease is diagnosed by urine organic acid analysis for N-acetylaspartic acid or by DNA mutation analysis. Basal ganglia anomalies may be suggestive of glutaric acidemia type 1, which is diagnosed by abnormalities on organic acid analysis or by assay for glutaryl–coenzyme A dehydrogenase deficiency in fibroblasts. Basal ganglia infarctions may also occur in methylmalonic acidemia, diagnosed by urine organic acid analysis. Basal ganglia calcifications might suggest a mitochondrial disorder, which will require specific enzymatic and DNA mutation analyses. Finally, a brain MRI scan may detect the leptomeningeal angiomatoses of Sturge-Weber syndrome and the intracranial manifestations of other neurocutaneous syndromes.

Evaluations of the spine by ultrasonography or MRI can prove useful in identifying spina bifida occulta or a tethered spinal cord, which may present with features of spastic diplegia. Peripheral nerve conduction slowing suggests a hereditary sensory and motor neuropathy or certain leukodystrophies. However, confirmatory diagnosis of type Ia Charcot-Marie-Tooth disease is based on testing for a duplication within the p arm of chromosome 17, either by molecular testing for a DNA junction fragment or by fluorescence in situ hybridization analysis using a probe for the PMP22 gene on interphase white blood cells. A nerve biopsy may prove useful in identifying the onion bulb structures of hereditary sensory and motor neuropathies or the axonal spheroids in neuroaxonal dystrophy.

Because various chromosomal abnormalities can present with features of diplegia or quadriplegia, a chromosome analysis would be part of the evaluation for these disorders, particularly if the patient has additional dysmorphic features. Plasma amino acid analysis is crucial for the diagnosis of the various urea cycle disorders, as the amino acid profile has characteristic elevations and depressions, depending on which cycle intermediates are affected by the various enzyme deficiencies; each urea cycle defect can be confirmed by particular enzyme assays (e.g., on red blood cells, white blood cells, fibroblasts, liver tissue). Plasma amino acid analysis also will detect elevations in phenylalanine (phenylketonuria, dihydropteridine reductase deficiency, and biopterin synthesis defects), sarcosine (sarcosinemia), and glycine (nonketotic hyperglycinemia [NKH]). However, the diagnosis of NKH often requires a concurrent CSF glycine level (CSF glycine–plasma glycine level is greater than 0.08 in NKH). Urine amino acid analysis would demonstrate neutral hyperaminoaciduria in Hartnup disease. Urine organic acid analysis would be helpful in the diagnosis of the organic acidurias, which may have features of quadriplegic cerebral palsy, particularly propionic aciduria and methylmalonic aciduria. Untreated medium-chain acyl–coenzyme A dehydrogenase (MCAD) deficiency may be mistaken for cerebral palsy but can be diagnosed by urine organic acid analysis with concurrent evaluation for the glycine conjugates that are typical markers for the condition; in addition, direct DNA mutation analysis for the common missense mutations that cause MCAD deficiency could be obtained.

Specific metabolic testing should be considered for evaluation of peroxisomal or mitochondrial disorders. Zellweger syndrome and X-linked adrenoleukodystrophy show a characteristic pattern on analysis of very-long-chain fatty acids, with elevations in 26-carbon and 24-carbon fatty acids relative to 22-carbon fatty acids. Refsum disease patients will have elevated serum levels of phytanic acid, which are also indicative of peroxisomal dysfunction. A mitochondrial disorder that mimics cerebral palsy might entail lactic acidosis, but confirming a mitochondrial abnormality often requires more extensive testing. A muscle biopsy may demonstrate ragged red fibers or mitochondrial proliferation, and ultrastructural studies on the muscle tissue might demonstrate abnormal mitochondrial configurations and inclusions suggestive of a primary mitochondrial abnormality. Muscle tissue can be analyzed for activities of the respiratory chain enzymes, with low activities suggesting mitochondrial dysfunction. Specific mitochondrial syndromes (e.g., Kearns-Sayre syndrome; MELAS; myoclonic epilepsy with ragged red fibers [MERRF]; neuropathy, ataxia, retinitis pigmentosa [NARP]) have mitochondrial DNA deletions or point mutations that are more often associated with certain phenotypes; direct DNA mutation analysis can be performed on various tissues but preferably is performed on muscle.

Leukodystrophies, lysosomal storage diseases, and neuroaxonal dystrophies should be distinguishable from cerebral palsy because of their progressive deteriorating course. However, late infantile, juvenile, and adult presentations of these disorders have been described that confound the diagnostic evaluation. As mentioned earlier, specific white blood cell enzyme assays are necessary to confirm a diagnosis of certain leukodystrophies (Krabbe's disease, metachromatic leukodystrophy). White blood cell enzyme assays are similarly confirmatory in lysosomal storage diseases that can mimic cerebral palsy (e.g., Tay-Sachs disease, Sandhoff disease, GM_1 gangliosidosis, Salla disease). Though neuroaxonal dystrophies have characteristic histopathologic abnormalities, the diagnosis of alpha-N-acetylgalactosaminidase deficiency can be confirmed by analysis of white blood cells or fibroblasts. The enzyme deficiencies in argininemia (arginase deficiency), Lesch-Nyhan syndrome (hypoxanthine phosphoribosyl transferase deficiency), and nucleoside phosphorylase deficiency generally are diagnosed on assay of red blood cells, contingent on the patient's not having undergone a recent blood transfusion.

An ophthalmologic examination can be a useful screening test for some disorders. Various lysosomal storage diseases may manifest a cherry-red spot. Telangiectasias may be present on the conjunctiva and the ear lobes in ataxia-telangiectasia. Other diagnostic features on ophthalmologic examination include retinitis pigmentosa (Refsum disease, NARP); cataracts (Marinesco-Sjögren's syndrome); abnormal eye movements, chorioretinal colobomas, and retinal dysplasia (Joubert syndrome); optic atrophy (Behr syndrome); aniridia (Gillespie syndrome); and blindness with macular degeneration and retinitis pigmentosa (neuronal ceroid lipofuscinosis [NCL]). Diagnosis of NCL can also be supported by finding "curvilinear bodies" on conjunctival biopsy or in white blood cells. An ophthalmologic examination may demonstrate the Kayser-Fleischer rings in Wilson's disease, although copper studies are indicated to confirm this diagnosis; serum ceruloplasmin is greatly reduced, and nonceruloplasmin copper is increased, giving a net reduction in serum copper, whereas urinary copper excretion is increased. Copper studies also are abnormal in Menke's syndrome, wherein serum copper and ceruloplasmin levels are very low.

Huntington's disease and several spinocerebellar ataxias (types 1 and 2, Machado-Joseph disease, and dentatorubral and pallidoluysian atrophy) are due to DNA triplet repeat expansions. Therefore, direct DNA mutation analysis is necessary for the confirmation of these diagnoses.

Carbohydrate-deficient glycoprotein syndrome has features of hypotonia, ataxia, peripheral neuropathy, and cerebellar hypoplasia. The biochemical defect is unknown, but carbohydrate or sialic acid content of various glycoproteins is reduced. Transferrin isoelectric focusing demonstrates increased amounts of carbohydrate-deficient transferrin.

FAMILIAL RECURRENCE OF CEREBRAL PALSY

Similarly affected relatives are uncommon in families of patients with cerebral palsy, but parents of a child with cerebral palsy will naturally be concerned about the recurrence in their other children or in a future pregnancy. Twin studies indicate that when a genetic or metabolic condition cannot be identified as the cause of the cerebral palsy phenotype, the genetic basis for the cerebral palsy is negligible and the recurrence risk would be low.[27,28]

In instances in which the cause of cerebral palsy clearly is a complication of pregnancy, the recurrence risk would be considered low unless similar circumstances were to occur. Similarly, if the cause of the cerebral palsy phenotype is determined to be the result of a genetic or metabolic condition, the recurrence risk would depend on the inheritance pattern of the condition.

Special consideration applies to families who have had a child with ataxic cerebral palsy because familial clustering has been reported for congenital ataxia and ataxic diplegia.[29,30] For children with cerebellar ataxia, in the absence of an identifiable condition, application of the empiric recurrence risk of 12.5% has been suggested.[31] Within the nonataxic forms of cerebral palsy, in which no etiologic clue is obtained from the history, physical examination, or investigations as to the cause of the phenotype, the recurrence risk of 10–20% is applied.[31] The lower risk (closer to 10%) may be used when there might have been an environmental influence, such as an influenzalike illness early during the pregnancy, whereas the higher risk (closer to 20%) would be used when the cerebral palsy phenotype is symmetric and minor congenital anomalies unrelated to the nervous system are present.

In general, thorough medical evaluations of children with cerebral palsy, often including the expertise of neurologists, ophthalmologists, and geneticists can help delineate the cause of the condition. A complete genetic evaluation would allow for the provision of appropriate genetic counseling, particularly regarding the recurrence risk in future pregnancies, prenatal diagnostic options, and assessment of other at-risk family members. Furthermore, the genetic evaluation of cerebral palsy often will provide an explanation as to the cause of a child's disabilities, in addition to the information that families require for future reproductive planning.

REFERENCES

1. Nelson KB, Ellenberg JH. Antecedents of cerebral palsy: multivariate analysis of risk. N Engl J Med 1986;315:81–86.
2. Stanley FJ. The changing face of cerebral palsy? Dev Med Child Neurol 1987; 29:263–265.
3. Blair E, Stanley FJ. Intrapartum asphyxia: a rare cause of cerebral palsy. J Pediatr 1988; 112:515–519.
4. Powell TG, Pharoah POD, Cooke RWI, et al. Cerebral palsy in low-birthweight infants: II. Spastic diplegia: associations with fetal immaturity. Dev Med Child Neurol 1988;30:19–25.
5. Naeye RL, Peters EC, Bartholomew M, et al. Origins of cerebral palsy. Am J Dis Child 1989;143:1154–1161.
6. Stanley F. Prenatal risk factors in the study of the cerebral palsies. Clin Dev Med 1984;87:87–97.
7. Blair E, Stanley F. Intrauterine growth and spastic cerebral palsy: I. Association with birth weight for gestational age. Am J Obstet Gynecol 1990;162:229–237.
8. Volpe JJ. Brain injury in the premature infant: is it preventable? Pediatr Res 1990; 27:528–533.

9. Koedea T, Suganuma I, Kohno Y. MR imaging of spastic diplegia. Comparative study between pre-term and term infants. Neuroradiology 1990;32:187–190.

10. Brusilow SW, Horwich AL. Urea Cycle Enzymes. In CR Scriver, AL Beaudet, WS Sly, et al. (eds), The Metabolic and Molecular Bases of Inherited Disease. New York: McGraw-Hill, 1995;1187–1232.

11. Scheuerle AE, McVie R, Beaudet AL, et al. Arginase deficiency presenting as cerebral palsy. Pediatrics 1993;91:995–996.

12. Gravel RA, Clarke JTR, Kaback MM, et al. The G_{M2} Gangliosidoses. In CR Scriver, AL Beaudet, WS Sly, et al. (eds), The Metabolic and Molecular Bases of Inherited Disease. New York: McGraw-Hill, 1995;2839–2879.

13. Hagberg B, Hagberg G. The changing panorama of infantile hydrocephalus and cerebral palsy over forty years: a Swedish survey. Brain Dev 1989;11:368–373.

14. Wiklund LM, Flodmark O, Uvebrant P. Periventricular leucomalacia: a common CT finding in fullterm infants with congenital hemiplegia. Neuroradiology 1991; 33:248–250.

15. Rosenbloom L. Diagnosis and management of cerebral palsy. Arch Dis Child 1995; 72:350–354.

16. Perlstein MA, Attola R. Neurologic sequelae of plumbism in children. Clin Pediatr 1966;5:292–297.

17. Hilburger AC, Willis JK, Bouldin E, et al. Familial schizencephaly. Brain Dev 1993; 15:234–236.

18. Shoffner JM, Wallace DC. Oxidative Phosphorylation Diseases. In CR Scriver, AL Beaudet, WS Sly, et al. (eds), The Metabolic and Molecular Bases of Inherited Disease. New York: McGraw-Hill, 1995;1535–1609.

19. Pasternak JF. Hypoxic-ischaemic brain damage in the term infant, lessons from the laboratory. Pediatr Clin North Am 1993;40:1061–1072.

20. Berman W, Haslam RHA, Konigsmark BW, et al. A new familial syndrome with ataxia, hearing loss, and mental retardation. Report of three brothers. Arch Neurol 1973;29:258–261.

21. Pfeiffer RA, Palm D, Jünemann G, et al. Nosology of congenital non-progressive cerebellar ataxia. Report on six cases in three families. Neuropädiatrie 1974;5: 91–102.

22. Schurig V, Orman AV, Bowen P. Nonprogressive cerebellar disorder with mental retardation and autosomal recessive inheritance in Hutterites. Am J Med Genet 1981;9:43–53.

23. Renier WO, Gabreels FJM, Hustinx TWJ, et al. Cerebellar hypoplasia, communicating hydrocephalus and mental retardation in two brothers and a maternal uncle. Brain Dev 1983;5:41–45.

24. Kvistad PM, Dahl A, Skre H. Autosomal recessive non-progressive ataxia with an early childhood debut. Acta Neurol Scand 1985;71:295–302.

25. Wichman A, Frank LM, Kelly TE. Autosomal recessive congenital cerebellar hypoplasia. Clin Genet 1985;27:373–382.

26. Young ID, Moore JR, Tripp JH. Sex-linked recessive congenital ataxia. J Neurol Neurosurg Psychiatry 1987;50:1230–1232.

27. Laplaza FJ, Root L, Tassanawipas A, et al. Cerebral palsy in twins. Dev Med Child Neurol 1992;34:1053–1063.

28. Goodman R, Alberman E. A twin study of congenital hemiplegia. Dev Med Child Neurol 1996;38:3–12.

29. Ingram TTS. Congenital ataxic syndromes in cerebral palsy. Acta Paediatr Scand 1962;51:209–221.

30. Gustavson KH, Hagberg B, Samver C. Identical syndromes of cerebral palsy in the same family. Acta Paediatr Scand 1969;58:330–340.

31. Hughes I, Newton R. Genetic aspects of cerebral palsy. Dev Med Child Neurol 1992;34:80–86.

7

Traumatic Brain Injury as a Cause of Cerebral Palsy

Michael J. Noetzel and Geoffrey Miller

Cerebral palsy acquired after the newborn period accounts for a surprisingly high percentage of children with this neurologic condition. Epidemiologic studies carried out since the 1970s both here in the United States and elsewhere have documented that of all children with cerebral palsy, between 10% and 26% of the cases result from an injury or illness occurring in infancy or childhood.[1–5] Head injury (including both accidental and nonaccidental trauma to the brain) is the second most common cause of postnatally acquired cerebral palsy (infections of the central nervous system [CNS] being the most common) and accounts for 20–30% of these cases.[1–5] Analyzed further, these data document that of all cases of cerebral palsy from any cause, head injury is the etiology for permanent motor disability in roughly 2.5–5.0% of the children.[1,3–5] In the metropolitan Atlanta area, the prevalence of cerebral palsy secondary to head injury is reported to be 1.1 per 10,000 children.[5]

The incidence of traumatic brain injury in childhood in the United States continues to increase.[6–8] Therefore, cerebral palsy resulting from head injury is likely to remain a significant medical concern to neurologists, pediatricians, and all those health professionals involved in the management of these children. We have developed a greater understanding of the typical clinical characteristics observed in children with traumatically induced cerebral palsy and of the changes in motor dysfunction that commonly occur during the process of recovery. Concomitant with this enhanced understanding have been improvements in our ability to provide medical and rehabilitative management for these children. Advances have also been made in determining the relationship between the motor disability characteristics of cerebral palsy and neuropathologic changes accompanying brain injury, both at a cellular level and as can be extrapolated from newer techniques of brain neuroimaging. These subjects are the focus of this chapter.

CLINICAL CHARACTERISTICS

Acute Stage

In children who experience moderate to severe head injury, the most frequent neuromuscular findings that accompany coma or obtundation are abnormalities in tone. Severe hypertonicity suggests a significant, often diffuse or multifocal, insult to the CNS or modest elevations of intracranial pressure (ICP) or both.[9] When accompanied by rigid dystonic posturing of both arms in flexion (decorticate rigidity), the deep gray and white matter structures, especially the thalamus, likely are involved. In contrast, decerebrate rigidity, in which the arms and legs are stiffly extended and internally rotated, appears in the condition of diencephalic-midbrain compression and suggests involvement of the upper pons. Severe generalized flaccidity indicates an even more severe injury that is a poor prognostic sign in terms of both mortality and recovery.[9,10]

As a child becomes minimally more responsive after severe head trauma (or in the initial stages of a moderate injury), the typical pattern of motor dysfunction is a selective or asymmetric increase in tone associated with an ipsilateral decrease in extremity movements. Over time, the findings on neurologic examination become more reproducible, resulting in rather clear-cut diagnoses of either spastic hemiparesis or quadriplegia that typically is asymmetric. The subsequent extent of improvement in neuromotor deficits is exceedingly variable. In patients with closed head injury, two very important factors appear to influence motor recovery: (1) the severity of the initial brain injury and (2) whether the initiating mechanical trauma elicits a series of pathologic responses that, in turn, result in further damage to the CNS, a phenomenon termed *secondary brain injury*.[10,11] Multiple studies have demonstrated that severity of initial head injury (as measured by the Glasgow Coma Scale at 6–72 hours and by the length of unconsciousness) directly correlates with the degree of acute motor dysfunction and long-term motor disability.[9-13] The most commonly implicated processes causing secondary injury after trauma are increased ICP, cerebral hypoperfusion, and hypoxia. The latter two typically reflect alterations in pulmonary function or the systemic circulation. Defining the extent to which secondary injury contributes to long-term motor disability is very difficult. Clearly, however, factors such as level of oxygenation, presence or absence of raised ICP, and clinical status in the field and in the emergency room (especially blood pressure) are related strongly to both survival and long-term outcome, including motor performance.[9,10,11,14]

Age at the time of head injury also appears to be an important factor in predicting eventual outcome and motor performance.[13-15] To some degree, the relation of age to outcome might reflect a greater vulnerability to diffuse injury in the very young child (see Pathogenesis and Neuropathology, below). However, this group of patients probably includes a high percentage of infants whose traumatic injury was nonaccidental (i.e., child abuse). In such cases, delay on the part of adults in seeking prompt medical treatment for the infant, for fear of exposure, and the high incidence of concomitant asphyxial injury in these unfortunate patients results in a population at significant risk for death and permanent neurologic disability, including a high incidence of cerebral palsy.[14,15] In one typical study, injury that resulted from abuse in children was the chief reason that young age at injury was associated with poor cognitive and motor outcomes.[15] Results such as this, in addition to our personal experience, indicate that nonaccidental head trauma is a particularly devastating form of injury.

In individuals with open head injuries, especially injuries secondary to gunshot wounds, the nature and extent of initial motor disability relates directly to the path of the missile. Of the eight patients with gunshot injury to the brain for whom we have provided inpatient neurorehabilitation services at St. Louis Children's Hospital from 1992–1997, six demonstrated moderate to severe flaccid hemiparesis at the time of their initial neurologic examination. Another adolescent was without any motor dysfunction, and the remaining patient had bilateral spasticity as a result of a significant midline missile injury that caused bihemispheric damage. In contrast to patients with closed head injury, the severity of initial cognitive impairment with open head injury may not parallel motor findings. In some cases, traumatic unconsciousness may be absent or, if present, of rather short duration.

Recovery Phase and Long-Term Outcome

Moderate Head Injury

After traumatic unconsciousness resolves, most patients with moderate closed head injury experience a gradual improvement in motor disability. The extent and rate of recovery varies greatly from child to child. In our experience, many children with moderate traumatic brain injury[16] demonstrate only generalized poor endurance and deficits in dynamic balance, without overt signs of abnormal tone or true weakness. The remainder of patients typically have mild to moderate hemiparesis or, less frequently, an asymmetric quadriparesis in which the less affected side predominantly exhibits hypertonicity without significant weakness. Over 2–6 weeks' time, the hemiplegia significantly improves or even resolves. Subsequent neurologic examinations in our patient population at between 6 and 12 months after injury usually demonstrate normal tone and strength, although persistent reflex abnormalities can occur.

Studies from other institutions have suggested that some patients or their parents may report concerns about incoordination or weakness after moderate head injury.[17] However, documenting functional limitations resulting from these concerns is difficult.

The long-term outlook for performance of motor activity in patients with moderate head injury is also relatively good. In a series of tests that assessed fine- and gross-motor skills, including strength and speed of motor response, significant gains in the reacquisition of previously learned motor skills were shown to take place during the first year after head injury.[16] Little further improvement of motor performance occurred between years 1 and 3 and, thus, normalization of motor performance in most subjects was believed to be unlikely ever to occur.[16] The functional impact of these deficits on daily living in children with moderate head injury is not clear. Cognitive impairment in areas such as performance IQ and adaptive problem solving are likely to have a much greater adverse affect on real-world and classroom performance of these patients than are mild motor problems.[16]

Severe Head Injury

Many patients with severe injury from trauma will require an extended inpatient program of neurorehabilitation, during which time continued recovery of motor function is likely to occur, even in children for whom the formal neurologic examination remains abnormal.[18,19] In one study, 16 (64%) of 25 children had spastic hemiplegia, and three others (12%) had tetraplegia at the time of discharge from a regional rehabilitation center after an average length of admission of 8.5 months.[18] Motor difficulties secondary to ataxia or dysmetria were noted in 11 children (44%), eight of whom also had spastic weakness. Despite these abnormal findings, 64% of the children could ambulate in the community, and another 16% could move about freely in their home.[18] Other studies have documented similar degrees of improvement over time in children with severe head injury.[14,19–23] Although the patients reported in these investigations likely represent a relatively heterogeneous group, a certain uniformity of results exists from which four broad conclusions can be derived.

First, *the period during which recovery of motor function occurs after severe traumatic brain injury is longer than previously was accepted.* One report documented resolution of cerebral palsy in five of 43 children (11.6%) based on normalization of the neurologic examination.[19] This resolution, on average, occurred sometime between the second and fifteenth month after injury, but recovery was seen at up to 34 months in rare patients. In another study involving 36 children representing the 5% of most severely damaged survivors of traumatic brain injury in Israel, improvement in motor function was noted in many of the patients for long periods after injury.[22] For example, four children progressed to ambulating independently after having been wheelchair-bound for at least 3 years after an accident.[22,23] Several other patients demonstrated progress from an abnormal to a normal gait during late stages of recovery.[23] Two other studies noted that while maximum gains in recovery of motor skills were achieved within the first 12 months after injury, continued improvement could be documented for as long as 2–3 years.[20,21]

Second, *despite the severity of head injury in these cases, a surprisingly high percentage of children progress to a normal neuromotor examination* (i.e., the resolution of cerebral palsy; Table 7.1). The most conservative figure was provided by a study of 344 patients admitted between 1959 and 1977 to Ranchos Los Amigos Hospital.[14] At 1-year follow-up, no residual motor deficits were identified in 10% of the children, whereas another 3% had only "soft signs." A similar figure of 12% of patients with normal examinations was noted at discharge from a regional pediatric rehabilitation referral unit, but the length

Table 7.1 Motor Findings at Follow-Up in Children with Severe Traumatic Brain Injury

Study	Brink et al.[14]	Emanuelson et al.[18]	Scott-Jupp et al.[19]	Costeff et al.[22]	Costeff et al.[23]
Number of patients	344	25	43	35	30
Average length of follow-up	12 mos	10.4 mos	15 mos	4 yrs	8 yrs
Normal	10%	12%	56%	20%	33%
Minimally abnormal	3%	—	—	20%	—
Spasticity	38%	44%	37%	26%	24%
Ataxia	8%	12%	—	—	10%
Both spasticity and ataxia	39%	32%	—	20%	17%
Movement disorder	—	—	7%	14%	13%
Other	2%	—	—	—	3%

Note: All patients in reference 23 were reported also in reference 22; in the later study (23), a longer follow-up period was provided in which changes in the motor examination were documented.

of follow-up was fairly short—on average, 10.5 months.[18] Other investigators reported a normal neurologic examination in 20% of severely head-injured patients and an equal percentage of children with only minimal findings after a 4-year follow-up[22]; at 8 years after injury, 33% of the children were reported to have no motor disability.[23] In a series from Johns Hopkins, 29.4% of the survivors were normal at a mean follow-up of 21 months posthospitalization,[21] whereas nearly 56% of the children receiving care at an English rehabilitation center for severe head injury were without abnormal neuromotor signs at an average follow-up of 15 months.[19]

It is likely that patterns of patient referral, length of follow-up, and initial severity of head injury account for at least some of the variability of outcome in these five studies. For example, average length of coma for children undergoing rehabilitation at Ranchos Los Amigos Hospital was between 5 and 6 weeks.[14] In two other studies, the duration was shorter, between 2 and 3 weeks.[21,23] In addition, the four most recent investigations among these describe outcomes in patients who had sustained their head injury between 1976 and 1989,[18,19,21,22] whereas some of the patients at Ranchos Los Amigos dated back to the late 1950s.[14] Improved emergency room and neurosurgical management of patients and the resultant decrease in secondary brain injury thus also likely contribute to differences documented in long-term motor outcome in these studies.

Third, *the residual* (presumably permanent) *motor deficits noted in these patient populations is fairly uniform.* In these children, the most common finding was spasticity, typically in the form of a spastic hemiplegia (Table 7.2).[14,19–23] Extracting an exact incidence of spastic hemiplegia from these studies is difficult, but spastic hemiplegia appears to account for between 50% and 67% of the cases of cerebral palsy after severe head injury. In nearly half of the

Table 7.2 Frequency of Cerebral Palsy and Other Motor Deficits Documented at Follow-Up in Children with Severe Traumatic Brain Injury

Study	Emanuelson et al.[18]	Scott-Jupp et al.[19]	Brink et al.[20]	Costeff et al.[23]
Number of patients	25	43	46	30
Average length of follow-up	10.4 mos	15 mos	1–7 yrs (range)	8 yrs
Hemiparesis	64%	21%	43%	40%
Quadriparesis	12%	5%	50%	3%
Diplegia	—	12%	—	—
Ataxia*	44%	—	60%	27%
Movement disorders	—	7%	—	13%

*Ataxia and cerebral palsy often were observed in the same child.

patients, the hemiparesis was minimal and unlikely to interfere in most motor activities. Those children with moderate hemiparesis had limited control of fine movements, especially in the hands. The resultant disability was greatest when the dominant hand was involved. Parietal lobe injury resulting in motor dyspraxia and disturbances in discriminatory sensation also might contribute to decreased fine-motor hand function. Bilateral spasticity, typically in the form of an asymmetric quadriparesis, was reported much less frequently,[19,22,23] except for one series in which it was noted in 50% of the children with cerebral palsy (see Table 7.2).[20]

Ataxia was the second most common persistent neuromotor abnormality in children with severe head injury, occurring in up to 60% of the patients who had an abnormal examination (see Table 7.2).[14,20,22,23] Not surprisingly, ataxia and hemiparesis often were noted in the same children, either on the same or on opposite sides. Less frequently, ataxia occurred in isolation.[14] In contrast to other post-traumatic movement disorders (described later), ataxia can be a prominent feature throughout the entire course of recovery, with onset often before discharge from the hospital. The degree of ataxia was minimal in two-thirds of cases in one reported series and did not interfere in movement.[20] Some improvement over time was noted in many children.[22]

Fourth, *most patients with severe head injury ultimately achieve a high level of motor performance despite the presence of cerebral palsy or other permanent forms of motor disability.* Most studies report that between 63% and 83% of injured persons are able to ambulate in the community,[14,18,22] with an additional 10–24% of the children able to ambulate independently over short distances. Even in the one study in which the prevalence of spastic cerebral palsy or ataxia was exceedingly high (93%), the vast majority of children (87%) achieved independence in ambulation and self-care.[20]

Using a different outcome measure, the Johns Hopkins study documented a return to normal level of motor and cognitive function in 29.4% of the survivors; in an additional 53% of the children, mild cognitive dysfunction but no functionally significant neuromotor deficits were noted.[21] In children who demonstrate good recovery of motor function and normalization of the neurologic examination, less obvious motor impairment still may persist. Such patients often find themselves unable to compete successfully in a sport in which they had previously demonstrated athletic talents.[22] Children with normal neurologic examinations but a history of significant traumatic brain injury performed less well than did age-matched controls on tests of motor performance in which speed was a component of either fine- or gross-motor tasks.[24] These deficits did appear to diminish over time, however, with recovery continuing even into the second year after injury.[24]

Overall, motor outcome after most cases of severe traumatic injury to the brain must be considered very good. Unfortunately, in many children so injured, more significant cognitive and behavioral sequelae from the head injury prove to be significant impediments for resumption of a normal family life and academic progress in school. A subset of infants and children with severe brain injury from trauma also exists for whom the outlook for motor performance is rather bleak. Several studies have demonstrated that prolonged unconsciousness, especially for longer than 90 days, is an ominous sign. In one study of 26 severely head-injured children who remained unconscious for more than 3 months, only four (15%) were able to achieve and maintain independent ambulation.[13] In contrast, three children (11.5%) died and another 14 (54%) had either no purposeful movement or exceedingly limited movement, such that ambulation was not possible and they were completely dependent on others for all activities of daily living.[13] Using a similar minimum duration of unconsciousness, slightly more optimistic outcomes were documented at Ranchos Los Amigos Hospital, where 38% of the patients became independent in ambulation and self-care.[14] Clearly, however, recovery of motor function is markedly diminished in patients with prolonged unconsciousness.

Minor Head Trauma

Motor dysfunction after minor head injury is not uncommon. However, it usually is very transient.[25] More long-term symptomatic complaints may continue for months to years, but the motor system typically is not involved.[25] In fact, most studies in the pediatric population suggest that virtually no true clinically significant long-term deficits result from mild traumatic brain injury.[26,27]

A clear exception to these findings is a unique syndrome of injury to the basal ganglia after minor, or even trivial, head injury.[28,29] In the typical case, a young child sustains a minor head injury often as a result of a fall, followed by transient loss of consciousness. Subsequently, unilateral mild to moderate weakness develops, affecting mainly the arm. Cranial imaging discloses a hypodense lesion in the basal ganglia contralateral to the weakness. This is postulated to represent ischemic injury secondary to an anterior stretch on the lateral branch of the perforator of the middle cerebral artery. The outlook for these children is uniformly good. Most commonly, the hemiparesis resolves rapidly and completely.[29]

Traumatic Movement Disorders

A variety of movement disorders has been described after traumatic injury to the brain during childhood.[30,31] A common feature of these disorders is the often long interval between injury and the development of the movement disturbance. On the basis of this typical delay in onset, a variety of pathophysiologic mechanisms have been postulated to underlie the development of post-traumatic movement disorders. These mechanisms include the development of lateral sprouting, remyelination, changes in sensitivity to neurotransmitters, ephaptic transmission, central motor synaptic reorganization, and heightened oxidative reactions as a result of hemorrhage.[30] At present, however, only a limited amount of evidence is available, most of it experimental in nature.

Dystonia   Head trauma is reported to account for slightly fewer than 10% of all cases of symptomatic hemidystonia.[32,33] Determining the actual incidence of dystonia as a consequence of head trauma is difficult: Some authors have suggested that it must be rare but likely is underreported.[31] In our unpublished series of 52 children and adolescents with traumatic brain injury (mainly severe), only a single patient developed dystonia. Other studies, also involving patients with severe head injury, have indicated that dystonia and other "basal ganglia syndromes" were noted in between 7% and 14%.[19,22,23] In a typical case, the predominant early neuromotor disturbance is spastic cerebral palsy, most usually hemiplegia. When the hemiplegia improves or resolves entirely, the dystonia appears; this most commonly transpires within the first 6 months after injury. However, in nearly one-third of the reported series, the interval between head trauma and the onset of dystonia was much longer, ranging from 3 to 9 years.[31,34] In either instance, the dystonia affects the same side of the body as did the hemiplegia and typically is found in a focal distribution involving predominantly the hand and arm.[31,34] With the passage of time, the dystonia progresses from focal dystonia to hemidystonia; more rarely, it evolves into a multifocal or generalized distribution. Treatment of pediatric post-traumatic dystonia has been somewhat disappointing, with most medications proving to be either ineffective or of minimum benefit.[30,31,35]

The origin of post-traumatic dystonia most likely is secondary to dysfunction within the lenticular nucleus or thalamus. In most reported series in patients of any age, evidence of traumatic damage to these structures is seen on imaging studies in between 60% and 90% of patients.[31,34] Abnormalities are especially common in those patients whose head injury occurred when they were younger than 18 years, even though computed tomography (CT) scans or magnetic resonance imaging (MRI) scans might not be obtained until years later.

In patients with normal imaging studies or minor nonspecific changes, microscopic damage might have occurred. Much less clear is why many other patients with thalamic or basal ganglia hemorrhage secondary to trauma never develop dystonia. Young age at time of injury appears to be a very important factor, perhaps reflecting the increased likelihood that mechanisms such as central synaptic reorganization or aberrant neuronal sprouting will take place. The common feature of resolution or improvement in hemiparesis suggests that the cortical spinal tract system must be functioning at normal or near-normal level before secondary dystonia can become manifest.

Other Post-Traumatic Movement Disturbances Tremor after head injury has been reported commonly in childhood. In one retrospective survey of 389 severely head-injured children, the prevalence of significant tremor as reported by parents was established to be at least 45%. By description, the tremor was of large amplitude and low frequency. It occurred with static maintenance of posture but was exaggerated by activity or anxiety.[36] The onset of tremor typically was within 18 months of the head injury. In more than 50% of the cases, the tremor spontaneously resolved. None of the patients appeared to have received any form of treatment for the tremor. Whether the tremor resulted in any degree of functional disability in these children cannot be determined on the basis of the information collected by the survey. Other post-traumatic movement disorders, including hemiballismus[22,37] and myoclonus,[37] have been described in pediatric patients, although much less frequently than tremor or dystonia. Typically, these occur in combination with tremor. As is the case with dystonia, these movement abnormalities often evolve unilaterally in the context of a resolving hemiparesis.[37] Long-term disability in severe cases is fairly common.

MANAGEMENT

Management issues for children with post-traumatic cerebral palsy overlap considerably with the therapeutic approaches used in other forms of cerebral palsy, especially as regards treatment of permanent motor disabilities (see Chapters 13 and 14). Some treatment considerations are specific to traumatically induced cerebral palsy. These are related mainly to the evolution of motor dysfunction observed acutely after injury to the brain and the subsequent typical pattern of recovery.

Acute Stage

The goal of early intervention in the traumatically brain-injured child is to prevent or minimize the development of physical deformities and other complications that otherwise will ensue as a result of abnormalities in tone and prolonged immobilization. Contractures in particular may take months to resolve if left unmanaged during the early stages of head injury.[38] Thus, neurorehabilitation of the traumatically brain-injured child should be instituted even while the child is comatose. During this stage, severe hypertonia and rigid dystonia of the extremities mandate passive exercises and range of motion to all limbs, supplemented by the use of splinting, all in an effort to reduce spasticity.[39] In more involved cases, inhibitive casting, especially of larger joints, may be required for further reduction of abnormal tone.[38] Neural disinhibition secondary to trauma often results in the re-emergence of developmentally primitive reflexes, such as the tonic labyrinthine and asymmetric tonic neck reflexes. Appropriate positioning decreases the adverse posturing that results from activation of these reflexes and, thus, allows more mature movement patterns to emerge.[40]

Recovery Phase

Once a child is medically stable and demonstrates increased awareness of the environment, including more directed movements, an intensive program of neurorehabilitation should be instituted. Typically, this program is provided by a multidisciplinary team composed of physicians, nurses, therapists, and other health professionals. Initially, motor, cognitive, and psychosocial deficits resulting from the trauma to the CNS are assessed within the framework of a clear understanding of normative development.[40] An integrated program of neurorehabilitation then is created. As regards motor disability, the program should focus on issues of functional significance and relate to practical management decisions. Continual reassessment of motor performance and dysfunction is mandatory in view of the differences in degree, extent, and rate of recovery among children and the variability of functioning from setting to setting and task to task in an individual child. In the early recovery period, therapy should be very aggressive and directed at increasing range of motion and at incorporating voluntary movements into appropriate developmental patterns. As the child's condition improves, the neurorehabilitation program shifts its focus from reacquisition of previously learned motor abilities to the learning of new skills required to compensate for deficits in motor function.[39]

Spasticity typically remains a problematic and often disabling feature during recovery from head injury. Aggressive physical therapy and appropriate splinting and casting are the cornerstone of treatment. In addition, pharmacologic management of spasticity may be indicated when physical modalities fail to halt the development of complications such as early contractures. Children, especially those with traumatic injury to the brain, are much more sensitive to the side effects of medications used to control spasticity, in particular sedation. Thus, possible adverse effects of medication on attention and cognitive and motor function should be monitored closely.[38]

Of the antispasticity agents most commonly used in children with head injury, dantrolene sodium has been suggested as the drug of choice, mainly due to the perception that its effects on attention and arousal are limited.[41] Because dantrolene can produce hepatic dysfunction, especially with prolonged use, liver function tests should be checked before initial administration of the drug. Baclofen is another useful antispasticity medication.[41] Our experience at St. Louis Children's Hospital indicates that the efficacy of baclofen is superior to dantrolene and, with careful and gradual titration, lethargy can be minimized. The duration of treatment with oral antispasticity medication in patients with post-traumatic cerebral palsy is relatively short. In most children, the natural history is one of gradual decline in spasticity and improvement in motor function; medication often is needed for only 2–6 months. For similar reasons, surgical interventions during the first year postinjury should be discouraged.[38]

In a small percentage of children, however, spasticity will increase progressively despite intensive therapy and use of oral agents. The potential for development of severe contractures and permanent bony deformities thus becomes significantly elevated. In these instances, intramuscular administration of botulinum toxin may be of benefit.[42] Typically, within 7–10 days, flaccid weakness of the injected muscle ensues, thus allowing for more intensive range-of-motion therapy or serial inhibitive casting.

PATHOGENESIS AND NEUROPATHOLOGY

Closed Head Injury

Closed head injury caused by blunt trauma can be subdivided further into two categories—impression injuries and acceleration injuries—on the basis of biomechanical considerations.[39] However, most cases of head trauma in children have components of both forms of injury, and so multiple types of damage to the CNS can be found in a single patient.

Impression Injury

Trauma delivered to a stationary head produces an impression injury that results in focal damage such as skull fractures, epidural hematomas, and contusions of the brain parenchyma. The extent of injury is determined primarily by the biomechanical forces generated at the time of injury. In older children and adolescents, moderate- to severe-impact trauma often causes contusions or bruising within the cortical surface, resulting from hemorrhaging of torn vessels. These lesions most commonly are located on the lateral surfaces of the cerebrum and over the convexity of the brain.[43] In severe injury, the contusions may extend through all of the cortical layer and down into the subcortical white matter. If the contusion is in close proximity to the site of impact, it is labeled *coup* injury. Some theorize that contusions are due to deformation of the skull or a depressed fracture. The ways in which energy generated at impact damages the underlying cortex while sparing the skull underlying the contusion (which often remains intact) is not entirely clear.[43]

Acceleration Injuries

Far more common are acceleration injuries, which result from impact to a moving head, causing the generation of rotational and shearing forces within the brain.[39] Differential displacement of the skull and cranial contents also takes place. As the brain rotates within the cranial cavity, the temporal and frontal regions of the brain are pushed against the bony prominences of the middle and anterior cranial fossae, producing *contrecoup* contusions.[43] In these instances, the damage typically is found along the ventral and lateral surfaces of the temporal lobes or over the orbital surface of the frontal lobes. Compared to other simple contusions, a contrecoup injury tends to be larger and to extend deeper, usually involving all of the cortex and a portion of the subcortical white matter. Coup and contrecoup contusions, however, are almost never seen in infants and are rare even in young children.[44] Apparently, a rigid cranium is required to transmit the kinetic forces of trauma into the parenchyma of the brain. In the absence of a completely ossified skull in the young individual, the impact forces are dissipated into the soft tissues of the head and neck. Traumatic intracranial hemorrhage also is relatively uncommon in infants and young children as compared to adolescents and adults.[44] Instead, lesions termed *contusional tears* are found, typically in the form of slitlike hemorrhages in the cerebral subcortical white matter, most commonly within the orbital and temporal lobes and the first and second frontal convolutions.[45] Differential movement of the cortical ribbon relative to the underlying immature white matter is believed to create a small cavity into which hemorrhaging occurs secondary to traction on bridging veins.

Subdural hematomas, another common injury that results from inertial acceleration and deceleration forces, are seen throughout the age spectrum of pediatric patients.[43,44] Most subdural hematomas result from the tearing of dural bridging veins near the venous sinuses. Size is typically a reflection of the severity of initial traumatic injury. Location, however, may relate more to etiology. Accidental impact injuries, such as those incurred in a motor vehicle accident, typically produce basilar or lateral hemorrhage. In child abuse, shaking tends to result in midline subdural hemorrhage.[44]

The prototypic acceleration injury in both children and adults is diffuse axonal injury, which is also the pathophysiologic process that underlies much of the long-term morbidity in child abuse, especially in shaken infants.[46] Linear and, more importantly, angular rotational forces generated in acceleration head injury causes various components of the brain to move in opposite directions. This, in turn, causes stretching, shearing, and tearing of both capillaries and axons of long passage.[43,44] More direct neuronal damage may be created as a result of avulsion or stretching injuries to dendrites or neurites.[44] In the early stages of diffuse axonal injury, the lesions consist of petechial-sized or small intraparenchymal hemorrhages. These lesions may be diffusely located, but favored areas of involvement include the corpus callosum, the rostral brain stem, subcortical white matter (often frontal or parietal), the corona radiata and internal capsule, and within the basal ganglia.[43] Bilateral cerebral swelling can be found in more extensive cases. Over time, the hemorrhagic lesions become sunken, cystic scars.[47] At the microscopic level, diffuse axonal injury initially consists of swollen axons and retraction balls, associated with chromolytic neurons. In cases of irreversible damage, wallerian degeneration ensues and a pattern of regional demyelination or dysmyelination can be observed.[44] The result, on gross inspection of the brain, is a reduction in the size of the white matter within the cerebral hemispheres and brain stem and ex vacuo dilatation of the ventricles. This type of permanent injury is seen far too often in cases of diffuse axonal injury secondary to child abuse. Possibly, shearing forces produce greater damage when acting within the less myelinated, immature brain.

Nonaccidental traumatic brain injury, an acceleration injury, is reported to be the most common cause of serious head injury in children aged less than 2 years[48] and is therefore an important cause of cerebral palsy. Clearly, such injury is a major public health problem that necessitates a high level of vigilance and action from social, educational, and health care agencies and more support for children's protective agencies. The parties inflicting the injuries often themselves are victims of child abuse and, although difficult socioeconomic circumstances are more likely to be part of the picture of child abuse, such abuse can occur at any level of social or education status.[44,49]

Nonaccidental injury should be suspected when the extent of injury found is not consistent with the reported history. The type of injury and the presence and pattern of associated injuries also provide evidence for abuse. For example, multiple bruises and fractures of different ages might be present, and burns or bites or subgaleal hemorrhages from forceful pulling of hair, the latter leading to the appearance of black eyes, might be seen.[50] Conversely, signs of external injury might be absent or slight and might not reflect the severity of internal damage.[44]

Nonaccidental head injuries are caused by direct blows, shaking, or a combination of the two.[44] If head injury is caused by direct impact from, for example, a punch or from striking of the head on or by a hard object or surface, epidural or subdural hemorrhage can occur, accompanied by underlying damage to the brain. Skull fractures may be absent but, if present, will not be the thin linear fractures seen in the parietal region after a low accidental fall.[44,50–52] The types of skull fractures that are more likely to be nonaccidental in origin are those that cross suture lines or are branching, stellate, bilateral, multiple, or more than 5 mm wide at presentation; alternatively, depressed occipital skull fractures may be seen in a child younger than 3 years.[50] Because of the relative pliancy of the infant skull, coup rather than contrecoup lesions occur.[44] These lesions may be associated with gray and white matter junction hemorrhages and whiter matter contusional tears.[45] Repeated trauma is associated with atrophic brain adherent to a chronic subdural membrane.[44]

When an infant is shaken vigorously, the whiplash movements of a relatively large head cause acceleration and deceleration forces that damage the brain, meninges, and eyes.[46,53–55] The typical findings in shaken baby syndrome are cerebral edema; subdural hemorrhage (which often includes interhemispheric bleeding); bilateral preretinal, subhyaloid, and intraretinal hemorrhage; optic nerve sheath hemorrhage[56]; epidural cervical hemorrhage, sometimes associated with cervical spine and cord injuries[44]; and characteristic rib fractures and periosteal metaphyseal damage.[50,55–57] Diffuse optic fundus involvement, vitreous hemorrhage, or large, subhyaloid hemorrhages are reported to be associated with more severe acute neurologic injury.[58] The acceleration and deceleration forces induced by shaking and impact cause cerebral interhemispheric hemorrhage by tearing the bridging veins that run from the surface of the brain to the sagittal sinus.[50,59] These same shearing forces can lead to axonal injury in the hemispheric white matter and lesions in the brain stem, corpus callosum, and superior cerebellar peduncles.[50] Haseler and colleagues[60] reported that, in infants with the shaken baby syndrome, the post-traumatic brain injury is a particularly severe form. They demonstrated that in these infants, examined by magnetic resonance spectroscopy, continuing abnormal biochemical changes occur in the brain as a result of neuronal injury. Furthermore, these changes could be used to predict outcome more accurately than could MRI findings alone.

After the assault, a spectrum of clinical events can occur. The baby may be rendered unconscious, probably due to a rotational shearing effect on the brain stem that may, in addition to loss of consciousness, cause tonic posturing, apnea, and autonomic dysfunction.[50] The infant then may become increasingly comatose or later regain consciousness and appear only lethargic or irritable, or even appear normal.[53,61] Several hours can pass before observers, who are not necessarily the perpetrators, notice undue lethargy or seizures. The most common presentation is a pale lethargic or irritable baby. Often, a history of seizures, extensor posturing, vomiting, and apneic episodes is elicited, and evidence of shock—hypotension, hypothermia, and tachycardia—may be present.[50]

Adverse neurologic and developmental outcomes after nonaccidental brain injury are common and often severe. Zimmerman and colleagues[62] found that all those who presented with interhemispheric hemorrhage developed cerebral atrophy, and half-developed brain infarcts. Outcomes include cognitive deficit, cerebral palsy, posthemorrhagic hydrocephalus, and visual deficits.[50,63,64] One group of young infants appears to be characterized by an absence of neurologic sequelae after the shaken baby syndrome. However, long-term follow-up of these infants reveals poor head growth, cognitive and language deficits, neurobehavioral difficulties, and, in some, the development of hemiparetic cerebral palsy.[65]

Open Head Injury

Although much less common than closed head injuries, open or penetrating head trauma statistically more often results in death or a poor neurologic outcome. Gunshot wounds can be particularly devastating, producing irreversible damage due to the maceration of brain tissue along the pathway of the bullet (Figures 7.1, 7.2). Once relatively uncommon in adolescents and children, gunshot injuries to the head are becoming increasingly more common.[66]

Secondary Injuries

Secondary injuries after head trauma can be divided into two main groups: damage related to the consequences of systemic or other extracranial trauma, and injuries resulting from pathophysiologic responses within the CNS that are initiated by the primary craniocerebral trauma. Examples within the first group include hypoxia or hypoperfusion, most commonly associated with pulmonary contusions, trauma-induced cardiac dysrhythmias, and clinical episodes of hypotension.[11,38,43] The resultant neuropathologic changes are those of ischemia (often in a watershed distribution) or hemorrhagic infarction.[43]

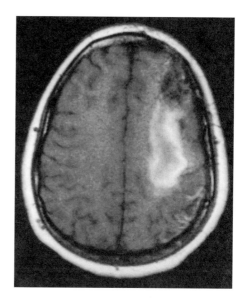

Figure 7.1 Axial T_1-weighted echo magnetic resonance imaging scan reveals a large parenchymal cerebral hematoma in the left frontoparietal region in an adolescent who sustained a penetrating gunshot injury. Within the hematoma is macerated tissue with subacute hemorrhage.

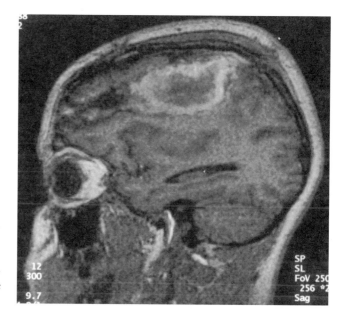

Figure 7.2 Sagittal T_1-weighted magnetic resonance imaging scan of the same patient as in Figure 7.1 again demonstrates extensive damage due to missile injury.

The cascade of pathophysiologic responses set in motion within the brain by purely biomechanical trauma is an exceedingly complex phenomenon, especially in the pediatric population, in which structural immaturity of the brain and developmentally regulated processes might actually diminish the resistance to mechanical injury. Increased ICP may be seen in patients of any age who have experienced a severe traumatic brain injury.[43] It is much more common, however, in younger patients owing to a greater incidence of cerebral edema.[44,67,68] In the pediatric population, cerebral edema can follow even relatively minimal head trauma, and it is notoriously difficult to treat.[67] Studies have suggested that in young children, especially those younger than 5 years, trauma produces a paradoxical increase in cerebral blood flow, whereas the adult brain responds to injury with a decrease in blood flow.[44] This cerebral hyperemia presumably is secondary to a lack of cerebrovascular autoregulation in young patients.[67–69] Some evidence also suggests that the capillary endothelial cell junction, the site of the blood-brain barrier, is more susceptible to injury in young children than in older individuals, thus resulting in a greater likelihood of vasogenic cerebral edema. As a result of these developmentally regulated responses to trauma, an infant or young child sustaining a head injury is at great risk for the secondary development of increased ICP and its adverse long-term effects on neurologic functioning.

CLINICOPATHOLOGIC CORRELATIONS

In the acute stage of head trauma, impairment in motor function can be attributed to a variety of pathophysiologic processes often acting diffusely within the brain but, most importantly, within the deep gray and white matter structures and often the brain stem.[43,44] In children, raised ICP contributes significantly to motor dysfunction.[9,67–69] Much of our knowledge in this area comes from neuropathologic studies of infants and children who have not survived their head injuries.[44] Neuroimaging studies of the brain after acute trauma have further increased our understanding of the consequences of head injury. In particular, imaging studies of the brain have resulted in more specific anatomic localization of damage in patients with longer-lasting motor impairment or permanent cerebral palsy.

Computed Tomographic Scans

A variety of reports have investigated the correlation between abnormal CT scans after head injury and long-term neurologic outcome.[12,14,23,70–73] In general, these studies have demonstrated that scans obtained after severe traumatic injury to the brain are better at predicting overall neurologic disability and cognitive impairment, as compared to deficits specific to motor performance, although some trends are apparent.[12,14,23] For example, a normal CT scan during the acute stages of injury was much more common in (but certainly not predictive of) minimal to absent motor disability.[23] In contrast, severely abnormal scans, especially those consisting of diffuse, often bilateral hypodensities of the cerebral hemispheres, almost always were noted in children with disabling spastic quadriparesis or, less commonly, hemiparesis.[70,71] CT scans obtained at times more remote from injury also appear to provide some prognostic information. The extent of cerebral atrophy, as manifested by ventricular enlargement, did correlate (but not strongly) with severity of motor deficits, including spasticity and weakness.[12,14]

Pathologically, this finding most likely represents a combination of neuronal loss and a reduced bulk of white matter, the latter secondary to shearing damage and diffuse axonal injury.[43,44] The general applicability of these findings is somewhat limited owing to the often retrospective nature of the studies, differences in local referral patterns, patient selection for scans, and the fact that, in some reports, not every patient actually underwent CT scanning. Several investigations have been carried out using much more appropriate study designs.[72,73] Outcome measures, however, were either global or limited to cognitive function; specific data regarding motor performance or disability were not provided.

Magnetic Resonance Imaging

In view of its greater sensitivity in detecting parenchymal damage after brain trauma, especially contusions and signs of shear injury,[74] it is not surprising that MRI can provide useful information concerning general neurologic outcome,[75,76] cognitive deficits,[77] and motor impairment.[70,78] One study in which 37% of the subjects had hemiparesis failed to demonstrate a statistical association of the hemiparesis with any particular pattern of brain damage as noted on MRI scans. However, the "localization groups" were defined only by extent of frontal lobe involvement.[75] In contrast, other investigators have documented that patients with lesions in deep central gray matter or brain stem experienced a higher incidence of long-term disability, including impairments in motor function.[76] Additional evidence correlates involvement of deep gray and white matter structures on MRI scan with long-term neuromotor disability, most predominantly spastic cerebral palsy. In one reported study, 100 patients were evaluated after head injury, including 63 adolescents and adults with spastic hemiplegia or quadriplegia.[78] Ten of the patients had only pyramidal tract signs; in the remaining 53, functional limitations such as difficulty with ambulation were noted. On MRI scans obtained more than 3 months after head injury, lesions in the deep white matter (Figures 7.3, 7.4), the corpus callosum, and the basal ganglia correlated to a highly significant degree with hemiplegia. In contrast, focal brain contusions documented in 33 cases did not correlate with hemiplegia. The study concluded that spastic hemiplegia after traumatic brain injury most likely is secondary to pyramidal tract damage either at the internal capsule or the corona radiata level.

Investigations carried out in children at St. Louis Children's Hospital tend to validate this conclusion. Of the 58 patients admitted to our acute neurorehabilitation service after severe closed head injury, 48 underwent both MRI and longitudinal neurologic assessment. The average interval between injury and MRI scans was 4.6 weeks. Spastic cerebral palsy was documented in 14 patients (29%), including two with asymmetric quadriparesis and 12 others with hemiplegia. Two distinct patterns of abnormal MRI scans correlated with motor disability in these children: Scans in eight of the 14 cases of permanent cerebral palsy revealed significant damage to the basal ganglia or deep white matter structures such as the internal capsule and cerebral peduncles (Figures 7.5, 7.6).

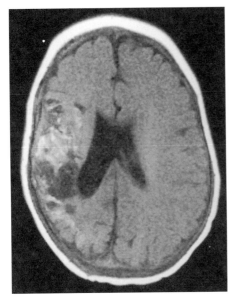 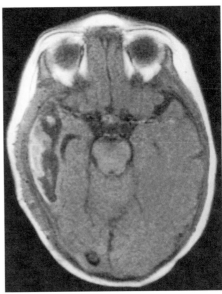

Figure 7.3 Axial T_1-weighted magnetic resonance imaging scans reveal extensive post-traumatic hemorrhagic infarction with cystic encephalomalacia in the right frontal, temporal, and parietal lobes in an infant with a severe left hemiparesis.

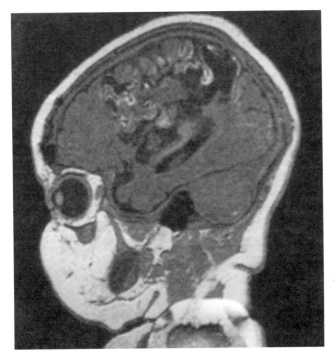

Figure 7.4 Sagittal T_1-weighted magnetic resonance imaging scan of the same patient as in Figure 7.3 again demonstrates extensive post-traumatic damage.

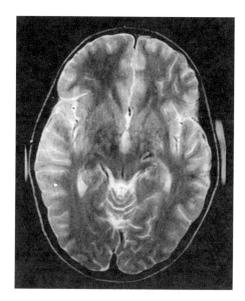

Figure 7.5 Axial T$_2$-weighted magnetic resonance imaging scan demonstrates hemorrhagic foci consistent with diffuse axonal injury in the left internal capsule posteriorly and the left cerebral peduncle in a child with a moderate right hemiparesis.

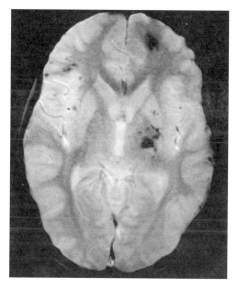 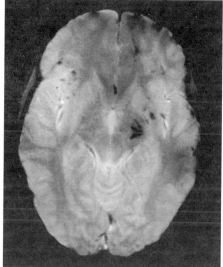

Figure 7.6 Axial gradient echo magnetic resonance imaging scans (which have a heightened sensitivity for blood products) of the same patient as in Figure 7.3 demonstrate the location of hemorrhage within deep white matter.

Involvement of either the basal ganglia or deep white matter was demonstrated in six other children, each of whom demonstrated early evidence of a spastic hemiparesis. These neuromotor deficits improved over time and resolved between 2 and 6 months after injury. In another five children with cerebral palsy, images revealed large areas of cystic encephalomalacia within the cerebral hemispheres, typically extending through the subcortical white matter (see Figures 7.3, 7.4). In two patients, gyral enhancement also was noted; CT scans obtained earlier in the course of injury revealed large areas of hypodensity within the cerebral hemispheres in all five cases. These imaging findings and the resultant permanent motor disability are thus very similar to the cases described by others.[70,71] In a single remaining child who has a mild spastic hemiparesis, MRI scans revealed only evidence of cortical contusions. Our findings suggest that, similar to adult cases, many cases of post-traumatic cerebral palsy in children result from damage to the deep white matter tracts, especially within the internal capsule.

However, a second mechanism of injury that results in cerebral palsy appears to be restricted to younger age groups. This mechanism involves trauma-induced cerebral ischemia that causes large areas of hemorrhagic infarction and, ultimately, extensive cystic encephalomalacia. The pathophysiologic basis of this form of injury is incompletely understood but likely reflects impairment of cerebrovascular autoregulation in the immature brain and the greatly increased incidence of raised ICP in children after head injury.

REFERENCES

1. O'Reilly DE, Walentynowicz JE. Etiological factors in cerebral palsy: an historical review. Dev Med Child Neurol 1981;23:633–642.
2. Holm VA. The causes of cerebral palsy. A contemporary perspective. JAMA 1982; 247:1473–1477.
3. Blair E, Stanley FJ. An epidemiological study of cerebral palsy in Western Australia, 1956–1975: III: Postnatal aetiology. Dev Med Child Neurol 1982;24:575–585.
4. Arens LJ, Molteno CD. A comparative study of postnatally acquired cerebral palsy in Cape Town. Dev Med Child Neurol 1989;31:246–254.
5. Murphy CC, Yeargin-Allsopp M, Decoufle P, Drews CD. Prevalence of cerebral palsy among ten-year-old children in metropolitan Atlanta, 1985 through 1987. J Pediatr 1993;123:S13–S20.
6. Kalsbeek WD, McLaurin RL, Harris BSH, Miller JD. The national head and spinal cord injury survey: major findings. J Neurosurg 1980;53:S19–S29.
7. Kraus JF, Fife D, Cox P, et al. Incidence, severity and external causes of pediatric brain injury. Am J Dis Child 1986;140:687–693.
8. DiScala C, Osberg JS, Gans BM, et al. Children with traumatic head injury: morbidity and postacute treatment. Arch Phys Med Rehabil 1991;72:662–666.
9. Bruce DA, Schut L, Bruno LA, et al. Outcome following severe head injuries in children. J Neurosurg 1978;48:679–688.
10. Berger MS, Pitts LH, Lovely M, et al. Outcome from severe head injury in children and adolescents. J Neurosurg 1985;62:194–199.
11. Michaud LJ, Rivara FP, Grady MS, et al. Predictors of survival and severity of disability after severe brain injury in children. Neurosurgery 1992;31:254–264.
12. Kriel RL, Krach LE, Sheehan M. Pediatric closed head injury: outcome following prolonged unconsciousness. Arch Phys Med Rehabil 1988;69:678–681.

13. Kriel RL, Krach LE, Jones-Saete C. Outcome of children with prolonged unconsciousness and vegetative states. Pediatr Neurol 1993;9:362–368.
14. Brink JD, Imbus C, Woo-Sam J. Physical recovery after severe closed head trauma in children and adolescents. J Pediatr 1980;97:721–727.
15. Kriel RL, Krach LE, Panser LA. Closed head injury: comparison of children younger and older than 6 years of age. Pediatr Neurol 1989;5:296–300.
16. Jaffe KM, Polissar NL, Fay GC, et al. Recovery trends over three years following pediatric traumatic brain injury. Arch Phys Med Rehabil 1995;76:17–26.
17. Greenspan AI, MacKenzie EJ. Functional outcome after pediatric head injury. Pediatrics 1994;94:425–432.
18. Emanuelson I, von Wendt L, Lundalv E, Larsson J. Rehabilitation and follow-up of children with severe traumatic brain injury. Childs Nerv Syst 1996;12:460–465.
19. Scott-Jupp R, Marlow N, Seddon N, Rosenbloom L. Rehabilitation and outcome after severe head injury. Arch Dis Child 1992;67:222–226.
20. Brink JD, Garrett AL, Hale WR, et al. Recovery of motor and intellectual function in children sustaining severe head injuries. Dev Med Child Neurol 1970;12:565–571.
21. Mahoney WJ, D'Souza JD, Haller JA, et al. Long-term outcome of children with severe head trauma and prolonged coma. Pediatrics 1983;71:756–762.
22. Costeff H, Groswasser Z, Landman Y, Brenner T. Survivors of severe traumatic brain injury in childhood: II. Late residual disability. Scand J Rehabil Med Suppl 1985;12:10–15.
23. Costeff H, Groswasser Z, Goldstein R. Long-term follow-up review of 31 children with severe closed head trauma. J Neurosurg 1990;73:684–687.
24. Chaplin D, Deitz J, Jaffe KM. Motor performance in children after traumatic brain injury. Arch Phys Med Rehabil 1993;74:161–164.
25. Alexander MP. Mild traumatic brain injury: pathophysiology, natural history, and clinical management. Neurology 1995;45:1253–1260.
26. Fay GC, Jaffe KM, Polissar NL, et al. Mild pediatric traumatic brain injury: a cohort study. Arch Phys Med Rehabil 1993;74:895–901.
27. Bijur PE, Haslum M, Golding J. Cognitive and behavioral sequelae of mild head injury in children. Pediatrics 1990;86:337–344.
28. Maki Y, Akimoto H, Enomoto T. Injuries of basal ganglia following head trauma in children. Childs Brain 1980;7:113–123.
29. Dharker SR, Mittal RS, Bhargava N. Ischemic lesions in basal ganglia in children after minor head injury. Neurosurgery 1993;33:863–865.
30. Jankovic J. Post-traumatic movement disorders: central and peripheral mechanisms. Neurology 1994;44:2006–2014.
31. Lee MS, Rinne JO, Ceballos-Baumann A, et al. Dystonia after head trauma. Neurology 1994;44:1374–1378.
32. Marsden CD, Obeso JA, Zarranz JJ, et al. The anatomical basis of symptomatic hemidystonia. Brain 1985;108:463–483.
33. Pettigrew LC, Jankovic J. Hemidystonia: a report of 22 patients and a review of the literature. J Neurol Neurosurg Psychiatry 1985;48:650–657.
34. Krauss JK, Mohadjer M, Braus DF, et al. Dystonia following head trauma: a report of nine patients and review of the literature. Mov Disord 1992;7:263–272.
35. Chandra V, Spunt AL, Rosinowitz MS. Treatment of post-traumatic choreoathetosis with sodium valproate. J Neurol Neurosurg Psychiatry 1983;46:963–965.
36. Johnson SL, Hall DM. Post-traumatic tremor in head injured children. Arch Dis Child 1992;67:227–228.
37. Andrew J, Fowler C, Harrison M. Tremor after head injury and its treatment by stereotaxic surgery. J Neurol Neurosurg Psychiatry 1982;45:815–819.
38. Gans BM, Mann NR, Ylvisaker M. Rehabilitation Management Approaches. In M Rosenthal, ER Griffith, MR Bond, JD Miller (eds), Rehabilitation of the Adult and Child with Traumatic Brain Injury. Philadelphia: FA Davis, 1990;593–615.

39. Molnar GE, Perrin JCS. Head Injury. In GE Molnar (ed), Pediatric Rehabilitation. Baltimore: Williams & Wilkins, 1992;245–292.
40. Ylvisaker M. Chorazy AJL, Cohen SB, et al. Rehabilitation Assessment Following Head Injury in Children. In M Rosenthal, ER Griffith, MR Bond, JD Miller (eds), Rehabilitation of the Adult and Child with Traumatic Brain Injury. Philadelphia: FA Davis, 1990;558–592.
41. Whyte J, Robinson KM. Pharmacologic Management. In MB Glenn, J Whyte (eds), The Practical Management of Spasticity in Children and Adults. Philadelphia: Lea & Febiger, 1990;201–226.
42. Yablon SA, Agana BT, Ivanhoe CB, Boake C. Botulinum toxin in severe upper extremity spasticity among patients with traumatic brain injury: an open-labeled trial. Neurology 1996;47:939–944.
43. Case MES. Central Nervous System Trauma. In JS Nelson, JE Parisi, SS Schochet (eds), Principles and Practice of Neuropathology. St. Louis: Mosby, 1993;470–504.
44. Leetsma JE. Forensic Neuropathology. In S Duckett (ed), Pediatric Neuropathology. Baltimore: Williams & Wilkins, 1995;243–283.
45. Lindenberg R, Freytag E. Morphology of brain lesions from blunt trauma in early infancy. Arch Pathol 1969;87:298–305.
46. Hadley MN, Sonntag VK, Rekate HL, Murphy A. The infant whiplash-shake injury syndrome: a clinical and pathological study. Neurosurgery 1989;24:536–540.
47. Adams JH, Graham DJ, Scott G, et al. Brain damage in fatal nonmissile head injury. J Clin Pathol 1980;33:1143–1145.
48. Billmore ME, Myers PA. Serious head injury in infants: accident or abuse? Pediatrics 1985;75:340–342.
49. Oates RK, Forest D, Peacock A. Mothers of abused children. A comparison study. Clin Pediatr 1985;24:9–13.
50. Brown JK, Minns RA. Non-accidental head injury, with particular reference to whiplash-shaking injury and medico-legal aspects. Dev Med Child Neurol 1993; 35:849–868.
51. Hobbs CJ. Skull fracture and the diagnosis of abuse. Arch Dis Child 1984;59: 246–252.
52. Hahn YS, Raimondi AJ, McLone DG, Yamanouchi Y. Traumatic mechanism of head injury in child abuse. Child Brain 1983;10:229–241.
53. Ludwig S, Warman M. Shaken baby syndrome: a review of 20 cases. Ann Emerg Med 1984;13:104–107.
54. Duhaime AC, Gennarelli TA, Thibault LE, et al. The shaken baby syndrome. A clinical, pathological, and biomechanical study. J Neurosurg 1987;66:409–415.
55. Caffey J. The whiplash shaken infant syndrome: manual shaking by the extremities with whiplash-induced intracranial and intraocular bleeding. Linked with residual permanent brain damage and mental retardation. Pediatrics 1974;54:396–403.
56. Lambert SR, Johnson TE, Hoyt CS. Optic nerve and retinal hemorrhage associated with shaken baby syndrome. Arch Ophthalmol 1986;104:1509–1512.
57. Caffey J. On the theory and practice of shaking infants. Am J Dis Child 1972; 124:161–169.
58. Wilkinson WS, Han DP, Rappley MD, Owings CL. Retinal hemorrhage predicts neurologic injury in the shaken baby syndrome. Arch Ophthalmol 1989;107:1472–1474.
59. Zimmerman RA, Russell EJ, Yarberg E, Leeds NE. Falx and interhemispheric fissure on axial CT: II. Recognition and differential of interhemispheric subarachnoid and subdural hemorrhage. Am J Neuroradiol 1982;3:635–642.
60. Haseler LJ, Arcinue E, Danielson ER, et al. Evidence from proton magnetic resonance spectroscopy for a metabolic cascade of neuronal damage in shaken baby syndrome. Pediatrics 1977;99:4–14.
61. Caldern IM, Hill I, Scholz CL. Primary brain trauma in non-accidental injury. J Clin Pathol 1984;37:1095–1100.

62. Zimmerman RA, Bruce D, Schut L, et al. Computerized tomography of craniocerebral injury in abused child. Radiology 1979;130:687–690.
63. Smith SM, Hanson R. 134 battered children: a medical and psychological study. Br Med J 1974;3:666–670.
64. Mushin AS, Morgan G. Ocular damage in the battered baby syndrome. Br J Ophthalmol 1971;55:34–47.
65. Bonnier C, Nassogne MC, Evrard P. Outcome and prognosis of whiplash shaken infant syndrome: late consequences after a symptom-free interval. Dev Med Child Neurol 1995;37:943–956.
66. Miner ME, Ewing-Cobbs L, Kopaniky DR, et al. The results of treatment of gunshot wounds to the brain in children. Neurosurgery 1990;20:20–24.
67. Snoek JW, Minderhoud JM, Wilmink JT. Delayed deterioration following mild head injury in children. Brain 1989;107:15–36.
68. Bruce DA, Alaui A, Bilaniu KL. Diffuse cerebral swelling following head injuries in children: the syndrome of "malignant brain edema." J Neurosurg 1981;54:170–178.
69. Obrist WD, Gennarelli TA, Segawa H. Relation of cerebral blood flow to neurological status and outcome in head-injured patients. J Neurosurg 1979;51:292–300.
70. Onuma T, Shimosegawa Y, Kameyama M, et al. Clinicopathological investigation of gyral high density on computerized tomography following severe head injury in children. J Neurosurg 1995;82:995–1001.
71. Duhaime AC, Christian C, Moss E, Seidl T. Long-term outcome in infants with the shaking-impact syndrome. Pediatr Neurosurg 1996;24:292–298.
72. Ruijs MB, Gabreels FJ, Thijssen HM. The utility of electroencephalography and cerebral computed tomography in children with mild and moderately severe closed head injuries. Neuropediatrics 1994;25:73–77.
73. Ong L, Selladurai BM, Dhillon MK, et al. The prognostic value of the Glasgow Coma Scale, hypoxia and computerised tomography in outcome prediction of pediatric head injury. Pediatr Neurosurg 1996;24:285–291.
74. Zimmerman RA, Bilaniuk LT. Pediatric head trauma. Neuroimaging Clin North Am 1994;4:349–366.
75. Mendelsohn D, Levin HS, Bruce D, et al. Late MRI after head injury in children: relationship to clinical features and outcome. Childs Nerv Syst 1992;8:445–452.
76. Levin HS, Williams D, Crofford MJ, et al. Relationship of depth of brain lesions to consciousness and outcome after closed head injury. J Neurosurg 1988;69:861–866.
77. Levin HS, Culhane KA, Mendelsohn D, et al. Cognition in relation to magnetic resonance imaging in head-injured children and adolescents. Arch Neurol 1993;50:897–905.
78. Masuzawa H, Kubo T, Kanazawa I, et al. Shearing injuries of parasagittal white matter, corpus callosum and basal ganglia: possible radiological evidences of hemiplegia in diffuse axonal injury. No Shinkei Geka 1997;25:689–694.

8

Prenatal and Perinatal Infectious Causes of Cerebral Palsy

James F. Bale, Jr., and William E. Bell

Despite safe, effective vaccines and potent, well-tolerated antimicrobial agents, infections remain major causes of cerebral palsy and other neurodevelopmental disabilities among children worldwide. Infants may acquire these infectious agents prenatally as a consequence of maternal infections, perinatally during their delivery, or postnatally via exposure to parents, siblings, or other persons who harbor the pathogens.[1] In this chapter, we summarize the epidemiology, clinical aspects, management, and sequelae of selected infections in humans that have the capacity adversely to affect early neurologic development.

VIRUSES

Women encounter numerous viruses during their pregnancies, and their offspring are potentially exposed to additional viral pathogens at the time of delivery or during the first several months of postnatal life.[1] Fortunately, most of these exposures do not result in serious infections of the developing central nervous system (CNS). Certain viruses, nonetheless, display neuroinvasiveness (i.e., the capacity to invade the CNS) or neurovirulence (i.e., the capacity to infect and perturb neural cell function) and therefore pose a potential threat to the young child's neurodevelopment.

Several neuroinvasive and neurovirulent pathogens are linked conceptually by the TORCH (toxoplasmosis, rubella, cytomegalovirus [CMV], herpes simplex virus [HSV]) acronym, a term coined in the early 1970s by investigators at Emory University and the Centers for Disease Control and Prevention in Atlanta, Georgia.[2] Although diagnostic "TORCH titers" have been replaced with more sensitive and precise molecular and virologic detection methods, this useful acronym reminds clinicians that these infectious agents tend to produce similar physical signs and laboratory abnormalities in infected infants. Clinicians must recognize also that several additional viral and nonviral agents,

This work was supported in part by National Institutes of Health grant HD22136.

including *Treponema pallidum* (syphilis), varicella zoster virus (VZV), human immunodeficiency virus (HIV), the nonpolio enteroviruses, lymphocytic chori-omeningitis virus, among others, must be considered in the differential diagnosis of TORCH infections.

Pathogenesis of TORCH Infections

The TORCH agents share several characteristics regarding the pathogenesis of their infections. First, severe CNS or systemic disease after congenital infection tends to be more likely during the primary, or first, maternal infection. Infants born to women who possess antibodies to CMV as a result of previous CMV infections, for example, have much lower rates of microcephaly, sensorineural hearing loss, developmental delay, and cerebral palsy[3] than do infants born to CMV-naive women who experience primary CMV infections during their pregnancies. Similarly, with exceedingly rare exceptions,[4] women who are immune to the rubella virus because of vaccination or natural infection do not give birth to infants with the congenital rubella syndrome (CRS). However, important exceptions to this dogma do exist. HIV-infected women, for example, may transmit HIV during subsequent pregnancies despite the presence of antibodies to this virus.[5]

Second, the chronology of maternal infection with certain viruses influences the probability or spectrum of damage to the developing CNS or other organs. Maternal rubella, for example, produces fetal cataracts and congenital heart lesions when infection occurs before the seventeenth gestational week,[6] whereas rubella infections after 20–24 weeks' gestation tend to be more benign. Similarly, the sequelae of fetal VZV infections are most severe after first-trimester maternal chickenpox, when the risk of fetal VZV embryopathy is 2–3%.[7] By contrast, HIV and HSV infections display little or no relationship among the timing of maternal infection, transmission of the virus to the fetus, and neurologic or systemic outcomes.

Finally, most infants infected with the TORCH pathogens lack physical signs of infection at birth, and so their infections carry favorable prognoses. The most frequent example of this principle is the absence of serious neurodevelopmental sequelae in approximately 90% of the infants with congenital CMV infections.[8] Again, however, exceptions do exist. Infants infected silently with HIV remain at risk for disease activation, and infants with silent CMV infections have a 10–15% risk of subsequent sensorineural hearing loss.[9]

Certain viruses, notably CMV and rubella, produce neurologic sequelae in infected infants as a consequence of congenital infection, whereas perinatal or postnatal infections with these agents typically are not associated with long-term neurologic consequences in full-term, immunocompetent infants. After exposure and infection of a susceptible woman, the viruses causing congenital infection replicate in such maternal tissues as the salivary glands, lymph nodes, liver, and spleen and induce an initial phase of maternal viremia. In nonimmune individuals, this wave of viremia seeds additional target organs, including the placenta, where the viruses replicate, thereby amplifying maternal viremia and facilitating fetal infection. Fetal infection and viremia, in turn, disseminate the virus to numerous fetal tissues, including the retina, cochlea, and brain, where viral replication and host immune responses may cause irreversible tissue damage.

Other viruses, although capable of inducing congenital infection, more typically infect and damage the CNS during perinatal or postnatal infections. Only 5% of neonatal HSV infections reflect congenital acquisition of the virus, whereas the vast majority occur perinatally, as the result of ascending infection during labor or direct contact with infected maternal secretions during delivery.[10] In the typical HSV infection, the virus replicates first at the site of inoculation (skin, conjunctiva, or other mucous membranes), inducing an initial wave of viremia that seeds the CNS or extraneural tissues, especially those of the reticuloendothelial system. Virus replication and host immune responses in the CNS, retina, or other organs may cause irreversible tissue damage, leading to permanent long-term sequelae, including cerebral palsy.

By contrast, HIV can be transmitted to the infant prenatally during maternal viremia, perinatally by contact with infected maternal blood or cervical secretions, or postnatally via breast milk or contaminated blood products, albeit rarely.[5] Each mode of HIV transmission has similar implications for the infected infant, producing HIV infection (i.e., symptomatic HIV disease with primary and secondary CNS complications).

Specific Agents

Cytomegalovirus

Epidemiology CMV infection, the most common congenital viral infection in many regions of the world, remains a major cause of virus-induced cerebral palsy, damaging as many as 1 in 1,000 live-born infants in the United States.[11] CMV, a beta-herpesvirus, resides in human reservoirs and infects humans through exposure to virus-contaminated human secretions or blood products. Annual infection rates range from 2–5% in the general population to 10–20% or more for toddlers in child care, the parents of such children, or persons with multiple sexual partners.[11]

After infection, immunocompetent CMV-infected persons experience a self-limited viremic phase and then shed CMV in saliva, urine, breast milk, semen, and cervical secretions. CMV-infected persons excrete the virus in remarkable quantities—as many as 10^6 infectious particles per milliliter of urine after congenital infection—and for prolonged periods—as long as 1 or more years after acquired infections and up to several years after congenital infections.[11] Reinfection with new CMV strains occurs among children in child-care environments[12] or persons with multiple sexual partners,[11] a process that prolongs virus excretion and enhances the potential for transmission to nonimmune individuals.

Although CMV seroprevalence varies greatly between geographic regions as a function of sociodemographic variables, approximately 40–60% of the women of childbearing age in the United States lack immunity to CMV, indicating that these women are at risk for transmitting the virus to their unborn infants

Table 8.1 Clinical and Laboratory Features of Congenital Cytomegalovirus Infection

Clinical manifestations
  Jaundice
  Petechiae or purpuric rash
  Hepatosplenomegaly
  Microcephaly
  Intrauterine growth retardation
  Chorioretinitis
  Hearing loss
  Seizures
Laboratory and radiographic manifestations
  Thrombocytopenia
  Direct hyperbilirubinemia
  Hemolytic anemia
  Elevated serum transaminases
  Intracranial calcifications
  Intracranial hemorrhage

during primary CMV infections. Such women acquire CMV from their sexual partners or young children. Toddlers, especially those in child-care environments, represent a major source of contagion for their parents and other care providers.[11,12] However, only 30–50% of the offspring become infected during maternal CMV infection,[13] a phenomenon that is not yet satisfactorily explained. Currently, maternal CMV infections cannot be prevented by vaccination.

Clinical Aspects Approximately 90% of congenitally infected infants excrete CMV in their saliva or urine but lack clinical signs of infection. The remaining infants have a constellation of physical and laboratory signs (Table 8.1) that reflect CMV replication in several target organs, including the spleen, liver, retina, cochlea, and brain. Common features consist of hepatosplenomegaly, jaundice, petechiae, direct hyperbilirubinemia, thrombocytopenia, and elevated serum transaminases.[14] Approximately 30–50% of the symptomatic, congenitally infected infants are microcephalic at birth, and 10–20% have ocular abnormalities in the form of chorioretinitis or optic atrophy.[14,15]

The diagnosis of congenital CMV infection is established best by isolating the virus from urine or saliva during the first 3 weeks of life using the shell vial assay.[11] CMV DNA can be detected also in fluids or tissues by using the polymerase chain reaction (PCR).[16] Detecting CMV in samples obtained after the third week of life can reflect congenital, perinatal, or postnatal acquisition of CMV, but these cannot be differentiated easily. Approximately 50% of the symptomatic, congenitally infected infants have intracranial calcifications (Figure 8.1) or other abnormalities, including periventricular leukomalacia, hemorrhage, or migration abnormalities that can be detected by computed tomography (CT), cranial sonography, or magnetic resonance imaging (MRI).[17,18]

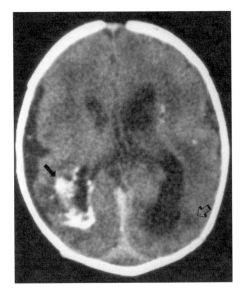

Figure 8.1 Unenhanced computed tomography scan of head of an infant with symptomatic congenital cytomegalovirus infection shows an area of dense periventricular calcifications adjacent to the occipital horn of the lateral ventricle (*solid arrow*), a more subtle area of periventricular leukomalacia (*open arrow*), and a small right cerebral hemisphere. Scattered calcifications also are present in the left hemisphere.

Sequelae Silently infected infants have a 10–15% rate of sensorineural hearing loss but have very low rates of other, more severe neurodevelopmental sequelae. In contrast, approximately 90% of the surviving CMV-infected infants who were symptomatic at birth have long-term neurologic sequelae affecting vision, hearing, intellect, or motor function.[17,19] Sensorineural hearing loss, a common and often progressive complication of congenital CMV infection, ranges from mild and unilateral to profound and bilateral, and approximately 20% of the infected infants have visual dysfunction because of chorioretinitis or optic atrophy. Approximately one-half of the infants who survive symptomatic CMV infections have cerebral palsy, ranging from mild hemiparesis to spastic quadriparesis, and an equivalent proportion suffer mental retardation (IQ <70). Microcephaly and seizures are additional potential sequelae.

In general, infants with abnormal CNS imaging studies, especially CT, are more likely to have severe neurodevelopmental sequelae.[17] However, the precise relationship between neuroimaging abnormalities (e.g., periventricular leukomalacia or migration disturbances) and specific neurologic outcomes (e.g., cerebral palsy) has not been elucidated. At present, no effective means have been developed to prevent or treat congenital CMV infection. Infants with congenital CMV infections should undergo periodic audiologic studies because of the potential for progressive or new-onset hearing loss.

Rubella

Epidemiology The 1964–1965 U.S. rubella epidemic poignantly illustrated the tragic public health consequences of maternal rubella virus infection and the CRS.[20,21] Approximately 20,000 cases of CRS occurred during that massive epi-

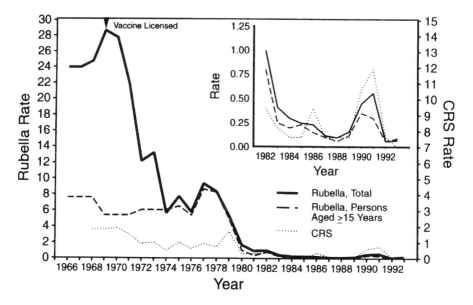

Figure 8.2 The incidence of rubella and congenital rubella syndrome (CRS) in the United States, 1966–1993. (Reprinted from the Centers for Disease Control and Prevention. Rubella and congenital rubella syndrome—United States, January 1, 1991–May 7, 1994. MMWR Morb Mortal Wkly Rep 1994;43:391,397–402.)

demic, and an additional 11,000 cases of fetal loss were attributed to maternal rubella virus infection. After the licensure and widespread use of the rubella vaccine in the late 1960s and early 1970s, however, the incidence of rubella virus infection and CRS in the United States declined dramatically (Figure 8.2). Only 20–70 cases were reported annually to the National CRS Registry during the 1970s and, during the decade of the 1980s, only 67 cases were reported in total.[22]

Despite the success of the vaccination programs, rubella virus remains a potential threat to women of childbearing age, as illustrated by a resurgence of CRS in 1990 and 1991, when 25 and 31 indigenous cases, respectively, were reported in the United States.[23] The indigenous cases occurred predominantly among the offspring of women who declined vaccination on religious grounds, and additional, imported cases were reported after maternal exposures in countries such as Mexico that do not routinely provide rubella vaccination.[22,23] After these outbreaks, the Centers for Disease Control re-emphasized the importance of vaccinating susceptible adolescents and adults in the United States, and many colleges and public school systems have instituted mandatory revaccination programs for students.

Clinical Aspects In general, the probability of sequelae and the severity of the neonatal clinical manifestations of CRS reflect the gestational chronology of maternal rubella virus infection.[6,20] Fetal cataracts or congenital heart disease (patent ductus arteriosus, pulmonary or aortic stenosis, septal defects) are more likely if maternal infection occurs before the twelfth gestational week, when the overall risk of CRS approaches 90%, whereas the critical period for sensorineural hearing loss, the final component of Gregg's original clinical triad,[24] extends through gestational week 24. Additional potential clinical features include intrauterine growth retardation, hepatosplenomegaly, petechial rash, osteopathy, jaundice, microcephaly, and pneumonitis.[20]

The diagnosis of CRS can be established by serologic studies, virus isolation, or reverse transcription-PCR (RT-PCR).[25] Direct hyperbilirubinemia, thrombocytopenia, and elevated serum transaminases are potential laboratory abnormalities. Neuroimaging abnormalities, common among symptomatic infants, consist of subependymal cystic degeneration, intracerebral calcification, cerebral atrophy, and periventricular leukomalacia.[26]

Sequelae Children and adults who survive CRS have substantial rates of cardiac, audiologic, ophthalmologic, and neurodevelopmental sequelae. Most have neurologic abnormalities consisting of mental retardation, microcephaly, language delays, autistic features, behavioral disturbances, or cerebral palsy.[27,28] In a long-term follow-up study, approximately 15% of CRS survivors had spastic diplegia, quadriplegia, or hemiparesis.[29] Two-thirds or more of the survivors have sensorineural hearing loss, the most frequent and, occasionally, progressive complication of CRS.[30] Additional late sequelae of CRS include diabetes, thyroid dysfunction, growth hormone deficiency, and post–rubella infection panencephalitis.[30] No specific antiviral drugs can successfully treat infants with CRS, but the condition can be prevented by vaccinating women of childbearing age.

Herpes Simplex Virus

Epidemiology The annual incidence of neonatal HSV infection in the United States ranges from 1 per 5,000 to 1 per 26,000 live-born infants, amounting to 400–1,000 cases per year.[31] HSV type 2 (HSV-2), typically associated with genital infections, causes approximately two-thirds of the neonatal cases, but only 20% of mothers report histories of genital HSV infection, and only 10% have active lesions at delivery. The remainder of perinatal infections are caused by HSV-1 acquired vertically or by postnatal exposure to individuals who harbor the virus.

Clinical Aspects The syndromes caused by perinatal HSV infections, categorized clinically as (1) skin-eye-mouth (SEM) infection; (2) disseminated infection; and (3) CNS disease, affect approximately 40%, 30%, and 20% of HSV-infected infants, respectively.[32] An additional 5% of HSV-infected infants have congenital disease, a relatively stereotypic disorder characterized by microcephaly, cataracts, intrauterine growth retardation, and vesicular skin lesions.[10] Perinatally infected infants can become symptomatic as early as the first day of life, although SEM and disseminated infections usually present dur-

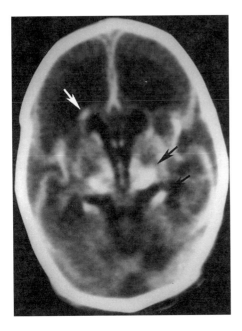

Figure 8.3 Unenhanced computed tomography scan of head of an infant with congenital herpes simplex virus infection shows diffuse encephalomalacia and areas of periventricular and deep calcifications (*black arrows*) as well as a periventricular hyperdensity that may represent hemorrhage or calcification (*white arrow*). (Reprinted with permission from IE Souza, JF Bale Jr. The diagnosis of congenital infection: contemporary strategies. J Child Neurol 1995;10:271–282.)

ing the second week of life, and CNS disease begins during the second and third weeks.

The early clinical manifestations of perinatal HSV infection—pallor, fever, irritability, high-pitched cry, jaundice, and respiratory distress—tend to be nonspecific, thus mimicking perinatal infections with bacteria or other viruses.[33] Skin lesions are common, although the absence of cutaneous abnormalities does not eliminate HSV from consideration. Progressive HSV disease causes multiorgan system dysfunction, including hepatitis, encephalitis, disseminated intravascular coagulopathy, pneumonitis, and death.

Infants with disseminated HSV infections frequently have elevated serum transaminases, direct hyperbilirubinemia, and clotting abnormalities indicative of disseminated intravascular coagulopathy. The cerebrospinal fluid (CSF) in encephalitis usually shows a lymphocytic pleocytosis and an elevated protein content. CT or MRI in acute perinatal HSV encephalitis cases may reveal focal or diffuse brain edema, whereas congenitally infected infants typically have intracranial calcifications and diffuse encephalomalacia (Figure 8.3). Sequential imaging studies frequently reveal cystic encephalomalacia in the survivors of perinatal HSV encephalitis. Electroencephalograms are nearly always abnormal in infants with acute perinatal HSV encephalitis.[34] The diagnosis can be confirmed by isolating HSV from skin, CSF, or mucous membranes, detecting HSV DNA in CSF or other samples, or identifying HSV antigens in skin lesions.

Sequelae Despite appropriate antiviral therapy with acyclovir, mortality rates for perinatal HSV encephalitis or disseminated disease range from 15% to 50%, and survivors have high rates of permanent neurodevelopmental sequelae, seizures, mental retardation, and cerebral palsy, as a consequence of necrotizing encephalitis. In the collaborative antiviral study of neonatal HSV infections, only 36% and 59%, respectively, of treated infants with encephalitis or disseminated disease were developing normally at 1 year of age.[35] By contrast, SEM infections rarely cause death, and nearly all infants affected with this form of the disease develop normally. However, infants with SEM disease and frequent skin relapses, a potential late complication of neonatal infection, have higher rates of neurologic sequelae than do infants with SEM infections who are without recurrent herpetic skin lesions.[35]

Human Immunodeficiency Virus

Epidemiology In the late 1970s and early 1980s, an unusual disease, known now as the acquired immunodeficiency syndrome (AIDS), appeared among homosexual men and intravenous drug users in certain regions of the United States.[36] As the epidemic broadened and heterosexual transmission of the causative agent, HIV, became more frequent, the condition was reported in numerous infants and young children.[5] By the late 1980s, the prevalence of HIV infection among women of childbearing age in the United States ranged from less than 0.2% to more than 3.0%. In certain regions of the world, notably sub-Saharan Africa, rates climbed considerably higher. Consequently, vertical HIV transmission contributes substantially to the morbidity and mortality among children worldwide. In untreated, HIV-infected women, vertical transmission averages 30%, whereas zidovudine treatment, as discussed subsequently, reduces the risk of transmission to approximately 8%.

Clinical Aspects Most HIV-infected infants do not display symptoms during the perinatal period; however, signs attributed to congenital HIV infection include hepatomegaly, splenomegaly, rash, thrombocytopenia, or neonatal meningoencephalitis.[5,37] The typical HIV-infected infant becomes symptomatic after 1 month of age, manifesting hepatomegaly, failure to thrive, interstitial pneumonitis, opportunistic infections, or neurologic disease, although the clinical manifestations often are modified by antimicrobial and antiretroviral therapy of high-risk infants and HIV-infected children.[38] Observations regarding the natural history of HIV infection suggest that a child born infected with HIV has a 50% chance of manifesting severe disease by 5 years of age but also a 75% chance of surviving to 5 years of age.[39]

The diagnosis of HIV infection can be supported in the perinatal period by virus culture, PCR, or p24 antigen assay.[38] Serologic studies have a low specificity in infants, because most infants born to HIV-positive mothers serorevert, indicating passive transfer of maternal antibody.[38] Serial HIV studies may be necessary to confirm infection of the young infant. Infection in the older child or adolescent can be established by HIV serologic tests, analogous to the diagnostic evaluation of adults in whom HIV infection is suspected.

Sequelae Therapeutic advances, such as improved management of opportunistic infections and combination antiretroviral therapy with zidovudine and protease inhibitors or other agents, have improved considerably the outlook for infants and children with perinatally acquired HIV infection. Moreover, perinatal transmission can be reduced substantially by zidovudine treatment of HIV-infected women before and during delivery and treatment of their infants postnatally.[40] Despite these advances, however, HIV infection remains an ominous potential cause of neurodevelopmental sequelae among young children.

Early case series from the United States suggested high rates of neurologic disease among HIV-infected children.[41,42] Progressive encephalopathy, the most distressing CNS complication, leads to acquired microcephaly and cognitive, behavioral, and motor dysfunction, including cerebral palsy. Belman[43] and others observed that HIV-related CNS disease in young children has several modes of clinical presentation, including static or progressive encephalopathy with paraparesis, spastic diplegia, and quadriparesis. CT or MRI scans of HIV-infected children frequently reveal cortical atrophy, white matter abnormalities, or cerebral calcifications involving the basal ganglia or frontal white matter.[44] Currently available data suggest that the prevalence of CNS disease, including motor dysfunction, among HIV-infected infants and children ranges from 10% to 50%,[43] although the spectrum and natural history of CNS disease among vertically infected children is highly variable.

Other Viral Pathogens

Varicella Zoster Virus Varicella embryopathy, an uncommon condition, develops in approximately 2–3% of infants born to nonimmune women who acquire chickenpox during the first trimester.[7,45] Clinical features of this disorder include skin scars (cicatrix), ophthalmologic abnormalities (cataracts, microphthalmia, chorioretinitis, or Horner's syndrome), limb hypoplasia, and cerebral lesions (hydranencephaly, hydrocephalus, or intracranial calcifications similar to those of congenital HSV infection).[45,46] Virologic diagnosis can be difficult postnatally, although VZV-specific IgM can be detected in fetal blood samples obtained by cordocentesis.[47] Infants with varicella embryopathy have high rates of cognitive and motor disabilities, including cerebral palsy.[45,46]

Lymphocytic Choriomeningitis Virus Lymphocytic choriomeningitis virus, a rodent-borne arenavirus, occasionally causes congenital infection in human infants.[48,49] Clinical features include chorioretinopathy, congenital hydrocephalus, microcephaly, or intracranial calcifications (Figure 8.4). The mortality rate among 26 reported cases was 35%, and approximately two-thirds of survivors had neurodevelopmental sequelae, consisting of seizures, visual loss, mental retardation, or cerebral palsy.[49] The incidence of congenital

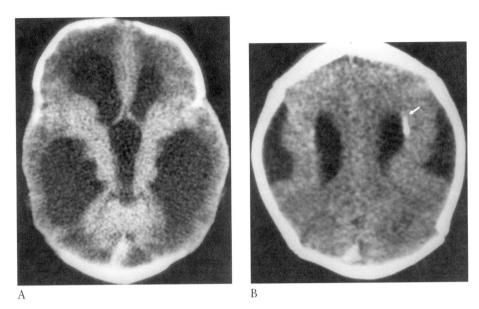

A   B

Figure 8.4 (A) Unenhanced computed tomography scan of head of an infant with congenital lymphocytic choriomeningitis virus infection and macrocephaly shows diffuse ventriculomegaly compatible with aqueductal obstruction. (B) Unenhanced computed tomography scan of head of another infant with congenital lymphocytic choriomeningitis virus infection and microcephaly shows periventricular calcifications (*arrow*) in the left hemisphere, subtle calcifications adjacent to the right lateral ventricle, and bilateral cortical abnormalities compatible with a disturbance of neuronal migration. (Reprinted with permission from R Wright, D Johnson, M Neumann, et al. Congenital lymphocytic choriomeningitis virus syndrome: a disease that mimics congenital toxoplasmosis or cytomegalovirus infection. Pediatrics 1997;100:91–96.)

lymphocytic choriomeningitis virus infection in endemic regions, such as the United States, is unknown and, currently, the diagnosis can be established only by serologic studies.

Nonpolio Enteroviruses During the annual summer and fall enterovirus outbreaks, as many as 10–15% of young infants may acquire enteroviral disease.[50] Although most infected infants are asymptomatic or have benign systemic illnesses or aseptic meningitis, nonpolio enteroviruses can cause life-threatening disease as a consequence of myocarditis, hepatitis, or encephalitis. Common clinical manifestations of enteroviral infections include fever, diarrhea, abdominal distention, irritability, and nonvesicular rash.[51] The diagnosis can be confirmed by isolating enteroviruses from stool or nasopharyngeal secretions or by detecting enteroviral RNA in CSF or stool by using RT-PCR.[52] Despite the potential acute neurologic complications, including seizures, survivors have very low rates of cerebral palsy or other neurodevelopmental sequelae.[53,54]

Parasites A limited number of parasites can infect and damage the CNS of the developing fetus and young infant. *Toxoplasma gondii*, the most notable of these, represents a major potential cause of permanent developmental and visual abnormalities and cerebral palsy among children born in many regions of the world. In certain highly endemic regions, such as France, screening and intervention programs have been instituted to reduce the neurodevelopmental sequelae of *T. gondii* infection. In addition, advances in postnatal therapy may improve outcome for infants with symptomatic congenital toxoplasmosis.

Trypanosoma cruzi, the causative agent of Chagas' disease, produces a congenital syndrome that resembles congenital infection with CMV or *T. gondii*.[55] Although this disorder appears to have adverse neurodevelopmental consequences for the young infant, the clinical spectrum and long-term outcome of congenital *T. cruzi* infection are less well-defined than for congenital toxoplasmosis.

Because of its prevalence worldwide, we will detail here the clinical spectrum and treatment options for *T. gondii* infection. *T. gondii*, an intracellular parasite, is maintained in mammal and bird reservoirs throughout the world. Infected domestic and wild felines, the definitive hosts, excrete immense quantities of oocysts, the extracorporeal and potentially infectious form of the parasite, which, depending on ambient conditions, can remain viable in soils for extended periods.[56,57]

Humans, an incidental but susceptible host, become infected by consuming contaminated foodstuffs (undercooked meats or unwashed raw fruits and vegetables) or by direct ingestion of sporulated oocysts (the infectious form) that were deposited in soils or other materials by cats harboring the parasite. Cat ownership has been highly associated with acquisition of *T. gondii* by children and adolescents,[58] whereas studies in other populations, such as those with AIDS, suggest that cat ownership may not increase the risk of *T. gondii* infection.[59] After human ingestion, infectious organisms, released during digestion in the gastrointestinal tract, penetrate the intestinal epithelium and enter blood vessels, which disseminate *Toxoplasma* to many tissues, including the placentas of pregnant women.

The incidence of maternal *T. gondii* infection during pregnancy ranges from approximately 1 per 1,000 or less in the United States and Norway,[60] which are low- to moderate-risk regions, to as great as 10 per 1,000 in France, a highly endemic area.[61] Most maternal infections occur without producing symptoms, although some immunocompetent women experience an infectious mononucleosis–like disorder with malaise, fever, lymphadenopathy, and hepatosplenomegaly.[57] Severe fetal infections result from primary maternal infections during the first or second trimesters, but women with AIDS can reactivate *T. gondii* and transmit the organism to the fetus. In the United States, as many as 3,000 infants with congenital toxoplasmosis are born annually.

Infants with congenital toxoplasmosis resemble those with congenital CMV infection (hence, the TORCH acronym) and display jaundice, hepatosplenomegaly, intrauterine growth retardation, and petechial or purpuric skin rash.[56] Chorioretinitis affects 30–75% of the infants with congenital toxoplasmosis, as compared to approximately 20% in congenital CMV.[15,62] Macrocrania due to communicating or obstructive hydrocephalus also occurs more commonly in congenital toxoplasmosis, whereas infants with congenital CMV more frequently exhibit microcephaly. Laboratory studies reveal thrombocytopenia, direct hyperbilirubinemia, and elevated levels of serum transaminases, analogous to those seen in disseminated viral infections.[56] Cranial CT in infants with congenital toxoplasmosis demonstrates intracranial calcifications, hydrocephalus, or cystic changes.[63]

The diagnosis of congenital toxoplasmosis currently depends on the detection of *T. gondii*–specific IgM in neonatal serum samples or persistently high levels of IgG in the infant's serum or CSF.[58] PCR can be used to detect *T. gondii* DNA in clinical samples, including amniotic fluid, although routine application of this technique to the diagnosis of congenital infection requires additional clinical evaluation of its sensitivity and specificity.[64] Prenatal diagnosis can be achieved by fetal serologic studies, PCR of amniotic fluid, and fetal ultrasonography.[65,66] Maternal antitoxoplasma therapy, using agents such as spiramycin (an investigational drug in the United States available from the U.S. Food and Drug Administration), or pregnancy termination has successfully prevented symptomatic congenital infection.[65,66] No vaccine is currently available to prevent maternal infection.

Prospective studies indicate that aggressive, prolonged postnatal therapy benefits infants with symptomatic congenital toxoplasmosis.[67,68] Current regimens suggest that infants with signs of congenital infection, especially those with neurologic abnormalities, should receive pyrimethamine and sulfadiazine for approximately 12 months postnatally. Progressive hydrocephalus requires ventriculoperitoneal diversion. Before current treatment regimens became available, 80%, 70%, and 85% of congenitally infected infants had seizures, motor abnormalities (including cerebral palsy), and mental retardation, respectively. Current management strategies reduce the proportion of infants with these sequelae to 30% or less per category.

NEONATAL BACTERIAL MENINGITIS

Bacterial meningitis in the first month after birth continues to be an important cause of chronic neurologic disability in the form of cerebral palsy. The remarkable virulence of the infection in this age group is accounted for by multiple factors, including the necrotizing effects of many of the causative organisms and their predisposition to provoke an intense vasculitis, the structural and chemical immaturity of the brain in early infancy, the immaturity of the immune mechanisms that protect against infection, and the nonspecific character of signs of sepsis and meningitis encountered at this age, which can delay diagnosis. Although the mortality rate of neonatal meningitis has declined gradually in the past three decades, approximately 30–50% of survivors will suffer some degree of permanent impairment of neurologic function.

In the vast majority of affected neonates, meningitis is a consequence of bacteremia or septicemia and thus, the suspicion or documentation of sepsis in the neonate warrants a search for meningitis by CSF examination. In an extensive study at Yale, the rate of occurrence of neonatal sepsis between 1979 and 1988 was found to be 2.7 cases per 1,000 live births, and the mortality rate from sepsis was 15.9%.[69] Bacterial sepsis in the neonate will be complicated by meningitis in at least 25% of cases.[70] Male infants are affected considerably more often than are female infants, and numerous predisposing conditions include low birth weight, maternal bacterial infection in the last month of pregnancy, and the need for intensive care management with respiratory support and indwelling vascular lines. The presence or absence of such protective techniques within a nursery as proper hand washing, appropriate isolation methods, and ongoing surveillance protocols are additional factors that can affect the incidence of nursery invasive infections.

Currently, *Staphylococcus epidermidis*, followed by group B streptococci, *Escherichia coli*, and *Klebsiella* species, is the leading cause of neonatal septic disease. Numerous other gram-negative enteric bacilli, *Enterococcus* species, *Listeria monocytogenes*, *Staphylococcus aureus*, and anaerobes, especially *Bacteroides fragilis*, account for occasional cases of neonatal sepsis or meningitis. The manner in which the etiologic causes of neonatal sepsis have changed over time reflects the impact of such medical measures as the introduction of antibiotics and, more recently, the development of neonatal intensive care. Freedman and colleagues,[71] at one large medical center, were able to study positive blood cultures obtained from neonates beginning as early as 1928. Their study revealed that in the 1930s and early 1940s, group A streptococci were the leading cause of sepsis in the infant, replaced by gram-negative coliform bacilli in the late 1940s and extending into the 1950s. Thus, the emergence of gram-negative organisms as a major cause of disease corresponded with the introduction of antibiotics into clinical medicine. This relationship was especially notable relative to *Pseudomonas aeruginosa*, which was virtually unrecognized as a pathogen before the mid-1940s. Between 1954 and 1958, *Staphylococcus* species emerged as a major neonatal pathogen, an event seemingly controlled by routine bathing of the neonate with hexachlorophene. Gram-negative organisms again became predominant until 1964, when group B streptococci were recognized as the leading cause of neonatal sepsis, a position that these organisms have retained to the present time.

Diagnosis of neonatal meningitis in most cases amounts to suspecting the possibility whenever sepsis is considered or is proved. Exceptions include the occurrence of seizures or the appearance of signs of raised intracranial pressure. Temperature instability is a frequent sign in the infant with sepsis or meningitis, especially with early-onset group B streptococcal sepsis, in which hypothermia is more common than fever. Fever, which is defined as temperature in excess of 37°C, should always suggest that a bacterial infection is present in neonates, as approximately 10% of febrile neonates will have positive bacterial cultures.[72] Age and degree of maturity of the infant at the onset of pyogenic meningitis are major determining factors relative to presenting clinical signs. The low-birth-weight neonate with early-onset group B streptococcal disease usually will exhibit respiratory distress, hypothermia, and neutropenia. The full-term infant with meningitis at 2–4 weeks of age is more likely to be febrile and to have signs recognizable as those of neurologic dysfunction. Irritability, lethargy, diminished feeding, vomiting, and seizures are common under these circumstances. The degree of tension at the anterior fontanelle is variable, whereas neck stiffness often is not part of the clinical presentation.

Neuropathologic Features

The neuropathologic features of neonatal meningitis vary, depending on numerous factors. The pathologic findings change, often dramatically, as the illness progresses.[73] When the offending organism is highly sensitive to antibiotics and with onset of treatment in the early stages of the condition, the neuropathologic changes may be minimal and consist only of a leptomeningeal exudate and brain swelling. However, this "mild" presentation is unusual with neonatal meningitis. The causative organism and the associated systemic complications, especially cardiorespiratory effects, can greatly affect the types of anatomic injury. For example, with early-onset group B streptococcal sepsis with meningitis, the meningeal inflammatory response may be relatively mild, but severe brain injury can result from shock and hypoxic-ischemic changes.

Certain organisms that cause neonatal meningitis are notable for their predisposition to cause an intense inflammatory vasculitis, leading to either small- or large-vessel obstruction and infarctions (Figure 8.5). These softened areas of brain are invaded rapidly by bacteria, causing the development of infected, necrotizing lesions that undergo liquefaction and then cavitation. This pathologic sequence is especially notable with meningitis caused by *Proteus*, *Enterobacter*, *Serratia*, and *Citrobacter* species. With any of the gram-negative bacillary organisms, ventriculitis and necrotizing destruction of the ependyma can lead to widespread subependymal necrosis, which often becomes hemorrhagic (Figure 8.6). Ventriculitis is characteristic of severe gram-negative bacillary meningitis and refers to abundant exudate within the ventricular system. The associated ependymal injury within the narrow aqueduct of Sylvius or the inflammatory exudate that leads to adhesive arachnoiditis at the outlet foramina of the posterior fossa compounds the process by inciting rapidly progressive hydrocephalus and further damage to the ventricular ependyma and the periventricular tissue. As a result of ventriculitis or ependymitis, septations will bridge the ependymal surfaces and can compartmentalize the ventricle.[74,75] With progressive hydrocephalus, ventricular loculations of this type make diversionary shunting very difficult, because multiple expanding cavities (rather than simply the two lateral ventricles) now are present that require decompression (Figure 8.7).

In particularly severe infections, the infected ventricular fluid can become frank pus, essentially forming an abscess within the ventricular lumen, a state referred to as *pyoventriculitis*. Survival is not common in the face of pyoventriculitis but, should patients survive, all will be left with sequelae, including hydrocephalus.

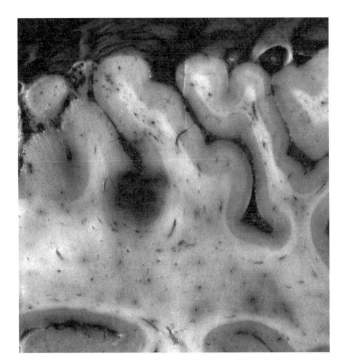

Figure 8.5 Septic cortical vein thrombosis complicating bacterial meningitis. The brain is congested, and a circular hemorrhagic cortical infarct is seen.

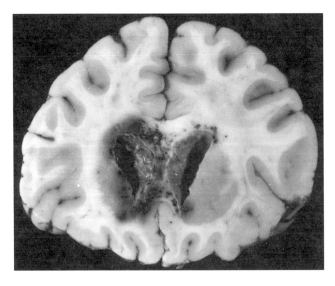

Figure 8.6 Periventricular hemorrhagic necrosis secondary to ventriculitis and ependymitis caused by gram-negative enteric bacilli.

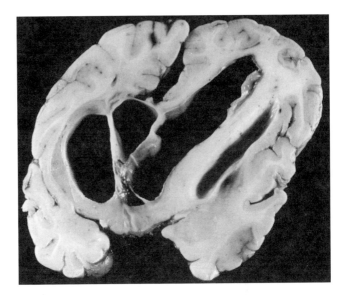

Figure 8.7 Late effects of neonatal gram-negative bacillary meningitis and ventriculitis. The lateral ventricles are enlarged owing to obstruction in the aqueduct. Fibrous septations have developed within one lateral ventricle, compartmentalizing its cavity.

Cerebral cortical and cerebellar changes can be mild in neonatal meningitis or, in more severe cases, can include extensive neuronal damage, sometimes to the point of cortical laminar necrosis followed by progressive gliosis. Whatever the pathologic findings in a given case, the primary causes of brain injury in neonatal meningitis include the abundant leptomeningeal and ventricular exudates, the pressure effects on brain and its major venous channels from hydrocephalus, the inflammatory vasculitis (which can affect both arterial and venous structures), the "toxic" encephalopathic injury to the cortex and subependymal tissues (stemming from the purulent exudate) and, in some instances, the associated cardiorespiratory effects brought about by systemic septicemia.

Neuroimaging

Neuroimaging examinations in the neonate with pyogenic meningitis can be useful in many ways and have enhanced our ability to anticipate sequelae after the illness. Ultrasonography in this setting has its greatest value in providing a rapid and noninvasive method of assessing ventricle size. Ultrasound study also can identify many types of intraventricular and periventricular pathologic processes that are far more common in the neonate with meningitis than in the older infant or child with this disease. Ongoing suppurative infection within the ventricle, so-called ventriculitis, can be visualized on the basis of ventricular septations, increased echogenicity of fluid within the ventricular space, and irregularity and increased echogenic appearance of the ependymal wall.[76] In some instances, with unyielding or relapsing infection, ultrasonographic findings of marked irregularity of the choroid plexus or increased echogenicity of the

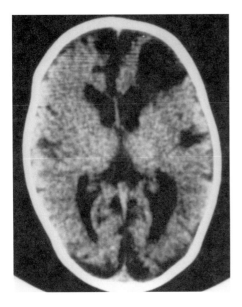

Figure 8.8 Computed tomography performed 8 weeks after onset of group B streptococcal meningitis. Mild ventricular enlargement is secondary to atrophic cerebral changes and not pressure-related hydrocephalus. Some surface subarachnoid spaces are enlarged, especially at the midline. The left frontal infarcted area is the site of a hemorrhagic, venous infarct seen during the acute stage of the illness.

subependymal brain parenchyma, indicating hemorrhagic necrosis, probably will explain the locus of the persisting infection.

CT in the early stage of neonatal meningitis often is normal or reveals some degree of cerebral swelling with small or collapsed lateral ventricles. Over time, in more severe cases, CT scans can reveal periventricular hemorrhagic necrosis or vascular complications in the form of either arterial or venous infarcts, the latter often being hemorrhagic in appearance (Figure 8.8). Occipital infarcts are especially common in severe cases of meningitis and usually predict the probability of some degree of cortical visual loss as a complication of the illness. CT rarely is diagnostic of either the presence of meningitis in the neonate or of the causative organism. The one exception is the presence of multiple, large abscesses with ring enhancement, seen on CT soon after meningitis has been diagnosed in a neonate; this finding usually predicts that the illness is caused by *Citrobacter* species. Less often, *Serratia marcescens*, *Enterobacter* species, or *Proteus* species will cause similar lesions (Figure 8.9).

Both CT and MRI generally will reveal similar findings, although whatever is seen on CT can usually be visualized better and in more detail by MRI. MRI with enhancement is especially effective at revealing so-called ependymal sheathing, which is seen commonly with pyogenic ventriculitis (Figure 8.10). MRI will demonstrate infarcts earlier than will CT and can reveal granulomatous changes in the subarachnoid space far better than can CT. Whereas both modalities can be important in some cases in the early stages of meningitis, their role in demonstrating the long-term anatomic sequelae of infection is at least as important.

Because CT is a more rapidly obtained study and allows for easier monitoring of the patient during its performance, this method usually is preferred in

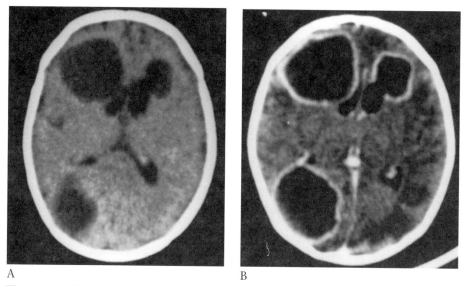

A   B

Figure 8.9   Computed tomography without (A) and with (B) contrast enhancement. Neonatal *Citrobacter* meningitis showing multiple, large, ring-enhancing abscesses.

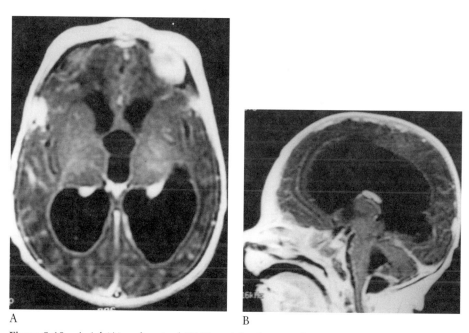

A   B

Figure 8.10   Axial (A) and sagittal (B) T$_1$-weighted magnetic resonance imaging in neonatal *Mycoplasma hominis* meningitis. The hyperintense signal arising from the ependyma on the axial view indicates ependymitis. The axial view shows a distended fourth ventricle immediately superior to an extra-axial fluid collection. Obstruction with granulomatous changes of the level of the outlet foramina of the fourth ventricle results in advanced hydrocephalus.

the early stages of neonatal meningitis. Later, when more detail is desired and the patient is more stable, MRI becomes preferable. Although all infants with meningitis do not absolutely require neuroimaging examinations, those who do not respond to treatment as expected, those with marked depression in state of responsiveness, infants with seizures or focal neurologic signs, and infants with obvious signs of increased intracranial pressure are candidates for such evaluations. Another important role played by neuroimaging techniques, especially MRI, is to allow discovery of anatomic defects that predispose to the occurrence of meningitis in infancy. These types of predisposing defects either are recognized on physical examination or are suspected when unusual organisms are found to be the cause of meningitis. Such unusual organisms include *S. aureus* in the nonshunted child or *Proteus* species in a person of any age. MRI is far more versatile than is CT in identifying lesions that allow CSF communication with the external environment or the intestinal tract. Among these lesions are congenital defects of the floor of the anterior fossa, basal meningoceles, a dermal sinus terminating in a posterior fossa dermoid cyst, neuroenteric sinuses extending to the CSF, and spinal dermal sinuses.

Sequelae

Somewhere between 30% and 50% of survivors of neonatal meningitis will experience permanent neurologic or visual sequelae. In general, the prognosis pertaining to both mortality and morbidity is better with gram-positive than with gram-negative neonatal meningitis, although exceptions are common when individual cases are considered. The outcome of early-onset group B streptococcal disease, predominantly a fulminating septic condition usually associated with pulmonary involvement, is less favorable as compared to late-onset disease, which is manifested chiefly by meningitis.[77]

Certain aspects of each case of meningitis in the newborn infant can have prognostic implications, although these vary widely. For example, septic shock in the neonate with meningitis portends a poor outcome. Outcome is generally poor also if depression of responsiveness is marked or if recurrent and unyielding seizures are seen during the illness. A very high CSF protein content (e.g., 500 mg/dl or greater) in the acute stage of disease indicates the presence of a severe inflammatory reaction that is likely to be complicated by hydrocephalus and ependymal injury. Definite parenchymal injury (including infarcts) seen on CT or MRI generally indicates a higher probability of some degree of permanent sequelae.

Postmeningitic hydrocephalus cannot always be managed successfully, in part because of high CSF protein content and in part because of ventricular septations and compartmentalization. Limbic, thalamic, and cerebral cortical injury leads to learning disabilities and behavioral abnormalities, which frequently are exacerbated by visual or hearing deficiencies. Shock from sepsis or vasculitis with infarction occasionally will cause hypothalamic damage, followed by a variety of clinical conditions such as hyperphagia and obesity, loss of the thirst mechanism with severe electrolyte disorder, abnormalities in antidiuretic hormone secretion, and precocious puberty.

Specific Pathogenic Types

Neonatal Gram-Negative Bacillary Meningitis

The etiologic picture of gram-negative bacillary meningitis is well-defined: This type of bacterial meningitis is seen in neonates, complicating neurosurgical operative procedures and craniocerebral trauma, secondary to dermal sinuses in the lumbosacral region and, less commonly, in chronically debilitated or immunosuppressed children or adults.[78] In the United States, its incidence in the newborn period is second only to group B streptococcal meningitis. In many parts of northern Europe, *E. coli* is the most common cause of neonatal meningitis, whereas in certain regions in the Middle East and northern Africa, *Salmonella* species are the leading cause of neonatal meningitis. Among the Enterobacteriaceae, *E. coli* is the prototype and the most common organism that gives rise to neonatal meningitis. In a large series of cases of gram-negative bacillary meningitis in infants and children reported by Unhanand and colleagues,[79] 53% were caused by *E. coli*, 16% by *Klebsiella-Enterobacter* species, 9% by *Citrobacter diversus*, 9% by *Salmonella* species, and 4% by *Proteus* species.

Other members of the Enterobacteriaceae that uncommonly can cause neonatal meningitis include *Pseudomonas* species, *S. marcescens*, and *Acinetobacter* calcoaceticus. Most cases of *E. coli* neonatal meningitis stem from vertical transmission of the organism from the mother. *Klebsiella* meningitis in the neonate usually has different epidemiologic factors compared to *E. coli*. As can *Proteus* and *Pseudomonas* species, *Klebsiella* species can contaminate suctioning and respiratory equipment, isolettes, and other neonatal intensive care unit equipment used to care for sick neonates. Clinically ill neonates who require ventilation, instrumentation, and antibiotic treatment, as well as those who have necrotizing enterocolitis, are predisposed to invasive infection by *Klebsiella* species.[80] Contaminated breast milk used to feed premature neonates has also been a source of this infection.[81]

E. coli is the most common of the gram-negative pathogens to cause meningitis in the neonate. More than 80% of *E. coli* strains that cause neonatal meningitis possess the K1 capsular polysaccharide antigen, as opposed to only 12% of *E. coli* strains isolated from stools of the normal neonate.[82] The presence of this capsular antigen confers increased virulence to the organism and, perhaps, enhances its ability to gain entrance into the CSF.

E. coli neonatal meningitis is usually a sporadic illness, although nursery outbreaks, in which the organism probably is transmitted from infant to infant by the hands of attendants, have been described.[83] Unlike the early-onset form of group B streptococcal meningitis, in which the neonate usually is clinically ill within 48 hours after birth, *E. coli* meningitis most often appears between 4 and 10 days after birth, although it can begin earlier or as late as 6 weeks. Delayed onset of meningitis until 3–5 weeks after birth is notable in sick neonates of very low birth weight, in whom the signs of meningeal infection can be especially deceptive.[84]

Risk factors predisposing a neonate to *E. coli* meningitis have been outlined by Mulder and colleagues[85] in their study of 132 cases. They found that risk factors were present in 63% of cases and included maternal urinary tract infections during the last month of gestation, prolonged rupture of membranes, obstetric abnormalities during delivery, congenital defects in the neonate and, especially, low birth weight. Among the infants in this series with neonatal *E. coli* meningitis, 42% weighed less than 2,500 g at birth. The case fatality rate was 36% among the low-birth-weight infected infants, as compared to a fatality rate of 18% in those born at term and weighing more than 2,500 g at birth. The other factor associated with an enhanced mortality rate was the onset of signs of meningitis in the first 2 days after birth.

Treatment of gram-negative bacillary meningitis in the neonate is determined by the specific organism isolated from blood, CSF, or urine, and the sensitivities of the organism. Cefotaxime, in combination with an aminoglycoside, is the usual initial choice, with alterations being made once the organism is identified and studied. Intrathecal or intraventricular antibiotics have not been shown to be beneficial and may contribute to sequelae. Three weeks of intravenous antibiotic therapy is the norm. The response to treatment is evaluated by periodic CSF examinations and, in some instances, by neuroimaging examinations. As with any type of neonatal pyogenic meningitis, evidence of progressive ventricular enlargement secondary to hydrocephalus must be sought, as this condition may require some form of diversionary treatment. The need for shunting depends not only on evidence of ventricular enlargement but also on some evidence that the enlargement is the result of increased intraventricular pressure. This evidence usually takes the form of an abnormal rate of head enlargement, progressive spreading of the cranial sutures, or increasing tension of the fontanelle. With severe meningitis, brain injury sometimes will be followed by ventricular enlargement in the absence of a pressure effect and need not be shunted.

Neonatal *Citrobacter* Meningitis

Citrobacter species are facultative gram-negative bacilli that, because of biochemical similarities, are grouped together as *Citrobacter-Salmonella-Arizona*. In past years, *Citrobacter* species, along with *Enterobacter* species, were included among an ill-defined group of gram-negative organisms called *paracolon bacilli*. *Citrobacter* species sometimes are found as part of the normal intestinal flora of humans but are infrequent causes of invasive disease in neonates or young infants. In adults, *Citrobacter* species occasionally are isolated from debilitated elderly patients and immunosuppressed persons with sepsis, urinary tract infection, osteomyelitis, and respiratory infection.[86] Most neonatal *Citrobacter* infections involve *Citrobacter diversus* and the remainder involve *Citrobacter freundii*.

Neonatal meningitis caused by *C. diversus* is a blood-borne infection; the neonate usually acquires the organism during the birth process or, less often, by nosocomial transmission in the nursery.[87] Infection in the infant in the initial weeks after birth usually takes the form of meningitis. The remarkable aspect of the illness, however, is the high frequency with which multiple large brain abscesses are found on neuroimaging examinations.[88] The clinical manifestations of this illness are those of acute meningitis beginning in the first few weeks of life; few signs are present to predict the multiple large lesions discovered on CT or MRI. Much less often, even the signs of sepsis or meningitis remain subtle, and the clinical presentation is that of rapidly progressive head enlargement days or weeks after birth.[89] Progressive hydrocephalus is assumed in such cases until neuroimaging examination reveals multiple, rim-enhancing abscesses. Graham and Band[90] reviewed 53 cases of neonatal *C. diversus* meningitis and found that brain abscess had developed in 41 (71%). This finding on CT or MRI is strongly suggestive of *Citrobacter* species infection, although similar lesions in the neonate have been seen with *S. marcescens* infection[91] and with *Enterobacter* species infection.[92]

The rapidity with which abscess formation in brain evolves in neonates with *Citrobacter* sepsis or meningitis suggests that localized areas of pus formation are preceded by infarctions followed by tissue necrosis which becomes infected and then liquefied.[93] As a result, infants with *C. diversus* meningitis have a fatality rate of at least 30%, and a high percentage of survivors are left with permanent and severe neurologic and visual disabilities.

Sepsis that provokes necrotizing cerebral vasculitis and leads to multiple areas of white matter necrosis also is postulated in the reported cases of neonatal brain abscesses attributed to *Proteus mirabilis*.[94,95] The literature makes clear that brain abscess in the neonate, as compared to brain abscess in the older child or adult, is more likely to be caused by gram-negative bacilli. The lesions are more likely to be multiple and to have become very large before they are identified. Most strikingly, brain abscess develops much more rapidly in the neonate than in the older child or the adult, which probably reflects the different pathogenesis of brain abscess in the neonate as compared to the more mature individual.

Group B Streptococcal Meningitis

In 1933, Rebecca Lancefield included group B streptococci among the five serogroups she recognized on the basis of cell wall carbohydrates.[96] The group B isolates were derived from cases of bovine mastitis, and the organism was assumed to be nonpathogenic to humans. In 1938, Fry[97] in London reported three fatal cases of puerperal sepsis caused by group B streptococci, thereby establishing its role as a human pathogen. The organism emerged as a decided menace to the neonate and young infant with the publication by Eickhoff and colleagues[98] in Boston in 1964. Over an 18-month period, these authors found that group B streptococci had become the single most common cause of neonatal sepsis, exceeding the role held before that time by *E. coli*.

Death and chronic encephalopathy with long-term neurologic disabilities have continued to be caused by this disease throughout the past three decades, even though the mortality rate has decreased considerably with advances in neonatal care. Preventive methods have been updated, which should further improve outcome.[99]

Incidence and Transmission Early-onset group B streptococcal sepsis is a consequence of vertical transmission of the organism from mother to child during parturition. Although the greatest degree of exposure of the fetus to the bacterium occurs during vaginal delivery, birth by cesarean section is not entirely protective.[100] The organism has been found to colonize the anogenital tract in 4–29% of women in the late stages of pregnancy, accounting for the frequent colonization of the neonate. Asymptomatic colonization of the neonate is estimated to be 100 times more common than neonatal invasive infection, assuming that the mother is asymptomatically colonized. Invasive maternal pelvic infection at the time of delivery has far greater consequences for the neonate. The incidence of neonatal invasive infection varies from 1.3 to 4 per 1,000 live births,[101] and the early-onset form of the illness is two to three times more common than is the late-onset type.

A variety of risk factors have been identified that predispose the neonate to the early-onset type of invasive disease. Among these factors are prematurity, prolonged rupture of the fetal membranes, high inoculum with the organism in the maternal anogenital tract, and low or absent levels of type-specific antibody in maternal serum.[102] Protection of the neonate against group B streptococcal infection is believed to be afforded by antibody-mediated phagocytosis. Although maternal asymptomatic colonization is associated with antibody production, titers often are low and, thus, nonprotective. Vogel and associates[103] found that only 9% of pregnant women had any measurable antibody against all four types of group B streptococci, and 45% had antibody against serogroup III, the type responsible for the great majority of cases of neonatal meningitis of either the early- or late-onset variety. Because IgG antibody is poorly transmitted across the placenta before 34 weeks' gestation, premature infants born before the thirty-fourth gestational week are predisposed to the illness, regardless of the level of the maternal antibody titer. Group B streptococci (*S. agalactiae*) have been divided into five serotypes (Ia, b, and c; II; III), any of which can cause neonatal disease, although most of the late-onset cases are due to serogroup III and most of the early-onset cases of sepsis with meningitis are the result of the same serotype.

Clinical Aspects Group B streptococcal infections in the neonate present in two reasonably distinguishable clinical patterns. The more common early-onset illness occurs between birth and 7 days and is primarily a septic infection with a potentially fulminating course. Clinical features often resemble gram-negative sepsis, suggesting an endotoxinlike pathogenesis. The incidence of meningitis among neonates with the early-onset illness was initially believed to be as high as 30%, although more recent data suggest that it might be as low as 6.3%.[104] The late-onset form is seen from 7 days up to 6–8 weeks after birth and is predominantly a meningitic infection, although occasionally a shocklike state will occur soon after the first symptoms appear. Thus, the clinical spectrum of group B streptococcal infection in infancy is the reverse of those infections caused by *Haemophilus influenzae* and *Neisseria meningitidis*, in which the infant is relatively protected by transplacental maternal antibody for the first 2 months of life and infection becomes more common thereafter. A partial explanation for this difference is provided by the frequent exposure of the neonate to group B streptococci during the birth process, an unlikely occurrence with the other organisms cited here.

Regardless of the time of onset of group B streptococcal infection, when meningitis occurs, it usually is caused by serogroup III organisms. Among those infants with early-onset disease, serogroup III accounted for 80% of cases associated with meningitis, whereas in the late-onset group with meningitis, 93% of cases were due to serogroup III organisms.[105] Infants with early-onset disease are almost always infected with the same serotype as is harbored by the mother, indicating direct transmission of the organism from the mother to the infant. Unlike those with late-onset disease, a high percentage of neonates with early-onset sepsis are born of mothers who experience obstetric complications, including maternal fever, chorioamnionitis, and prolonged rupture of membranes.[106] The mean age at onset of clinical signs in the early-onset type of disease is 20 hours after birth, although some neonates are ill almost immediately after birth and most show signs of illness by 48 hours.[101]

Progressive respiratory compromise, apnea, lethargy, and signs of poor tissue perfusion are usual initial features of the septic illness. Some infants will be febrile, although hypothermia is more typical and frequently is accompanied by neutropenia. In those with respiratory distress, the chest radiograph can be indistinguishable from respiratory distress syndrome (hyaline membrane disease) or can show localized infiltrates that are more suggestive of pneumonia. A subset of infants with early-onset infection will present with progressive cyanosis, apnea, hypoxemia, and metabolic acidosis, manifestations indicative of persistent fetal circulation with sustained increase in pulmonary vascular resistance.[107] Among infants with meningitis, the process sometimes is identified by the finding of abnormal CSF obtained because of clinical evidence of sepsis or because of signs suggestive of meningeal involvement, such as seizures or a full fontanelle.

Early-onset group B streptococcal sepsis, with or without meningitis, is always assumed to be a potentially serious illness. During the 1960s and 1970s, the case fatality rate generally was placed at approximately 50%,[108] whereas more recent studies indicate a much better outcome, with mortality as low as 14%.[104]

Late-onset group B streptococcal infection presents after 7 days postnatally, with a mean age of onset of 3 weeks. This illness infrequently is preceded by maternal obstetric complications and, though a blood-borne infection, usually presents with manifestations of acute meningitis. The source of the infectious agent is less clear as compared to the early-onset form of disease, although nosocomial and community transmission are believed to be responsible.[109]

Infants with late-onset group B streptococcal meningitis generally are less ill at onset than are their early-onset counterparts. Fever, irritability, poor feeding, vomiting, lethargy, full fontanelle, and the occurrence of a seizure are the common initial manifestations of this form of the disease. The survival rate is higher with the late-onset type, although the risk of mortality or permanent sequelae increases in those who present with coma, shock, or prolonged seizures.

An infrequent but widely recognized danger in treating an infant with meningitis caused by group B streptococci is the possibility of relapsing infection during or soon after antibiotic therapy. Relapsing infection probably increases the risk of long-term sequelae, although this is not well documented. With both the early- and late-onset forms, diagnosis is confirmed by isolation of the organism from blood or CSF. The latex agglutination test applied to urine, blood, or CSF has a useful role, although false-positive results diminish its value.

Long-Term Sequelae Although the mortality rate associated with group B streptococcal meningitis has been lower over the past three decades than that associated with gram-negative bacillary meningitis in the neonate, comparison of the incidence of neurologic sequelae in survivors is difficult. With either type of infection, similar neurologic disabilities ensue. In the early years after group B streptococcal meningitis became prevalent, survivors with group B streptococcal meningitis were reported to suffer fewer permanent neurologic sequelae than did those with gram-negative bacillary meningitis.[110] This claim became less supportable over time.

More recent follow-up evaluations show that the outcomes are comparable or that, perhaps, infants with group B streptococcal meningitis experience a higher rate of sequelae than do those with gram-negative bacillary meningitis. Among 38 survivors of meningitis caused by group B streptococci, Edwards and colleagues[111] found that only 50% had no disabilities, whereas 21% had mild or moderate neurologic deficits and 29% had major neurologic sequelae. As expected, coma, shock, or neutropenia in the acute stage were risk factors for a poor outcome.

Lasting neurologic disabilities vary in both pattern and severity. The most common long-term abnormalities include mental retardation, behavior problems, seizures, vision loss, deafness, spastic quadriparesis, and hydrocephalus. One interesting and unusual type of disability stems from severe hypothalamic-pituitary injury,[112] secondary to either inflammatory damage or hypoperfusion as part of the shock state. Infants affected in this fashion can exhibit diabetes insipidus during the acute illness, to be followed by pituitary hormonal insufficiency, profound temperature dysregulation, disturbances of the thirst mechanism that result in serum hyperosmolarity, and hyperphagia, which leads to overt obesity. Infants with severe hypothalamic-pituitary injury can be expected to have other diffuse and multifocal brain injuries, usually associated with visual loss, mental retardation, and microcephaly.

Neonatal Listeriosis

Listeria monocytogenes is a gram-positive rod that has variable gram-staining characteristics and has been confused with nonpathogenic diphtheroids on Gram's staining of clinical specimens. The organism is widely distributed in nature, being present in a variety of food substances such as raw vegetables, milk, poultry, fish, and cheeses. Human infection from consumption of contaminated foods has become widely recognized in the past decade. Invasive infection with *L. monocytogenes* usually occurs at the extremes of life (i.e., the elderly, the fetus, and the neonate). The illness also is encountered in immunosuppressed or chronically debilitated individuals and in pregnant women. Listerial infection in the healthy older child or the healthy, nonpregnant adult is unusual. The organism has a strong predisposition to invade the CNS in septic-borne fashion and also tends to be an intracellular pathogen. Intracellular location of the infectious agent diminishes the effectiveness of body defense mechanisms and the effectiveness of antibiotics.

During the last trimester of pregnancy, the heightened risk for bloodstream invasion after exposure to *L. monocytogenes* is attributed to mild impairment of cell-mediated immunity, which is characteristic of this period. Maternal bacteremia can remain asymptomatic but, more often, is associated with flulike symptoms, including fever, headache, anorexia, myalgia, and diarrhea. The maternal illness usually is self-limited, whereas transplacental transmission that results in fetal infection has far greater potential consequences. Fetal infection with *L. monocytogenes* can lead to spontaneous abortion, stillbirth, or the premature birth of a live infant seriously affected with widespread visceral granulomas and microabscess formation. This rare, overwhelming pyogenic condition is called *granulomatosis infantisepticum* and usually is rapidly fatal.

The more common expressions of *L. monocytogenes* infection in the neonate somewhat resemble group B streptococcal infection (both early- and late-onset forms). However, unlike early-onset group B streptococcal infection, in which bacterial contamination of the fetus is by direct contact in the birth canal, *Listeria* is most likely a blood-borne, transplacentally transmitted infection. The mother usually has experienced a symptomatically febrile illness before delivery. Amniotic fluid is usually stained brown, and premature delivery is common. Fever, early onset of respiratory distress, lethargy, rash, and hepatosplenomegaly are common features on the first or second day after birth.[113] The illness is predominantly a septic one, although evidence of meningitis occasionally is found on CSF examination.[114] Shock, so commonly seen with early-onset group B streptococcal sepsis, is far less common with the listerial counterpart and, thus, mortality is considerably lower in *Listeria* infection. Placental involvement with villitis and multiple microabscesses is characteristic of these cases and can be useful diagnostically to indicate prenatal infection.[115]

Late-onset neonatal *Listeria* infection most often begins after 2 weeks of age. In such cases, the organism is believed to be acquired by either direct exposure in the birth canal during delivery or by nosocomial exposure. The infant with the late-onset type infection is more likely to have been born at term, usually is a product of an uncomplicated birth, is less ill at onset of symptoms, and is much more likely to have a meningitic illness than is the infant affected immediately after birth. Initial symptoms include fever, irritability, poor feeding, and lethargy. Unlike the adult with *Listeria* meningitis in whom CSF often reveals a normal glucose content and a cellular response that is mainly mononuclear, the infant with late-onset neonatal infection usually has CSF abnormalities that are more typical of bacterial meningitis. Even in this group, however, the CSF glucose is not always markedly reduced. Mortality rate is lower and permanent neurologic sequelae are believed to be considerably less among infants with the late-onset type of *Listeria* infection as compared to infants with other types of bacterial meningitis in the first month of life.[116]

Neonatal *Mycoplasma hominis* Meningitis

The *Mycoplasma* and *Ureaplasma* species are the smallest organisms capable of survival and multiplication in an extracellular environment. The mycoplasmas lack a cell wall, rendering them insensitive to beta-lactam antibiotics. They stain poorly with the customary stains used to demonstrate the common bacteria and are smaller in diameter than are some of the larger viruses.

Species that are most important as a cause of human infection include *Mycoplasma pneumoniae*, *M. hominis*, and *Ureaplasma urealyticum*, the latter two being referred to as *genital mycoplasmas*, owing to their frequent colonization of the female urogenital tract. In some studies, up to 55% of postpubertal women will harbor *M. hominis* in the genital tract, whereas up to 70% can be found to be colonized with *U. urealyticum*.[117] Exposure to these organisms during the birth process results in colonization in a high percentage of neonates born vaginally of colonized mothers. Despite this high frequency of exposure, invasive neonatal infections caused by these organisms are, surprisingly, relatively uncommon.[118] Although *M. hominis* generally is accepted to be a cause of postpartum maternal fever, its role as a cause of neonatal disease has been questioned. Certain reports raise doubt about the pathogenicity of the organism, even when it is isolated from clinical specimens such as CSF.[119]

Although some authors have doubted any association of *M. hominis* with neonatal disease,[120] others have attributed to this organism a variety of lesions, such as scalp abscess,[121] ocular infection,[122] and suppurative adenitis.[123] The general consensus now is that *M. hominis* can be a cause of neonatal infection, although the spectrum of illnesses, the incidence of such infections, and the significance in terms of organ damage therefrom remain questionable.

Over the last several years, observations have come to support the concept that *M. hominis* can be a cause of CNS disease in the neonate and that the infant acquires the infection either during the birth process or from aspiration of infected amniotic fluid. The infection frequently is not recognized and its incidence is underestimated because CSF from an infected neonate does not always reveal a cellular response, Gram's staining does not identify the pathogen, and growth (if it occurs) is poor on media customarily used to isolate common bacteria.[124] Consequently, evidence that might raise suspicion of *M. hominis* as a cause of neonatal meningitis is sparse, and requests usually are not made for use of the special methods needed to culture and identify this underrecognized pathogen. The laboratory use of broth or media that will allow identification of *M. hominis* should be requested in the face of evidence of neonatal meningitis and CSF findings compatible with pyogenic meningitis but negative Gram's stain and bacteriologic cultures. Another finding that might support this approach is MRI evidence of a granulomatous meningeal reaction, sometimes with meningeal loculations, in addition to ependymitis.

Few reports exist of *M. hominis* meningitis in the neonate and, collectively, they describe relatively few cases of the illness.[125–129] Despite the small number of cases described thus far, a common, although markedly variable, pattern appears to emerge. Maternal intrapartum or postpartum fever signals a potential problem for the neonate in most cases. Low-birth-weight infants are overrepresented numerically in the available reports, and infants with neural tube defects also appear to be predisposed to neonatal *M. hominis* CNS infection.[127,129] Fever, irritability, lethargy, and hypotonia are the usual initial signs in the neonate, and these usually evolve between 1 and 3 weeks after birth. This infection can be relatively mild and followed by recovery or more severe with seizures and coma. Meningitis is the usual expression of the illness, although parenchymal involvement with brain abscess formation has been described.[128] CSF findings are highly variable, but the most common pattern is a polymorphonuclear pleocytosis, possibly amounting to several thousand cells per cubic millimeter, a moderate reduction in glucose content, and a progressive rise in the protein content, characteristics resembling those of bacterial pyogenic meningitis but notable for a negative CSF Gram's stain.

The limited number of reported cases of neonatal *M. hominis* meningitis precludes accurate information about prognosis or sequelae. Hydrocephalus can complicate the infection, possibly necessitating a shunting procedure.[125,127] The value of antibiotic therapy for CNS infection provoked by this organism also is unclear. Beta-lactam antimicrobials are not useful, and many antimicrobials that are believed to be effective do not readily gain entrance into CSF. Chloramphenicol is an exception in this regard but is of concern when administered to the low-birth-weight neonate. Clindamycin and doxycycline are effective against *M. hominis*, but neither penetrate CSF well, even in the presence of meningovascular inflammation.

Neonatal Staphylococcal Meningitis

By the latter part of the nineteenth century, staphylococci were known to cause pyogenic disease. At that time, the organisms producing a gold-colored pigment in culture were recognized for their virulence and were called *S. aureus*, whereas those generating a white pigment were assumed not to be pathogenic in humans and were designated as *Staphylococcus albus*. Later, *S. aureus* was found to be coagulase-positive, whereas other organisms were separated because of their coagulase-negative characteristics.

By the early 1980s, reports began to appear of the increasing prevalence of invasive infections by coagulase-negative organisms in neonatal intensive care units. By this time, such organisms, previously known as *S. albus*, had been renamed *Staphylococcus epidermidis*. In the last decade, *S. epidermidis* has emerged as the most common cause of nosocomial bacterial infection in most neonatal intensive care nurseries, especially among low-birth-weight and very low–birth-weight neonates.

Now at least 31 species of coagulase-negative staphylococci are known, *S. epidermidis* being by far the most important as a cause of invasive infection. Predisposing factors that lead to neonatal infection with this organism include low birth weight, prolonged confinement in an intensive care unit, and long-term indwelling vascular catheters. Low-birth-weight neonates are much more susceptible to this infection than are their full-term counterparts because of the much higher frequency of multiple medical complications that necessitate life-supporting measures (e.g., intravenous parenteral alimentation), the prolonged need for such measures, and the well-known immunodeficiencies associated with advanced prematurity.[130]

Clinical features of neonatal *S. epidermidis* sepsis vary widely but generally are more subtle and less explosive than those that characterize infection resulting from gram-negative bacillary organisms or group B streptococci. Episodes of apnea and bradycardia, irritability, and temperature instability are among the common manifestations.[131] Despite the common occurrence of sepsis, *S. epidermidis* is an infrequent cause of blood-borne neonatal meningitis. Most occurrences of *S. epidermidis* meningitis in early infancy complicate ventriculoperitoneal shunting or the placement of indwelling intraventricular reservoirs. When shunts are placed in the first week of life, the infection can still be seen in the neonatal period because most infections occur within 2–4 weeks of the operation.

Among some neonates without ventricular shunts who develop blood-borne *S. epidermidis* meningitis, symptoms such as lethargy, high-pitched cry, vomiting, or seizures can suggest the possibility of meningeal infection, which should lead the practitioner to order CSF examination. In most sick, low-birth-weight infants, however, symptoms are nonspecific, and the diagnosis of meningitis is made because the CSF examination is included in the workup when sepsis is suspected in the neonate. The immature neonate with *S. epidermidis* meningitis sometimes will generate little meningeal inflammatory response to this infection and the CSF findings, except for the positive culture, may not provide evidence of meningitis.[132] This is true also of the older infant with *S. epidermidis* shunt infection and probably diminishes the effectiveness of intravenous antibiotics, most of which depend on meningovascular inflammation to gain entrance into the CSF.

Another complicating aspect of treatment of neonatal staphylococcal meningitis is the expected resistance of the organism to the beta-lactam antibiotics, the aminoglycosides, and numerous other antimicrobials. For this reason, treatment is usually with vancomycin, with or without the addition of rifampin. Although death in neonates with *S. epidermidis* sepsis is infrequent, the development of meningitis compounds the seriousness of the infection and can be complicated by progressive hydrocephalus and other sequelae, including seizures, mental retardation, spastic signs, and visual and hearing loss.

S. aureus meningitis can, on rare occasion, complicate sepsis in the neonate,[133] although the majority of cases occur in association with CNS malformations.[134] This relationship is sufficiently strong that whenever *S. aureus* meningitis occurs in the neonate (other than in the very low–birth-weight neonate), a search, including the performance of MRI, should be made for CSF fistulas such as a congenital dermal sinus, a nasal encephalocele, or a neuroenteric sinus that communicates with the subarachnoid space. *S. aureus* meningitis can also ensue after neurosurgical such procedures as a ventricular shunt but is much less common than infection with *S. epidermidis* in such cases.

REFERENCES

1. Bale JF Jr, Murphy JR. Infections of the central nervous system of the newborn. Clin Perinatol 1997;24:6-1–6-19.
2. Nahmias AJ, Walls KW, Stewart JA, et al. The TORCH complex. Pediatr Res 1971; 5:405.
3. Fowler KB, Stagno S, Pass RF, et al. The outcome of congenital cytomegalovirus infection in relation to maternal antibody status. N Engl J Med 1992;326:663–667.
4. Robinson J, Lemay M, Vaudry WL. Congenital rubella after anticipated maternal immunity: two cases and a review of the literature. Pediatr Infect Dis J 1994;13: 812–815.
5. Fallon J, Eddy J, Wiener L, Pizzo PA. Human immunodeficiency virus infection in children. J Pediatr 1989;114:1–30.
6. Ueda K, Nishida Y, Oshima K, Shepard TH. Congenital rubella syndrome: correlation of gestational age at time of maternal rubella with type of defect. J Pediatr 1979;94:763–765.
7. Brunell PA. Varicella in pregnancy, the fetus and the newborn: problems in management. J Infect Dis 1992;166:S42–S47.
8. Conboy TJ, Pass RF, Stagno S, et al. Intellectual development in school-aged children with asymptomatic congenital cytomegalovirus infection. Pediatrics 1986; 77:801–806.
9. Williamson WD, Demmler GJ, Percy AK, Catlin FI. Progressive hearing loss in infants with asymptomatic congenital cytomegalovirus infection. Pediatrics 1992;90:862–866.
10. Hutto C, Arvin A, Jacobs R, et al. Intrauterine herpes simplex virus infections. J Pediatr 1987;110:97–101.
11. Demmler GJ. Summary of a workshop on surveillance for congenital cytomegalovirus disease. Rev Infect Dis 1991;13:315–329.
12. Bale JF Jr, Petheram SJ, Souza IE, Murph JR. Cytomegalovirus reinfection in young children. J Pediatr 1996;128:347–352.
13. Stagno S, Pass RF, Cloud G, et al. Primary cytomegalovirus infection in pregnancy. JAMA 1986;256:1904–1908.
14. Istas AS, Demmler GJ, Dobbins JG, et al. Surveillance for congenital cytomegalovirus disease: a report from the National Congenital Cytomegalovirus Disease Registry. Clin Infect Dis 1995;20:665–670.
15. Boppana SB, Pass RF, Britt WJ, et al. Symptomatic congenital cytomegalovirus infection: neonatal morbidity and mortality. Pediatr Infect Dis J 1992;11:93–99.
16. Demmler GJ, Buffone GJ, Schimbor CM, et al. Detection of cytomegalovirus in urine from newborns by using polymerase chain reaction DNA amplification. J Infect Dis 1988;158:1177–1184.
17. Boppana SB, Fowler KB, Vaid Y, et al. Neuroradiographic findings in the newborn period and long term outcome in children with symptomatic congenital cytomegalovirus infection. Pediatrics 1997;99:409–414.
18. Barkovich AJ, Lindan CE. Congenital cytomegalovirus infection of the brain: imaging analysis and embryologic considerations. AJNR Am J Neuroradiol 1994;15:703–715.

19. Pass RF, Stagno S, Myers GJ, Alford CA. Outcome of symptomatic congenital cytomegalovirus infection: results of long-term longitudinal follow-up. Pediatrics 1980;66:758–762.
20. Dudgeon JA. Congenital rubella. J Pediatr 1975;87:1078–1086.
21. Cochi SL, Edmonds LE, Dyer K, et al. Congenital rubella syndrome in the United States, 1970–1985. Am J Epidemiol 1989;129:349–361.
22. Centers for Disease Control and Prevention. Rubella and congenital rubella syndrome—United States, 1994–1997. MMWR Morb Mortal Wkly Rep 1997;46:350–354.
23. Centers for Disease Control and Prevention. Rubella and congenital rubella syndrome—United States, January 1, 1991–May 7, 1994. MMWR Morb Mortal Wkly Rep 1994;43:391,397–402.
24. Gregg NM. Congenital cataract following German measles in the mother. Trans Ophthalmol Soc Aust 1941;3:35.
25. Bosma TJ, Corbett KM, Eckstein MB, et al. Use of PCR for prenatal and postnatal diagnosis of congenital rubella. J Clin Microbiol 1995;33:2881–2887.
26. Yamashita U, Matsuishi T, Muarkami Y, et al. Neuroimaging findings (ultrasonography, CT, MRI) in 3 infants with congenital rubella syndrome. Pediatr Radiol 1991;21:547–549.
27. Givens KT, Less DA, Jones T, Ilstrup DM. Congenital rubella syndrome: ophthalmic manifestations and associated systemic disorders. Br J Ophthalmol 1993;77:358–363.
28. Desmond MM, Fisher ES, Voderman AL, et al. The longitudinal course of congenital rubella encephalitis in nonretarded children. J Pediatr 1978;93:584–591.
29. Wild JN, Sheppard S, Smithells RW, et al. Onset and severity of hearing loss due to congenital rubella infection. Arch Dis Child 1989;64:1280–1283.
30. Sever J, South MA, Shaver KA. Delayed manifestations of congenital rubella. Rev Infect Dis 1985;7:2164–2169.
31. Stone KM, Brooks CA, Guinan ME, Alexander ER. National surveillance for neonatal herpes simplex virus infections. Sex Transm Dis 1989;16:152–156.
32. Whitley RJ, Corey L, Arvin A, et al. Changing presentation of herpes simplex virus infection in neonates. J Infect Dis 1988;158:109–116.
33. Koskiniemi M, Happonen JM, Jarvenpaa AL, et al. Neonatal herpes simplex virus infection: a report of 43 patients. Pediatr Infect Dis 1989;8:30–35.
34. Mikati MA, Feraru I, Krishnamoorthy K, Lombroso CT. Neonatal herpes simplex meningoencephalitis. Neurology 1990;40:1433–1437.
35. Whitley R, Arvin A, Prober C, et al. Predictors of morbidity and mortality in neonates with herpes simplex virus infections. N Engl J Med 1991;324:450–454.
36. Centers for Disease Control. Kaposi's sarcoma and pneumocystis pneumonia among homosexual men—New York City and California. MMWR Morb Mortal Wkly Rep 1981;30:305–308.
37. Srugo I, Wittek AE, Israele V, Brunell PA. Meningoencephalitis in a neonate congenitally infected with human immunodeficiency virus type 1. J Pediatr 1992;120:93–95.
38. Committee on Infectious Diseases, American Academy of Pediatrics. Report of the Committee on Infectious Diseases: HIV Infection and AIDS. Elk Grove Village, IL: American Academy of Pediatrics, 1994;258–261.
39. Barnhart HX, Caldwell MB, Thomas P, et al. Natural history of human immunodeficiency virus disease in perinatally infected children: an analysis from the pediatric spectrum of disease project. Pediatrics 1996;97:710–716.
40. Connor EM, Sperling RS, Gelber R, et al. Reduction of maternal-infant transmission of human immunodeficiency virus type 1 with zidovudine treatment. N Engl J Med 1994;331:1172–1180.
41. Epstein LG, Sharer KR, Joshi VV, et al. Progressive encephalopathy in children with acquired immune deficiency syndrome. Ann Neurol 1985;17:488–496.

42. Belman AL, Ultmann MH, Horoupian D, et al. Neurological complications in infants and children with acquired immune deficiency syndrome. Ann Neurol 1985;18: 560–566.
43. Belman AL. Central nervous system involvement in pediatric HIV-1 infection: an overview. Int Pediatr 1992;7:126–135.
44. DeCarli C, Civitello LA, Brouwers P, Pizzo PA. The prevalence of computed tomographic abnormalities of the cerebrum in 100 consecutive children symptomatic with the human immune deficiency virus. Ann Neurol 1993;34:198–205.
45. Grose C. Congenital infections caused by varicella zoster virus and herpes simplex virus. Semin Pediatr Neurol 1994;1:43–49.
46. Alkalay AL, Pomerance JJ, Rimoin DL. Fetal varicella syndrome. J Pediatr 1987;111:320–323.
47. Cuthbertson G, Weiner CP, Giller RH, et al. Prenatal diagnosis of second trimester congenital varicella syndrome by virus-specific IgM. J Pediatr 1987;111:592–595.
48. Sheinbergas M. Hydrocephalus due to prenatal infection with the lymphocytic choriomeningitis virus. Infection 1976;4:185–191.
49. Wright R, Johnson D, Neumann M, et al. Congenital lymphocytic choriomeningitis virus syndrome: a disease that mimics congenital toxoplasmosis or cytomegalovirus infection. Pediatrics 1997;100:91–96.
50. Jenista JA, Powell KR, Menegus MA. Epidemiology of neonatal enterovirus infection. J Pediatr 1984;104:685–690.
51. Morens DM. Enterovirus disease in early infancy. J Pediatr 1978;92:374–377.
52. Schlesinger Y, Sawyer MA, Storch GA. Enteroviral meningitis in infancy: potential role for polymerase chain reaction in patient management. Pediatrics 1994;94: 157–162.
53. Bergman I, Painter MJ, Wald ER, et al. Outcome in children with enteroviral meningitis during the first year of life. J Pediatr 1987;110:705–709.
54. Rorabaugh LM, Berlin LE, Heldrich R, et al. Aseptic meningitis in infants younger than 2 years of age: acute illness and neurologic complications. Pediatrics 1992; 92:206–211.
55. Bittencourt AL. Congenital Chagas disease. Am J Dis Child 1976;130:97–103.
56. Koskiniemi M, Lappalainen M, Hedman K. Toxoplasmosis needs evaluation: an overview and proposals. Am J Dis Child 1989;143:724–728.
57. Dukes CS, Luft BJ, Durack DT. Toxoplasmosis. In WM Scheld, RJ Whitley, DJ Ducak (eds), Infections of the Central Nervous System. Philadelphia: Lippincott–Raven, 1997;785–806.
58. Pereira LH, Staudt M, Tanner CE, Embil JA. Exposure to *Toxoplasma gondii* and cat ownership in Nova Scotia. Pediatrics 1992;89:1169–1172.
59. Wallace MR, Rossetti RJ, Olson PE. Cats and toxoplasmosis risk in HIV-infected adults. JAMA 1993;269:76–77.
60. Stray-Pedersen B. A prospective study of acquired toxoplasmosis among 8,043 pregnant women in the Oslo area. Am J Obstet Gynecol 1980;136:399–406.
61. Desmonts G, Couvreur J. Congenital toxoplasmosis: a prospective study of 378 pregnancies. N Engl J Med 1974;290:1110–1116.
62. Couvreur J, Desmonts G. Congenital and maternal toxoplasmosis: a review of 300 congenital cases. Dev Med Child Neurol 1962;4:519–530.
63. Diebler C, Dusser A, Dulac O. Congenital toxoplasmosis. Clinical and neuroradiological evaluation of the cerebral lesions. Neuroradiology 1985;27:125–130.
64. Johnson JD, Butcher PD, Savva D, Holliman RE. Application of the polymerase chain reaction to the diagnosis of human toxoplasmosis. J Infect Dis 1993;26:147–158.
65. Daffos F, Forestier F, Capella-Pavlovsky M, et al. Prenatal management of 746 pregnancies at risk for congenital toxoplasmosis. N Engl J Med 1985;318:271–275.
66. Hohlfeld R, Daffos F, Thulliez P, et al. Fetal toxoplasmosis: outcome of pregnancy and infant follow-up after in utero treatment. J Pediatr 1989;115:765–769.

67. Guerina NG, Hsu H-W, Ceissner C, et al. Neonatal screening and early treatment for congenital *Toxoplasma gondii* infection. N Engl J Med 1994;330:1858–1863.
68. Roizen N, Swisher C, Stein M, et al. Neurologic and developmental outcome in treated congenital toxoplasmosis. Pediatrics 1995;95:11–20.
69. Gladstone IM, Ehrenkranz RA, Edberg SC, Baltimore RS. A ten-year review of neonatal sepsis and comparison with the previous fifty-year experience. Pediatr Infect Dis J 1990;9:819–825.
70. Siegel JD, McCracken GH. Sepsis neonatorum. N Engl J Med 1981;304:642–647.
71. Freedman RM, Ingram DL, Gross I, et al. A half century of neonatal sepsis at Yale. Am J Dis Child 1981;135:140–144.
72. Voora S, Srinivassan G, Lilien LD, et al. Fever in full-term newborns in the first four days of life. Pediatrics 1982;69:40–44.
73. Berman PH, Banker BQ. Neonatal meningitis: a clinical and pathological study of 29 cases. Pediatrics 1966;38:6–24.
74. Kalsbeck JE, DeSousa AL, Kleiman MB, et al. Compartmentalization of the cerebral ventricles as a sequelae of neonatal meningitis. J Neurosurg 1980;52:547–552.
75. Schultz P, Leeds NE. Intraventricular septations complicating neonatal meningitis. J Neurosurg 1973;38:620–626.
76. Reeder JD, Sanders RC. Ventriculitis in the neonate. Recognition by sonography. Am J Neuroradiol 1983;4:37–41.
77. Franco SM, Cornelius VE, Andrews BF. Long-term outcome of neonatal meningitis. Am J Dis Child 1992;146:567–571.
78. Berk SL, McCabe WR. Meningitis caused by Gram-negative bacilli. Ann Intern Med 1980;93:253–260.
79. Unhanand M, Mustafa MM, McCracken GH Jr, Nelson JD. Gram-negative enteric bacillary meningitis: a twenty-one–year experience. J Pediatr 1983;122:15–21.
80. Hill HR, Hunt CE, Matsen JM. Nosocomial colonization with *Klebsiella*, type 25, in a neonatal intensive-care unit associated with an outbreak of sepsis, meningitis, and necrotizing enterocolitis. J Pediatr 1974;85:415–419.
81. Donowitz LG, Marsik FJ, Fisher KA, Wenzel RP. Contaminated breast milk: a source of *Klebsiella* bacteremia in a newborn intensive care unit. Rev Infect Dis 1981;3:716–720.
82. Robbins JB, McCracken GH Jr, Gotschlich EC, et al. *Escherichia coli* K1 capsular polysaccharide associated with neonatal meningitis. N Engl J Med 1974;290:1216–1220.
83. Headings DL, Overall JC Jr. Outbreak of meningitis in a newborn intensive care unit caused by a single *Escherichia coli* K1 serotype. J Pediatr 1977;90:99–102.
84. Perlman JM, Rollins N, Sanchez PJ. Late-onset meningitis in sick, very-low-birth-weight infants. Clinical and sonographic observations. Am J Dis Child 1992;146:1297–1301.
85. Mulder CJJ, Van Alphen L, Zanen HC. Neonatal meningitis caused by *Escherichia coli* in the Netherlands. J Infect Dis 1984;150:935–940.
86. Lipsky BA, Hook EW III, Smith AA, Plorde JJ. *Citrobacter* infections in humans: experience of the Seattle veterans administration medical center and a review of the literature. Rev Infect Dis 1980;2:746–760.
87. Graham DR, Anderson RL, Ariel FE, et al. Epidemic nosocomial meningitis due to *Citrobacter diversus* in neonates. J Infect Dis 1981;144:203–209.
88. Kline MW. *Citrobacter* meningitis and brain abscess in infancy: epidemiology, pathogenesis, and treatment. J Pediatr 1988;113:430–434.
89. Vogel LC, Ferguson L, Gotoff SP. *Citrobacter* infections of the central nervous system in early infancy. J Pediatr 1978;93:86–88.
90. Graham DR, Band JD. *Citrobacter diversus* brain abscess and meningitis in neonates. JAMA 1981;245:1923–1925.

91. Campbell JR, Diacovo T, Baker CJ. *Serratia marcescens* meningitis in neonates. Pediatr Infect Dis J 1992;11:881–886.
92. Willis J, Robinson JE. *Enterobacter sakazakii* meningitis in neonates. Pediatr Infect Dis J 1988;7:196–199.
93. Foreman SD, Smith EE, Ryan NJ, Hogan GR. Neonatal *Citrobacter* meningitis: pathogenesis of cerebral abscess formation. Ann Neurol 1984;16:655–659.
94. Renier D, Flandin C, Hirsch E, Hirsch JF. Brain abscess in neonates. A study of 30 cases. J Neurosurg 1988;69:877–882.
95. Smith ML, Mellor D. *Proteus mirabilis* meningitis and cerebral abscess in the newborn period. Arch Dis Child 1980;55:308–309.
96. Lancefield RC. A serological differentiation of human and other groups of hemolytic streptococci. J Exp Med 1993;57:571–595.
97. Fry RM. Fatal infections by haemolytic streptococcus group B. Lancet 1938;1:199–201.
98. Eickhoff TC, Klein JO, Daly K, et al. Neonatal sepsis and other infections due to group B beta-hemolytic streptococci. N Engl J Med 1964;271:1221–1228.
99. Committee on Infectious Diseases, American Academy of Pediatrics. Revised guidelines for prevention of early-onset group B streptococcal (GBS) infection. Pediatrics 1997;99:489–496.
100. Pass MA, Gray BM, Dillon HC Jr. Puerperal and perinatal infections with group B streptococci. Am J Obstet Gynecol 1982;143:147–152.
101. Baker CJ. Group B streptococcal infections in neonates. Pediatr Rev 1979;1:5–14.
102. Baker CJ, Kasper DL. Correlation of maternal antibody deficiency with susceptibility to neonatal group B streptococcal infection. N Engl J Med 1976;294: 753–756.
103. Vogel LC, Boyer KM, Gadzala CA, Gotoff SP. Prevalence of type-specific group B streptococcal antibody in pregnant women. J Pediatr 1980;96:1047–1051.
104. Weisman LE, Stoll BJ, Cruess DF, et al. Early-onset group B streptococcal sepsis: a current assessment. J Pediatr 1992;121:428–433.
105. Baker CJ, Barrett FF. Group B streptococcal infections in infants. The importance of the various serotypes. JAMA 1974;230:1158–1160.
106. Baker CJ, Barrett FF, Gordon RC, Yow M. Suppurative meningitis due to streptococci of Lancefield group B: a study of 33 infants. J Pediatr 1973;82:724–729.
107. Shankaran S, Farooki ZQ, Desai R. Beta-hemolytic streptococcal infection appearing as persistent fetal circulation. Am J Dis Child 1982;136:725–727.
108. Vollman JH, Smith HL, Ballard ET, Light IJ. Early onset group B streptococcal disease: clinical roentgenographic, and pathologic features. J Pediatr 1976;89: 199–203.
109. Paredes A, Wong P, Mason EO Jr, et al. Nosocomial transmission of group B streptococci in a newborn nursery. Pediatrics 1977;59:679–682.
110. Haslam RH, Allen JR, Dorsen MM, et al. The sequelae of group B beta-hemolytic streptococcal meningitis in early infancy. Am J Dis Child 1977;131:845–849.
111. Edwards MS, Rench MA, Haffar AAM, et al. Long-term sequelae of group B streptococcal meningitis in infants. J Pediatr 1985;106:717–722.
112. Pai KG, Rubin HM, Wedemeyer PP, Linarelli LG. Hypothalamic-pituitary dysfunction following group B beta hemolytic streptococcal meningitis in a neonate. J Pediatr 1976;88:289–291.
113. Halliday HL, Hirata T. Perinatal listeriosis—a review of twelve patients. Am J Obstet Gynecol 1979;133:405–410.
114. Teberg AJ, Yonekura ML, Salminen C, Pavlova Z. Clinical manifestations of epidemic neonatal listeriosis. Pediatr Infect Dis J 1987;6:817–820.
115. Topalovski M, Yang SS, Boonpasat Y. Listeriosis of the placenta: clinicopathologic study of seven cases. Am J Obstet Gynecol 1993;169:616–620.

116. Nichols W Jr, Wooley PV Sr. *Listeria monocytogenes* meningitis. Observations based on 13 case reports and a consideration of recent literature. J Pediatr 1962; 61:337–350.

117. Dinsmoor JJ, Ramamurthy RS, Gibbs RS. Transmission of genital mycoplasmas from mother to neonate in women with prolonged membrane rupture. Pediatr Infect Dis J 1989;8:483–487.

118. Likitnukel S, Kusmiesz H, Nelson JD, McCracken GH Jr. Role of genital mycoplasma in young infants with suspected sepsis. J Pediatr 1986;109:971–974.

119. Valencia GB, Banzon F, Cummings M, et al. *Mycoplasma hominis* and *Ureaplasma urealyticum* in neonates with suspected infection. Pediatr Infect Dis J 1993;12: 571–573.

120. Klein JO, Buckland D, Finland M. Colonization of newborn infants by mycoplasmas. N Engl J Med 1969;280:1025–1030.

121. Glaser JB, Engelberg M, Hammerschlag M. Scalp abscess associated with *Mycoplasma hominis* infection complicating intrapartum monitoring. Pediatr Infect Dis J 1983;2:468–470.

122. Jones DM, Tobin B. Neonatal eye infections due to *Mycoplasma hominis*. BMJ 1968;3:467–468.

123. Powell DA, Miller K, Clyde WA Jr. Submandibular adenitis in a newborn caused by *Mycoplasma hominis*. Pediatrics 1979;63:798–799.

124. Waites KB, Duffy LB, Crouse DT, et al. Mycoplasmal infections of cerebrospinal fluid in newborn infants from a community hospital population. Pediatr Infect Dis J 1990;9:241–245.

125. Boe O, Diderichsen J, Matre R. Isolation of *Mycoplasma hominis* from cerebrospinal fluid. Scand J Infect Dis 1973;5:285–288.

126. Gewitz M, Dinwiddie R, Rees L, et al. *Mycoplasma hominis*. A case of neonatal meningitis. Arch Dis Child 1979;54:231–239.

127. McDonald JC, Moore DL. *Mycoplasma hominis* meningitis in a premature infant. Pediatr Infect Dis J 1988;7:795–798.

128. Siber GR, Alpert S, Smith AL, et al. Neonatal central nervous system infection due to *Mycoplasma hominis*. J Pediatr 1977;90:625–627.

129. Wealthall SR. *Mycoplasma* meningitis in infants with spina bifida. Dev Med Child Neurol 1975;17(suppl 35):117–122.

130. Hall SL. Coagulase-negative staphylococcal infections in neonates. Pediatr Infect Dis J 1991;10:57–67.

131. Patrick CC. Coagulase-negative staphylococci. Pathogens with increasing clinical significance. J Pediatr 1990;116:497–507.

132. Gruskay J, Harris MC, Costarino AT, et al. Neonatal *Staphylococcus epidermidis* meningitis with unremarkable CSF examination results. Am J Dis Child 1989; 143:580–582.

133. Schlesinger LS, Ross SC, Schalberg DR. *Staphylococcus aureus* meningitis: a broad-based epidemiologic study. Medicine 1987;66:148–156.

134. Givner LB, Kaplan SL. Meningitis due to *Staphylococcus aureus* in children. Clin Infect Dis 1993;16:766–771.

9

Perinatal Cerebrovascular Causes of Cerebral Palsy

Van S. Miller

Cerebral palsy is a group of disorders in which movement, coordination, posture, and cognition are affected to varying degrees and for which onset is during brain development. Cerebrovascular disorders in neonates are among the most important causes of cerebral palsy,[1] and they occur in both preterm and full-term infants. Neonatal cerebrovascular disorders are classified anatomically in Table 9.1. The most familiar of these disorders is periventricular/intraventricular hemorrhage (PIVH), seen frequently in preterm infants. However, cerebrovascular injury in the full-term or preterm newborn that later leads to cerebral palsy may also result from trauma during labor or delivery, hypoxia-ischemia, cerebrovascular malformations, metabolic disorders, acquired or inherited coagulopathies, and other causes.

PERIVENTRICULAR/INTRAVENTRICULAR HEMORRHAGE

Periventricular Vascular Anatomy of the Neonatal Brain

The subependymal (periventricular) germinal matrix is the site of cortical neuronal and glial proliferation in the mid- and late-gestation fetal brain. It is also the location for intraventricular hemorrhage, the most common type of intracranial hemorrhage in the premature infant. Several interesting and distinctive maturational, structural, and hemodynamic features of this area make it especially vulnerable to hemorrhage. The size of the germinal matrix is maximal at 20–27 weeks' gestation, after which it undergoes progressive involution and becomes essentially vestigial by term. During this time, the periventricular matrix zone is hypercellular and hypervascularized. Blood vessels are surrounded by the end-feet of local astrocytes and are continuously in the process of remodeling.[2] The endothelium of these blood vessels is vulnerable to hypoxia-ischemia, which leads to focal hemorrhage. Between 28 and 32 weeks' gestation, the germinal matrix is most prominent at the head of the caudate nucleus at the thalamostriate notch. Consequently, PIVH before 28 weeks' gestation tends to occur along

Table 9.1 Cerebrovascular Disorders in Neonates

Intracranial hemorrhage
    Periventricular or intraventricular
    Subdural
    Subarachnoid
    Epidural
    Parenchymal
    Posterior fossa

Cerebral infarction
    Embolic
    Thrombotic

Congenital vascular defects
    Aneurysms
    Vein of Galen arteriovenous malformations

the body of the caudate nucleus, whereas between 28 and 32 weeks, the most common site of PIVH is more anteriorly, at the head of the caudate at the level of the foramen of Monro. PIVH in full-term infants tends to originate from the choroid plexus, which is an uncommon site of this disorder in premature infants. Hence, an understanding of the vascular anatomy of the subependymal germinal matrix is necessary to appreciate the pathogenesis of PIVH.

The arterial vascular anatomy of the fetal brain changes from a predominantly basal ganglia–oriented pattern at 24 weeks' gestation to a cortically oriented pattern by term. Arterial blood supply to the subependymal germinal matrix is via the anterior circulation: Deep penetrating vessels from the anterior and middle cerebral arteries and from the internal carotid artery feed an elaborate capillary network that, during late gestation, becomes more complex even as the germinal matrix involutes. Vascular anatomy of the venous drainage of the subependymal region is particularly important in the pathogenesis of PIVH. Cortical veins (the medullary, choroidal, and thalamostriate veins) join the subependymal venules to empty into the terminal vein, which courses anteriorly until it makes an abrupt hairpin turn at the head of the caudate nucleus and then runs posteriorly as the internal cerebral vein. This peculiar reversal of direction predisposes the thin-walled veins at this site to rupture if cerebral blood flow suddenly increases or venous pressure rises downstream, as often happens in the ill, premature newborn. Further, the relatively larger diameter of germinal matrix blood vessels as compared with cortical vessels may lead to greater pressure on the walls of the germinal matrix vasculature,[3] predisposing them to rupture during periods of high cerebral blood flow.

PIVH is graded according to the location and size of the bleed and to whether it distends the cerebral ventricles. Grade 1 PIVH is defined as hemorrhage restricted to the germinal matrix; in grade 2 PIVH, hemorrhage occurs inside the lateral ventricle without ventricular distention; and in grade 3 PIVH,

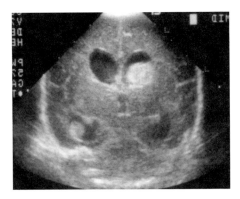

Figure 9.1 Cranial ultrasound scan from a premature infant shows a left grade 3 periventricular-intraventricular hemorrhage. The ventricles are enlarged.

the ventricular system is enlarged. The most severe type of PIVH in neonates is periventricular hemorrhagic infarction, which has been designated as grade 4. The early assumption that grade 4 hemorrhage was simply an extension of grade 3 hemorrhage out into the cortical parenchyma has been refuted by several lines of evidence.[4] These periventricular lesions, which typically are adjacent to the lateral ventricle and often are very large, probably are due to venous infarction of the medullary veins in the periventricular white matter. Periventricular hemorrhagic infarctions typically are unilateral, are strikingly asymmetric when bilateral, and appear to be due to obstruction of the ventriculofugal veins by intraventricular and germinal matrix blood clot, although injurious vasoactive compounds such as lactic acid, iron, and glutamate may play a role.[5]

Intraventricular blood impairs periventricular blood flow, leading first to local venous congestion and then to hemorrhagic infarction. However, some premature infants have an apparent periventricular hemorrhagic infarction without an ipsilateral PIVH; presumably, in these infants, the initial tissue injury is due to hypoxia-ischemia, which then develops into periventricular hemorrhagic leukomalacia.

Cranial ultrasonography (US) is the most common imaging modality used in the neonatal intensive care unit because it is portable and can be combined with Doppler imaging to evaluate cerebral blood flow. Because the neurologic outcome of PIVH depends strongly on severity of the hemorrhage (as discussed next), grades 1 and 2 PIVH will be referred to here as *mild PIVH*, and grade 3 PIVH and intraparenchymal hemorrhage will be termed *severe PIVH*. Figure 9.1 illustrates a cranial US image of a grade 3 PIVH in an infant born prematurely.

The major neuropathologic consequences of PIVH include obstructive hydrocephalus, porencephaly, cystic encephalomalacia, and periventricular leukomalacia, which are all large-scale disruptions of cerebral development. A more subtle, though not unimportant, consequence of PIVH is a disturbance of neuronal and glial migration from the germinal matrix into the cortex. Radial glial cells that guide the migration of neuronal and glial precursors are destroyed or injured at the site of the hemorrhage, thereby altering normal development of the synaptic structure of the cortex. A role for injury to subplate neurons by damage to the germinal matrix has been proposed by Volpe,[6] on the basis of observations that the subplate neuron layer in human frontal cortex reaches a peak between 23 and 34 weeks' gestation, with subsequent regression due to programmed cell death of these neurons by the sixth month of postnatal life. However, no direct evidence is available currently to confirm that disruption of subplate neuron maturation plays a causal role in the cognitive or motor sequelae of PIVH.

Intraventricular Hemorrhagic Clinical Syndromes

Neonatal intracranial hemorrhage may present in an infant with an impressively sudden and severe decline in neurologic function that evolves over 1–2 hours. Infants with this catastrophic syndrome, due to a large intracranial hemorrhage with subsequent obstructive hydrocephalus and increased intracranial pressure, typically become unresponsive and develop tonic posturing, loss of normal spontaneous movement, and brain stem dysfunction as evidenced by apnea and loss of corneal and gag reflexes and pupillary response to light. Often, the fontanelle becomes full, and the infant becomes hypotensive, bradycardic, and hypothermic. Metabolic acidosis, anemia, and hyponatremia may accompany the hemorrhage. The speed of evolution and severity of this syndrome depends, in part, on the swiftness with which the hydrocephalus ensues but may also reflect the size of the hemorrhage.

The catastrophic syndrome is uncommon and, in fact, intracranial hemorrhage usually is either initially asymptomatic or associated with subtle clinical signs. In some infants symptoms evolve gradually over several hours (*saltatory syndrome*). Irritability, poor feeding, slightly decreased spontaneous movement or subtle changes in eye movements (staring, nystagmus, anisocoria, absent oculocephalic response), and disturbances in sleep patterns in premature infants with PIVH have been noted. An abnormally tight popliteal angle has been described as a sensitive physical finding in infants with PIVH, but this requires experience of what is normal in preterm infants of varying gestational ages.[7]

Epidemiology, Timing, and Risk Factors

Most studies indicate an incidence of PIVH of 30–40% in infants born at less than 35 weeks' gestation.[8-11] A study of nearly 3,000 premature infants found that 45% (1,350) sustained PIVH.[12] In general, the risk of PIVH increases with decreases in gestational age and weight at birth, although gestational age may be a more reliable predictor than weight.[13] In a prospective study of 309 premature infants born between 23 and 34 weeks and followed with serial head US, no relationship could be ascertained between gestational age and timing of onset of PIVH,[14] although the overall incidence of hemorrhage was related to gestational age. A declining incidence of intraventricular hemorrhage over the last decade or so has been noted in several studies.[15-17] This decline is unexplained, though improvements in prenatal care of the mother and in peripartum care of the immature infant may be responsible.

The risk of PIVH is highest in the immediate peripartum period. A study of nearly 1,000 infants weighing less than 2,000 g at birth found that 25% of the infants had PIVH in the first week of life.[18] In more than one-third of these infants, the hemorrhage was evident on cranial US by 5 hours of life, indicating either intrapartum or early postnatal onset. PIVH occurs on the second postnatal day in approximately 25% of infants and on the third postnatal day in nearly 10%. Perhaps 5% of premature infants with PIVH undergo hemorrhage beyond the third day of life, and PIVH occurs in a few infants even after the first postnatal week, indicating the value of a routine cranial imaging study after the first week of life in premature infants. Intracranial hemorrhage occurring before labor or delivery is very uncommon, even in very premature infants, and should prompt a search for a bleeding diathesis such as alloimmune thrombocytopenia[19] or deficiency of factors VII, X, or XIII,[20–22] though in most infants with antenatal hemorrhage, no definite coagulopathy can be shown. Alloimmune thrombocytopenia is also a common cause of severe PIVH in full-term infants.[23] The predilection of PIVH to occur during the first few days after delivery is most likely due to the events attendant on labor (if present), delivery, and the stabilization period immediately after birth. However, intriguing evidence that maturation of the germinal matrix (and reduced likelihood of PIVH) is induced postnatally has been presented in beagle puppies.[24]

Analyses of perinatal risk factors for PIVH are presented in Table 9.2. Some studies have not found strong correlations between maternal obstetric factors and PIVH.[25–28] One careful study of risk factors for PIVH in premature infants born at Parkland Hospital reviewed records of 463 infants and found that respiratory distress syndrome, ventilator requirement, hypercapnia, hypoxia, low Apgar scores at 1 and 5 minutes, and pneumothorax significantly increased the risk of PIVH.[29] Other studies have identified antenatal risk factors such as maternal smoking and aspirin and alcohol use.[30–33] Cocaine use has been inconsistently shown to increase the risk of PIVH.[34–37] Whether cesarean section delivery reduces the incidence or severity of intracranial hemorrhage in premature infants is controversial, but a protective effect might be offered by cesarean delivery if performed prior to the onset of labor.[38–42]

Abnormal regulation of cerebral blood flow is strongly related to an increased risk of PIVH. In the premature infant, impaired autoregulation of cerebral blood flow is common, so that increases in systemic blood pressure tend to be transferred directly to blood vessels in the germinal matrix. Probably for this reason, sudden elevations of systemic blood pressure in premature infants that are induced by painful procedures, rapid colloid infusion, tracheal suctioning, and even routine handling are associated with an increased risk of PIVH.[43–45] Blood pressure fluctuations correlated with pneumothorax have also been implicated in the pathogenesis of PIVH[46,47] and, in some studies, are the most important identified risk factors.[48] Seizures sharply increase cerebral blood

Table 9.2   Risk Factors for Periventricular-Intraventricular Hemorrhage

Antenatal risk factors
Increased risk
    Maternal smoking
    Maternal aspirin use
    Maternal alcohol use
    Cesarean section before labor begins
    Ominous fetal heart rate patterns
    Early cord clamping

Decreased risk
    Toxemia
    Surfactant
    African-American race, female gender
    Epidural anesthesia
    Intrauterine growth retardation

Postnatal risk factors
Fluctuations in blood pressure
Seizures
Low Apgar scores
Elevated creatine kinase–BB in serum
Elevated cross-linked fibrin degradation products
Assisted ventilation, neonatal depression
Acidosis
Pneumothorax with hypotension
Heparin administration
Benzyl alcohol administration
High umbilical artery placement

flow and thus may also be an important risk factor for PIVH,[49] although seizures may be a result of PIVH rather than a cause.

Episodes of systemic hypotension that lead to decreased cerebral perfusion pressure and are followed by abrupt elevations in arterial blood pressure may be particularly harmful, inciting reperfusion injury.[50] Hypoxia-ischemia may impair the already poor autoregulatory ability of the premature brain, so that cerebral blood flow becomes even more pressure-passive than in the normal state. If the endothelial wall of germinal matrix blood vessels sustains hypoxic-ischemic injury during the low-flow state, vessels may rupture when cerebral blood flow is re-established.[51] Hypotension has been demonstrated to be a risk factor for PIVH in a number of animal and human studies.[52,53] Surfactant treatment for respiratory distress syndrome appears to be complexly related to the risk of PIVH, but a meta-analysis of approximately 1,700 premature infants treated with surfactant showed no increased risk of PIVH.[54]

Increased central venous pressure may also play a role in the pathogenesis of PIVH by impairing cerebral blood flow. Respiratory distress syndrome and its complications are accompanied by elevated central venous pressure and are strongly associated with PIVH,[29,55] perhaps due to the requirement for high-pressure ventilation in infants with this syndrome. Labor and delivery are accompanied by fetal head compression, which in turn leads to increased central venous pressure. Therefore, one might expect higher rates of PIVH in infants born vaginally than in those born by cesarean section but, as mentioned earlier, studies addressing this issue have produced conflicting results. Studies have shown that prolonged labor is associated with an increased risk of PIVH[56] and that early PIVH (within the first hour of life) is more likely in infants born vaginally than in those born abdominally, even though the overall incidence of PIVH was the same in the two groups.[39]

Complications and Neurodevelopmental Outcome

Mortality clearly is related to the severity of intracranial hemorrhage. Of 75 infants with a parenchymal hemorrhage, only 41% survived, as compared to only 8% of infants with grade 3 PIVH.[57] Similar survival rates were obtained in an analysis of 169 infants born between 24 and 30 weeks' gestation, in which 64% of infants with PIVH survived, as compared to 90% of infants without PIVH.[58] In this latter study, infants with grade 3 or 4 PIVH had a survival rate of only 51%, whereas infants with grade 1 or 2 PIVH were as likely to survive as were those infants without cranial hemorrhage.

A prominent and sometimes serious complication of PIVH is progressive hydrocephalus, which may occur acutely or in a more indolent fashion, depending generally on the amount of blood present in the ventricular system. Acute obstructive hydrocephalus develops within a few days of the PIVH, especially if the intracranial bleed is large, presumably due to the prevention, by particulate blood, of circulation of cerebrospinal fluid (CSF). Subacute hydrocephalus is more common and may develop over a few weeks after the PIVH, although rarely it may remain unrecognized for many months.[59] An obliterative arachnoiditis involving the arachnoid granulations or, less commonly, the cerebral aqueduct or foramina of Magendie and Luschka in the posterior fossa, occurs in subacute hydrocephalus. Thus, subacute posthemorrhagic hydrocephalus is often a communicating hydrocephalus.

Approximately half of infants with PIVH develop ventriculomegaly,[60] but only 10% or so of these neonates develop posthemorrhagic hydrocephalus, with rapidly increasing head circumference and increased intracranial pressure.[61] In nearly half of affected infants, the posthemorraghic hydrocephalus will resolve or become stable without intervention. In those infants with progressive ventriculomegaly after PIVH, a variety of temporary measures for controlling increased intracranial pressure can be used: Among these are serial spinal taps, external ventriculostomy, ventriculogaleal shunt, and the administration of

Table 9.3 Neurodevelopmental Correlates of Periventricular/Intraventricular
Hemorrhage

Adverse neurodevelopmental outcomes in premature infants with periventricular/intra-
ventricular hemorrhage (PIVH) are associated most closely with parenchymal lesions
and ventriculomegaly.

Grades 1 and 2 PIVH infrequently are associated with severe motor or cognitive deficits.

Obstructive hydrocephalus often accompanies severe PIVH but does not add significantly
to the risk of severe neurodevelopmental deficits.

Cystic periventricular leukomalacia correlates more closely with subsequent cerebral
palsy than does PIVH, and both may occur in the same infant.

Parenchymal hemorrhagic lesions often evolve into porencephalic cysts, with a contralateral hemiparesis.

Periventricular leukomalacia is associated with a high incidence of spastic cerebral palsy,
especially if the cerebral ventricles are enlarged and irregular.

drugs to decrease CSF production. However, ventriculoperitoneal shunting of
CSF often is ultimately necessary.

Follow-up studies that began in the 1980s are contributing to a clearer
understanding of neurodevelopmental sequelae of PIVH (Table 9.3). In most of
these studies, severity and location of PIVH was determined by bedside cranial
US, generally through the anterior fontanelle, although some researchers used
computed tomography (CT) or magnetic resonance imaging (MRI). Although
MRI generally is superior to cranial US and CT in most neonatal neurologic disorders,[62] cranial US in the neonatal period may be more predictive of neurodevelopmental outcome than is MRI done at 44 weeks' postmenstrual age.[63]
Nonetheless, MRI is more sensitive than CT or US for detection of subtle
periventricular lesions, and probably cranial MRI will be more predictive of
long-term neurodevelopmental outcome than will other imaging techniques,
especially in patients with mild cognitive or motor deficits.

The degree of parenchymal involvement by PIVH is a critical determinant of
neurodevelopmental outcome, as was recognized in early reports of short-term
outcome and was confirmed in subsequent studies.[8,64,65] For example, all 33
infants born weighing less than 2,250 g who had large parenchymal hemorrhages
also had either moderate or severe neurologic deficits,[10] though some studies
emphasized that infants with even severe PIVH might develop without serious
neurologic sequelae.[66] In another study of 198 surviving premature infants, major
neurologic deficits at 2 years of age were seen in 9% with grade 1 PIVH, 11%
with grade 2 PIVH, 36% with grade 3 PIVH, and 76% with parenchymal hemorrhage.[67] Of 10 infants with grade 3 PIVH, 8 had identifiable neurologic deficits at
12 months of age, compared to only 3 of 10 infants without PIVH.[68] One
prospective study evaluated 90 preterm infants with PIVH whose birth weight
was not more than 1,750 g and whose gestational age was less than 35 weeks and

compared the data to 22 full-term control infants.[69] Twenty-nine preterm infants had mild (grade 1 or 2) PIVH, 34 preterm infants had severe PIVH, and 27 infants had no intracranial hemorrhage. Evaluations by standard neurodevelopmental assessments at 3, 7, 12, and 24 months of age showed that although infants with severe PIVH had neurologic sequelae at every time point, improvement tended to occur over time, an important point that is not often recognized.

Even in infants with parenchymal hemorrhagic infarction, a range of neurologic outcome can be seen. Clearly, the size of the bleed is an important determinant of the likelihood of severe motor and cognitive deficits. Infants with extensive cortical hemorrhage nearly always have motor deficits such as hemiparesis or diparesis and cognitive impairment.[57] In comparison, infants with localized, especially unilateral, parenchymal hemorrhage may have a much better outcome, with approximately 10% being apparently normal. The most common motor deficit patterns seen in children with severe PIVH are hemiparesis and dystonia.[70]

Degree of ventriculomegaly is also related to neurodevelopmental outcome of infants with PIVH. Bozynski and colleagues[71,72] studied neurodevelopmental outcome of premature infants with PIVH at 1 and 2 years. Almost half of these infants had a history of PIVH; evaluations at 12 months using Bayley Scales found that infants with PIVH and ventriculomegaly had poorer motor performance than did infants with PIVH without ventriculomegaly and control patients without PIVH. An important finding was that those infants whose ventricles had decreased to normal size by term fared significantly better than did those infants with persistent ventriculomegaly, though less favorable outcomes overall have been reported in other series. Persistent ventriculomegaly increased the risk of poorer neurologic outcome in another study: A fivefold increase in the risk of cerebral palsy and a threefold risk for hypertonia and hyperreflexia were found at 18 months in infants with enlarged ventricles, although none of five infants with parenchymal hemorrhage had cerebral palsy.[73] Although one might expect that development of posthemorrhagic hydrocephalus that ultimately requires shunting significantly worsens neurodevelopmental outcome, independent of ventricular size, this has not been demonstrated consistently.[74]

In addition to ventricular size, the shape of the cerebral ventricles on MRI correlates with neurodevelopmental outcome in premature infants. In one study, 42 prematurely born children were matched with term-born children and studied with MRI at school age.[75] Four premature infants developed cerebral palsy. Of these children, three had enlarged ventricles, two had irregularly shaped ventricles, and all had periventricular leukomalacia (PVL) on MRI. However, six of 24 neurologically normal children born prematurely in this study also had PVL, and five had enlarged ventricles, but none had irregularly shaped cerebral ventricles. This observation suggests that ventricular configuration is a more specific predictor of cerebral palsy than is either cerebral ventricle size or PVL.

Another feature predictive of long-term neurologic outcome of PIVH on cranial US is whether midline shift is present at the time of the hemorrhage. In a study of 44 premature infants with PIVH, a shift of the midline by 3 mm or more was associated with an increased risk of major neurologic deficit in infants.[76] Only 3 of 12 infants in this series who had PIVH without midline shift had a major neurologic deficit at follow-up, but all 22 infants with PIVH that caused a midline shift had at least one major developmental deficit.

Whereas short-term outcome studies have been very useful in assessing the impact of PIVH on motor function, long-term neurodevelopmental studies with follow-up to school age are needed to evaluate effects on cognitive performance. Unfortunately, few such studies are available. Two-year-old children who were born prematurely with or without mild PIVH and control 2-year-old children born at term were assessed on a battery of cognitive tests.[77] On most cognitive measures, prematurely born children with PIVH did not differ from those without PIVH, although both groups of premature infants performed less well than did the full-term, control children. In another study, poor perceptual-motor skills and impairment on selected memory tests were noted in 6 of 15 infants with PIVH who were tested at 5 years of age and who were believed to be neurologically normal at 30 months of age.[78] Lowe and Papile[79] followed 11 infants with mild PIVH and 27 without PIVH who were born weighing less than 1,501 g; all were developmentally normal at 1–2 years of age. Neurodevelopmental assessment at 5–6 years showed that infants with PIVH scored lower than did premature infants without PIVH on a combined battery of tests.

Prevention

Prevention of premature birth is clearly the optimal strategy for reducing the incidence of PIVH, although this is not always possible. Advances in the obstetric care of high-risk pregnancies, such as transport of the mother before delivery to hospitals with appropriate perinatal care facilities and expertise, have also been important.

Significant interest has been expressed in pharmacologic interventions for PIVH prophylaxis.[80] Of the available drugs, the most promising appear to be corticosteroids administered before delivery. Numerous small- and large-scale studies have demonstrated the efficacy of antenatal corticosteroids in reducing the incidence of PIVH.[81–83] A National Institutes of Health consensus statement has recommended that antenatal corticosteroid administration be strongly considered in all mothers with impending preterm delivery.[84] Indomethacin administered postnatally also has been shown to reduce the incidence and severity of PIVH; the incidence of severe PIVH especially has been favorably affected.[85,86] Indomethacin markedly reduces cerebral blood flow, and so widespread use of this agent has been limited by fears that indomethacin would cause ischemic injury to cerebral white matter in premature infants. However, serial cranial US scans in indomethacin-treated infants have not revealed evidence of cerebral ischemic injury and, in a follow-up study at 36 months, no adverse effects of indomethacin on cognitive function were noted.[87]

Other drugs to prevent or ameliorate the cerebral damage caused by PIVH include antenatal (but not postnatal) phenobarbital administration,[88–90] ethamsylate,[91–93] vitamin E,[94–96] and vitamin K.[97,98] None of these agents is in routine use for PIVH prophylaxis currently, because of concern about the toxicity of such agents, but indomethacin and phenobarbital appear to be the most likely to gain wider acceptance in the near future.

SUBDURAL HEMORRHAGE

Subdural hemorrhage in neonates is associated with traumatic tearing of the great cerebral veins, a cerebral venous sinus, or the bridging superficial cerebral veins, especially in premature infants. During labor and delivery, excessive traction, compression, or rotation of the pliable neonatal skull causes tearing of intracranial blood vessels. Accordingly, risk factors for subdural hemorrhage include large size at birth, small birth canal, prolonged delivery, breech presentation, vacuum extraction, and extreme head molding,[99–101] but subdural hemorrhage might occur in infants with none of these risk factors. Rarely, a subdural hemorrhage may be a clue to an inborn coagulopathy or thrombocytopenia.[102]

Clinical signs of subdural hemorrhage are related to whether the subdural hemorrhage is located within the posterior fossa or above the tentorium. Neurologic symptoms are due to (1) direct mass effect of the hematoma, (2) obstruction of CSF flow, and (3) irritative effects of blood, causing seizures. Posterior fossa subdural hematomas tend to present with apnea, arching, and brain stem signs such as skew deviation, tongue fasciculations, facial weakness, and oculomotor paresis. Bradycardia is an ominous sign because it indicates serious brain stem compromise. Cortical subdural hemorrhage is seen most frequently as an extension over the occipital and posterior temporal lobes of a hematoma that results from a tentorial tear, though such a hemorrhage can occur alone over the cerebral convexity. Cortical subdural hemorrhage may be asymptomatic or might cause seizures, conjugate lateral eye deviation, and hemiparesis. Obstructive hydrocephalus can result from either infratentorial or supratentorial subdural hemorrhage, owing to subarachnoid inflammation. As with other types of intracranial hemorrhage in newborns, subdural hemorrhage in infants should prompt a search for evidence of thrombocytopenia and coagulopathy.[103]

Clinical features and neurologic outcome of 48 infants with subdural hematomas detected during the first 10 days of life have been reported.[104] Three-fourths of these infants were born at term. On the basis of CT findings, nearly half of the subdural hematomas occurred along the posterior interhemispheric fissure and approximately one-third extended from the incisura to the posterior fossa. Subdural hematoma accompanied intracerebral hemorrhage in three (7%) neonates. Increased intracranial pressure, as measured through the anterior fontanelle, correlated inversely with neurologic outcome. All six infants with intracranial pressure of less than 300 mm H_2O were normal at follow-up at 6 months to 3 years, but only four of seven infants with intracranial pressure greater than 300 mm H_2O were classified as normal. The location of the subdural hematoma did not appear to affect neurodevelopmental outcome significantly.

Somewhat longer follow-up evaluations were presented in a review of 15 infants born at or later than 36 weeks' gestation who had a posterior fossa subdural hematoma.[105] At follow-up ranging from 2 to 10 years, seven children were believed to be neurologically normal with age-appropriate skills. Three children had mild neurologic deficits, two were moderately affected, and three were profoundly impaired. The pattern of neurologic deficits related to location of the subdural hemorrhage was not consistent. One child was hemiplegic with language delay, one was cortically blind and hemiplegic with motor and cognitive deficits, and one had delayed walking and dysarthric speech. Rather, evidence of supratentorial injury (porencephaly, cerebral atrophy, and cerebral calcifications) was observed in the children with the worst functional outcomes.

SUBARACHNOID HEMORRHAGE

The incidence of isolated subarachnoid hemorrhage in newborns is variably estimated but probably is very high, as determined by both autopsy and cranial CT imaging studies.[106,107] In preterm infants, the pathogenesis of subarachnoid hemorrhage may be due to rupture of immature leptomeningeal blood vessels (analogous to the pathogenesis of germinal matrix hemorrhage), whereas in full-term infants, subarachnoid hemorrhage is believed to result primarily from the trauma of labor and birth (analogous to the pathogenesis of subdural bleeds). However, the cause in most instances is unknown. Nearly always, the amount of subarachnoid blood is small and the infant is asymptomatic. Seizures and apnea are the most common neurologic manifestations in symptomatic, full-term infants, who usually have a moderate amount of subarachnoid blood.[108] Large collections of subarachnoid blood may lead to acute or delayed obstructive hydrocephalus. Fortunately, long-term neurodevelopmental sequelae may be avoided and probably are more closely related to concomitant hypoxic-ischemic injury than to adverse effects of the subarachnoid bleed itself. However, in one study, only 50% of full-term infants with subarachnoid hemorrhage had an apparently normal outcome, and outcome did not differ between infants whose disorder had a presumed traumatic etiology and those whose disorder had a hypoxic-ischemic etiology.[108]

CEREBELLAR HEMORRHAGE

Cerebellar hemorrhage is an uncommon but potentially devastating disorder seen primarily in premature infants. Four major types of cerebellar hemorrhage occur in infants: (1) primary intracerebellar hemorrhage, (2) venous hemorrhagic infarction, (3) extension of PIVH or subarachnoid hemorrhage into the cerebellum, and (4) traumatic laceration of the cerebellum or major cerebral veins or sinuses.[5] Several interrelated causal factors are associated with cerebellar hemorrhage in newborns, with trauma to the pliant newborn skull being probably the most important pathogenetic factor. During breech delivery or difficult forceps extraction, the premature skull is subjected to shear forces that can push the occipital bone up underneath the parietal skull, thereby lacerating the tentorium, the cerebellum, or the occipital sinus. Even if direct laceration does not occur, displacement of the occipital bone can raise venous pressure in the occipital sinus and create a hemorrhagic venous infarction in the cerebellum. Upward cerebellar herniation could occur through similar mechanisms. In premature infants, cerebellar hemorrhage may be seen in the absence of trauma, but risk factors are not well established owing to the rarity of this type of hemorrhage. Concurrent supratentorial intraventricular hemorrhage and hypoxic-ischemic injury may be present as well. Nontraumatic causes of intracerebellar hemorrhage include rupture of the cerebellar germinal matrix, which tends to outlive its cortical homolog, the subependymal germinal matrix.

Small intracerebellar hemorrhages may be asymptomatic. However, infants with large hemorrhages may present with rapid onset of obstructive hydrocephalus owing to interruption of CSF flow through the fourth ventricle. Signs of brain stem compression such as apnea, vertical or horizontal dysconjugate gaze, bifacial weakness, and loss of the corneal reflex are present. Bradycardia suggests that immediate surgical intervention—either posterior fossa decompression or ventricular shunting—may be necessary.[109] Cranial CT or MRI is superior to head US in recognizing cerebellar hemorrhage because of the difficulty in imaging the posterior fossa with US, though US viewing through the posterior fontanelle may improve diagnostic accuracy in such cases.

The neurodevelopmental prognosis for infants with cerebellar hemorrhage varies. Mortality is high, especially in premature infants. In survivors, cerebellar function is nearly always impaired, as one might expect, but severe global cognitive deficits also are seen in some premature and full-term infants. In one report of six full-term infants with cerebellar hemorrhage examined at an average of 32 months, five had hypotonia, truncal ataxia, and intention tremor, and two had nystagmus. Only one child walked independently, and intellectual performance was impaired in all six patients.[110] In the acute phase, surgical decompression is indicated for large hemorrhages that interfere with brain stem function, but smaller hemorrhages are best followed conservatively.

EPIDURAL HEMORRHAGE

Epidural hemorrhage is unusual in newborns and occurs when the middle meningeal artery or large veins are injured, such as from a skull fracture. An overlying cephalhematoma often is present. Initial neurologic symptoms include lethargy and seizures. Later, signs of increased intracranial pressure, such as a bulging fontanelle and an ipsilateral dilated pupil, may occur. Emergent drainage of an epidural hematoma may be necessary, but three of four infants in one series were treated successfully with drainage of the associated cephalhematoma, and all made a complete recovery. The fourth infant, whose course was complicated by intraventricular and subarachnoid hemorrhage and disseminated intravascular coagulation, recovered without surgical intervention but had residual motor deficits.[111]

CEREBRAL INFARCTION AND HEMORRHAGE

Focal infarctions of the cerebral cortex are far less common in neonates than are intracranial hemorrhagic lesions. Cerebral infarctions may have an intrauterine or a peripartum onset. Although a variety of etiologies have been reported, in a particular infant a specific cause often cannot be identified.

Focal cerebral infarction is much more likely to occur in full-term than in preterm infants. In a large autopsy series, the incidence of cerebral infarction was 5%.[112] The middle cerebral artery territory is affected more often than are the anterior or posterior artery territories,[113] and involvement of more than one artery in a given patient is uncommon. The left middle cerebral artery alone is involved in 63% of infants with cerebral infarction.[5] The presence of multifocal cerebral infarctions strongly suggests embolism or a diffuse vasculopathy.

Embolism is most often cited as the cause of cerebral infarction, although definitive evidence usually is lacking. Emboli may arise from cardiac, placental, or other organ sources and are particularly likely in the context of sepsis and disseminated intravascular coagulation.[112] Elevated maternal antiphospholipid antibodies have been implicated in a few neonates with cerebral infarction,[114,115] but this author has been unable to identify these antibodies in neonates with cerebral infarctions. Embolic arterial occlusion may be evident in the peripheral vasculature of an otherwise well-appearing child, though this is very unusual. Although perinatal hypoxia-ischemia has been postulated as a frequent cause of neonatal cerebral infarction, little evidence supports this claim.[116]

Cortical infarctions often are asymptomatic in the neonatal period and are discovered usually during the first year of life on cranial imaging performed to evaluate a hemiparesis. In the newborn period, seizures are the most common presenting symptom of cortical infarctions, though apnea, lethargy, and hypotonia can also be seen.[117] Seizures typically are focal and clonic, with onset during the first 2 days of life. Surprisingly, major focal motor deficits during the early postnatal period are uncommon, even in infants with large infarctions; this observation has been assumed as evidence that the control of movement in the neonate is mediated primarily through subcortical and cerebellar structures. Nonetheless, subtle motor deficits usually are present in full-term infants, detection of which may require careful comparison of the spontaneous movements of the affected and unaffected sides.

Neonatal cortical infarctions appear on head US as loss of gyral definition, focal increased echogenicity, and mass effect if the infarct is large.[118] Other imaging techniques such as proton- and diffusion-weighted MRI[119,120] can demonstrate clearly the area of infarcted cerebral tissue in infants. Doppler evaluation may show decreased or absent cerebral artery flow in the affected vascular distribution.[121] Not surprisingly, cranial MRI is superior to US and CT in the diagnosis of cortical infarction,[62] especially in identifying early or small infarc-

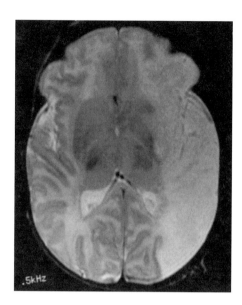

Figure 9.2 Neonatal cortical infarction. A left middle cerebral artery infarction is shown on this magnetic resonance image. The infant was born at term and presented with focal seizures.

tions. An MRI scan demonstrating an infarction of the left middle cerebral artery in a full-term infant is shown in Figure 9.2. In some cases, MRI is useful also in establishing the approximate timing of an intrauterine infarction. Absence of gliosis around the infarct site indicates that the infarction occurred before 23 weeks' gestation, because reactive gliosis in the brain develops at approximately this time.

Limited data exist regarding the long-term neurologic outcome of infants with neonatal ischemic stroke. Contralateral hemiparesis is common but not universal, and nearly 10% of children will have a hemiparesis *ipsilateral* to the cerebral infarction. In one series of 16 children born at term with neonatal infarction, 11 of 15 survivors had an apparently normal outcome, although detailed neurodevelopmental evaluations were not conducted.[117] Of nine infants with neonatal stroke involving the corticospinal tract in another study, five developed hemiplegia,[113] and similar findings were obtained in another small series.[122] Of 29 infants with a single cerebral infarction in one series, 21 had a hemiparesis, but intelligence testing at a mean of 44 months of age was normal in all children.[123] Whereas severe motor and cognitive disabilities are not always apparent after neonatal cerebral infarction, careful neurodevelopmental testing may reveal significant abnormalities not evident on cursory examination.[123,124] The incidence of seizures in children with spastic hemiparesis is high, and such children may be more difficult to taper off anticonvulsant therapy than are children with other types of cerebral palsy and seizures.[125]

Isolated cerebral parenchymal hemorrhage in full-term infants is not uncommon and may occur in any lobe of the cerebral cortex or in the thalamus or basal ganglia (Figure 9.3). Certainly, a large proportion of these hemorrhages

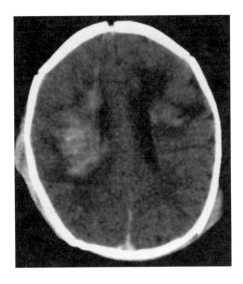

Figure 9.3 Neonatal parenchymal hemorrhage. This computed tomographic image shows multiple, focal parenchymal hemorrhages in a 1-day-old full-term infant with alloimmune thrombocytopenia. (Courtesy of Dr. Darryl Crisp.)

are secondary to a focal cerebral infarction or cerebral venous thrombosis, and the incidence of primary parenchymal hemorrhage is unknown but probably low. As with cerebral infarction, the most common presenting symptom is seizures. All four children with lobar cortical hemorrhages in one series presented with seizures beginning on or before the second day of life.[103,126] At follow-up ranging from 1 to 6 years, three of these children were normal. One child, who had a left occipital lobe hemorrhage, had severe developmental delay at 3 years of age. In this series, the location of the hemorrhage did not seem related to outcome because another child with a left occipital lobe hemorrhage was normal at 1 year of age.

Thalamic hemorrhage is an uncommon but potentially serious type of intracranial hemorrhage in the newborn, occurring in nearly 4% of full-term infants who have intracranial hemorrhage,[127] and may be associated with intraventricular hemorrhage.[128] Some studies report that thalamic hemorrhage occurs after severe perinatal asphyxia.[129] The most common presenting symptom is seizures, although apnea, lethargy, and brain stem findings are seen if the hemorrhage is large enough either to produce an obstructive hydrocephalus or to cause direct compression of the brain stem. Rarely, the hemorrhage is so massive that the infant dies, but in the more common small thalamic bleeds, the infants do fairly well.[127]

Cerebral venous sinus thrombosis once was believed to be rare, but advances in cranial imaging have revealed this disorder with increasing frequency. Slow blood flow through the cerebral sinuses and great veins secondary to intravascular clot can be demonstrated by Doppler US, and the thrombus can easily be visualized by MRI. The posterior part of the superior sagittal sinus and the transverse sinus are the most frequently involved cerebral blood vessels, although thrombus originating in the superior sagittal sinus may spread to involve other blood vessels, and thrombus may occur in the transverse sinus or deep cerebral veins alone. Cerebral venous sinus thrombosis may lead to hemorrhagic infarction of the parasagittal cortex or thalamus and basal ganglia or to diffuse cerebral edema.[130] Seizures or lethargy are the most common symptoms, and the neurologic prognosis may be good.[131] In my experience, seven infants with cerebral sinus thrombosis who presented with seizures and who were treated conservatively without systemic anticoagulants all had normal short-term neurodevelopmental outcome. In contrast, thalamic hemorrhage associated with cerebral venous thrombosis is associated with severe neurologic deficits.[130]

PERIVENTRICULAR LEUKOMALACIA

Necrosis of the periventricular cerebral white matter appearing weeks or months after birth is a serious neurologic complication primarily (though not exclusively) of premature birth. Although the pathogenesis of PVL still is unknown, the neurodevelopmental implications of PVL have become clearer, and several clinical risk factors have been identified. PVL occurs in a characteristic distribution, involving the white matter adjacent to the external angle of the lateral ventricle and the posterior cerebral white matter in the peritrigonal area. The white matter adjacent to the ventricular wall usually is spared. Lesions in the periventricular area tend to affect the centrum semiovale and the optic and temporal radiations. Thus, lesions in the periventricular area affect association and commissural axons that connect adjacent cortical gyri to each other, and homologous cortical areas across the midline. Further, through the periventricular area pass axons of ascending sensory fibers from the spinal cord and descending motor fibers from the cortex to the spinal cord. Microscopic examination of PVL lesions reveals coagulative necrosis and swollen and encrusted axons, with proliferation of reactive astrocytes, macrophages, and microglia. Oligodendroglial damage leads to impairment of subsequent myelination.[132]

PVL usually is bilateral, though it often is asymmetric.[133] It can be classified according to size of the white matter cysts noted on cranial US. Cystic PVL refers to large areas of necrosis in the periventricular white matter (Figure 9.4), whereas microcystic PVL is characterized by ventricular dilation in the absence of large cysts. PVL often is seen in association with PIVH: Of infants with pathologically proved PVL, 50–75% also have PIVH,[134,135] suggesting common causal factors, but both disorders can occur independently. The importance of systemic hypotension in the pathogenesis of PVL has been emphasized by observations in experimental animals and in human premature infants. PVL is more common in infants with hypovolemia, patent ductus arteriosus, transient systemic hypotension, and infants with hypoplastic left heart syndrome.[136–138] Not all studies have found hypotension to be related to risk of PVL. In a study involving 69 premature infants with cystic PVL, researchers found that intra-

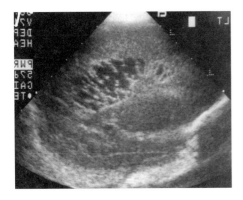

Figure 9.4 This cranial ultrasound scan shows extensive, severe cystic periventricular leukomalacia in a premature infant who had repeated episodes of hypotension and bradycardia after delivery.

uterine infection days or weeks before pregnancy and prolonged rupture of membranes were the best predictors of PVL.[139] Similarly, chorioamnionitis significantly increased the risk of subsequent PVL in another study.[140]

PVL carries a high risk of mortality, especially if PIVH is present. Nearly half of the infants born at less than 33 weeks' gestation who had PVL died, compared with two-thirds of infants with both PVL and PIVH.[138] In very low–birth-weight infants, the mortality rate associated with PVL is even higher.

PVL usually is unrecognizable clinically during the first few weeks after birth, although in some infants lower-extremity weakness can be detected.[5] Long-term neurodevelopmental outcome of PVL, as with PIVH, depends greatly on the size and site of the cerebral white matter lesions and on whether other lesions, such as PIVH or cortical infarction, are present. As might be expected, motor and cognitive deficits are more severe if the white matter injury involves both anterior and posterior cortex.[141] Similarly, infants with frontal PVL fared better neurologically at 18 months than did infants with extensive PVL.[142]

Cranial imaging findings in children with cerebral palsy are markedly different in infants born prematurely and infants born at term.[143] In one large study, MRI was obtained in 40 infant patients with cerebral palsy, 29 of whom were born at term and 11 of whom were premature.[144] All 11 premature infants had deep white matter atrophy, especially in the peritrigonal area, and abnormally enlarged ventricles with irregular borders (Figure 9.5). In contrast, full-term infants had more varied abnormalities on MRI, and 34% of patients had normal periventricular cerebral white matter. Six of the full-term infants with white matter lesions had overlying neuronal migration anomalies, and fewer than half had ventricular enlargement or irregular ventricular borders. Neuronal migration abnormalities were not seen in any infants born before term.

VASCULAR MALFORMATIONS

Vascular malformations and aneurysms do not commonly present in the newborn period except for vein of Galen malformations, in which there is an

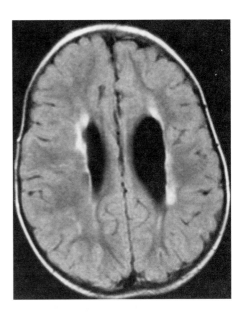

Figure 9.5 Cranial magnetic resonance image of an infant born at 30 weeks' gestation who has spastic diparesis and a right hemiparesis at 12 months of age. Note the high-signal lesions around the lateral ventricles and that the ventricles are enlarged with irregular borders.

anastomotic connection between branches of the carotid or vertebral circulation and the vein of Galen, a major draining vein of the cerebrum, or its embryologic precursor, the medial vein of the prosencephalon. In newborns, vein of Galen malformations most often present with high-output cardiac failure due to left-to-right shunting of blood through the malformation or, less commonly, with obstructive hydrocephalus due to interruption of CSF flow by the dilated vascular malformation. Clinically, infants with this malformation may have signs of increased intracranial pressure, seizures, and obtundation, in addition to a cranial bruit, hepatomegaly, tachycardia, and respiratory distress. Cranial US with Doppler can show blood flow through the dilated vein of Galen, and diagnosis can be confirmed with contrast-enhanced CT or MRI, although cerebral arteriography is needed to define the feeding and draining blood vessels (Figure 9.6).

Survival rates are poor in untreated patients, especially in infants with severe heart failure. If heart failure does not dominate the clinical picture, then ventriculoperitoneal shunting can relieve the hydrocephalus, if present, and intravascular embolization of the vascular malformation can dramatically reduce mortality.[145] Surgical removal of the malformation is associated with very high mortality rates unless the malformation can be reduced by prior embolization. Intravascular embolization via arterial or venous approaches can be carried out, often in stages to effect a gradual reduction in cerebral blood flow through the arteriovenous malformation. Embolization can improve both mortality and neurologic morbidity in these patients. Approximately 30–50% of the survivors of vein of Galen malformations who underwent intravascular embolization in the newborn period are neurologically normal on follow-up.[146,147]

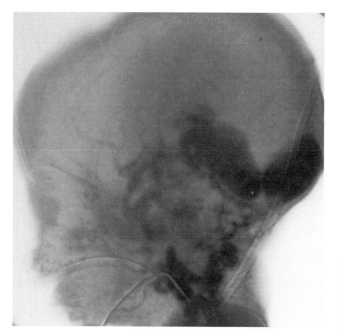

Figure 9.6 This cerebral arteriogram shows a vein of Galen malformation in a young infant.

Cerebral arterial aneurysms and arteriovenous malformations other than vein of Galen malformations are rare causes of intracranial hemorrhage in the newborn (Figure 9.7). The choroid plexus, cerebral hemispheres, and third ventricle are the most common sites for symptomatic hemorrhage of these vascular defects in newborns. Neurologic symptoms are the same as are seen in intracranial hemorrhage from other causes and include seizures, hydrocephalus, and apnea. MRI and magnetic resonance angiography are useful adjuncts to cranial US in the diagnosis of these vascular defects, but conventional arteriography still is required to delineate fully the anatomy and extent of the abnormal cerebral blood vessels. Other rare causes of intracranial hemorrhage include bleeding associated with tumors in the posterior fossa (e.g., medulloblastoma) or in the cerebral cortex (e.g., choroid plexus papilloma). Coarctation of the aorta is associated with intracranial vascular anomalies, but these very rarely present in neonates. In patients with tumors that present with hemorrhage in the neonatal period, the long-term neurologic outcome is unknown because of the rarity of such tumors.

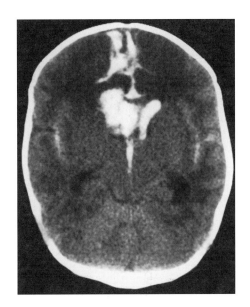

Figure 9.7 Cranial computed tomography shows a focal hemorrhage in the right caudate nucleus with intraventricular extension in a young infant. Edema is present also in both frontal lobes; arteriography demonstrated an anterior cerebral artery aneurysm.

REFERENCES

1. Kuban KCK, Leviton A. Medical progress. Cerebral palsy. N Engl J Med 1994; 330:188–195.
2. Marin-Padilla M. Review of perinatal brain damage, repair, and neurologic sequelae in the prematurely born infant. Int Pediatr 1995;10:26–33.
3. Burger PC, Graham DG, Burch JG, et al. Hemorrhagic cerebral white matter: infarction with cerebral deep venous thrombosis and hypoxia. Arch Pathol Lab Med 1978;102:40–42.
4. Volpe JJ. Intraventricular hemorrhage in the premature infant—current concepts (pt 1). Ann Neurol 1989;25:3–11.
5. Volpe JJ. Neurology of the Newborn. Philadelphia: Saunders, 1995.
6. Volpe JJ. Subplate neurons—missing link in brain injury of the premature infant? Pediatrics 1996;97:112–113.
7. Dubowitz LM, Levene MI, Morante A, et al. Neurologic signs in neonatal intraventricular hemorrhage: a correlation with real-time ultrasound. J Pediatr 1981;99: 127–133.
8. Ahmann PA, Lazzara A, Dykes FD, et al. Intraventricular hemorrhage in the high-risk preterm infant: incidence and outcome. Ann Neurol 1980;7:118–124.
9. Hawgood S, Spong J, Yu VY. Intraventricular hemorrhage. Incidence and outcome in a population of very-low-birth-weight infants. Am J Dis Child 1984;138:136–139.
10. McMenamin JB, Shackelford GD, Volpe JJ. Outcome of neonatal intraventricular hemorrhage with periventricular echodense lesions. Ann Neurol 1984;15:285–290.
11. Shankaran S, Bauer CR, Bain R, et al. Prenatal and perinatal risk and protective factors for neonatal intracranial hemorrhage. National Institute of Child Health and Human Development Neonatal Research Network. Arch Pediatr Adolesc Med 1996;150:491–497.

12. Shankaran S, Bauer C, Bandstra E, et al. Intracranial hemorrhage (ICH) in 2928 <1500 g neonates [abstract]. Pediatr Res 1991;29:266A.
13. Claris O, Besnier S, Lapillonne A, et al. Incidence of ischemic-hemorrhagic cerebral lesions in premature infants of gestational age ≤28 weeks: a prospective ultrasound study. Biol Neonate 1996;70:29–34.
14. Ment LR, Oh W, Ehrenkranz RA, et al. Risk period for intraventricular hemorrhage of the preterm neonate is independent of gestational age. Semin Perinatol 1993;17:338–341.
15. Cooke RW. Trends in preterm survival and incidence of cerebral haemorrhage 1980–9. Arch Dis Child 1991;66:403–407.
16. Hanigan WC, Morgan AM, Anderson RJ, et al. Incidence and neurodevelopmental outcome of periventricular hemorrhage and hydrocephalus in a regional population of very low birth weight infants. Neurosurgery 1991;29:701–706.
17. Philip AG, Allan WC, Tito AM, et al. Intraventricular hemorrhage in preterm infants. Declining incidence in the 1980s. Pediatrics 1989;84:797–801.
18. Paneth N, Pinto-Martin J, Gardiner J, et al. Incidence and timing of germinal matrix/intraventricular hemorrhage in low birth weight infants. Am J Epidemiol 1993;137:1167–1176.
19. Burrows RF, Caco CC, Kelton JG. Neonatal alloimmune thrombocytopenia: spontaneous in utero intracranial hemorrhage. Am J Hematol 1988;28:98–102.
20. Horng YC, Chou YH, Chen RL, et al. Congenital factor VII deficiency complicated with hemoperitoneum and intracranial hemorrhage: report of a case. J Formos Med Assoc 1993;92:85–87.
21. Sandler E, Gross S. Prevention of recurrent intracranial hemorrhage in a factor X-deficient infant. Am J Pediatr Hematol Oncol 1992;14:163–165.
22. Abbondanzo SL, Gootenberg JE, Lofts RS, McPherson RA. Intracranial hemorrhage in congenital deficiency of factor XIII. Am J Pediatr Hematol Oncol 1988;10:65–68.
23. Jocelyn LJ, Casiro OG. Neurodevelopmental outcome of term infants with intraventricular hemorrhage. Am J Dis Child 1992;146:194–197.
24. Ment LR, Stewart WB, Ardito TA, et al. Germinal matrix microvascular maturation correlates inversely with the risk period for neonatal intraventricular hemorrhage. Brain Res Dev Brain Res 1995;84:142–149.
25. Van de Bor M, Van Bel F, Lineman R, et al. Perinatal factors and periventricular-intraventricular hemorrhage in preterm infants. Am J Dis Child 1986;140:1125–1130.
26. Bada HS, Korones SB, Anderson GD, et al. Obstetric factors and relative risk of neonatal germinal layer/intraventricular hemorrhage. Am J Obstet Gynecol 1984;148:798–804.
27. Rayburn WF, Donn SM, Kolin MG, et al. Obstetric care and intraventricular hemorrhage in the low birth weight infant. Obstet Gynecol 1983;62:408–413.
28. Adhikari M, Gouws E, Desai PK. Periventricular hemorrhage in a developing world. Is drug intervention appropriate? Brain Dev 1995;17:164–168.
29. Wallin LA, Rosenfeld CR, Laptook AR, et al. Neonatal intracranial hemorrhage: II. Risk factor analysis in an inborn population. Early Hum Dev 1990;23:129–137.
30. Spinillo A, Ometto A, Bottino R, et al. Antenatal risk factors for germinal matrix hemorrhage and intraventricular hemorrhage in preterm infants. Eur J Obstet Gynecol Rep Biol 1995;60:13–19.
31. Spinillo A, Ometto A, Stronati M, et al. Epidemiologic association between maternal smoking during pregnancy and intracranial hemorrhage in preterm infants. J Pediatr 1995;127:472–478.
32. Holzman C, Paneth N, Little R, et al. Perinatal brain injury in premature infants born to mothers using alcohol in pregnancy. Neonatal Brain Hemorrhage Study Team. Pediatrics 1995;95:66–73.

33. Bada HS, Korones SB, Perry EH, et al. Frequent handling in the neonatal intensive care unit and intraventricular hemorrhage. J Pediatr 1990;117:126–131.
34. Singer LT, Yamashita TS, Hawkins S, et al. Increased incidence of intraventricular hemorrhage and developmental delay in cocaine-exposed, very low birth weight infants. J Pediatr 1994;124:765–771.
35. Dusick AM, Covert RF, Schreiber MD, et al. Risk of intracranial hemorrhage and other adverse outcomes after cocaine exposure in a cohort of 323 very low birth weight infants. J Pediatr 1993;122:438–445.
36. Spires MC, Gordon EF, Choudhuri M, et al. Intracranial hemorrhage in a neonate following prenatal cocaine exposure. Pediatr Neurol 1989;5:324–326.
37. McLenan DA, Ajayi OA, Rydman RJ, et al. Evaluation of the relationship between cocaine and intraventricular hemorrhage. J Natl Med Assoc 1994;86:281–287.
38. Anderson GD, Bada HS, Shaver DC, et al. The effect of cesarean section on intraventricular hemorrhage in the preterm infant. Am J Obstet Gynecol 1992;166:1091–1099.
39. Shaver DC, Bada HS, Korones SB, et al. Early and late intraventricular hemorrhage: the role of obstetric factors. Obstet Gynecol 1992;80:831–837.
40. Ment LR, Oh W, Philip AG, et al. Risk factors for early intraventricular hemorrhage in low birth weight infants. J Pediatr 1992;121:776–783.
41. O'Shea M, Savitz DA, Hage ML, et al. Prenatal events and the risk of subependymal/intraventricular haemorrhage in very low birthweight neonates. Paediatr Perinat Epidemiol 1992;6:352–362.
42. Leviton A, Fenton T, Kuban KC, et al. Labor and delivery characteristics and the risk of germinal matrix hemorrhage in low birth weight infants. J Child Neurol 1991;6:35–40.
43. Wimberley PD, Lou HC, Pedersen H, et al. Hypertensive peaks in the pathogenesis of intraventricular hemorrhage in the newborn. Abolition by phenobarbitone sedation. Acta Paediatr Scand 1982;71:537–542.
44. McDonald MM, Koops BL, Johnson ML, et al. Timing and antecedents of intracranial hemorrhage in the newborn. Pediatrics 1984;74:32–36.
45. Goldberg RN, Chung D, Goldman SL, et al. The association of rapid volume expansion and intraventricular hemorrhage in the preterm infant. J Pediatr 1980;96:1060–1063.
46. Lipscomb AP, Thorburn RJ, Reynolds EO, et al. Pneumothorax and cerebral haemorrhage in preterm infants. Lancet 1981;1:414–416.
47. Hill A, Perlman JM, Volpe JJ. Relationship of pneumothorax to occurrence of intraventricular hemorrhage in the premature newborn. Pediatrics 1982;69:144–149.
48. Thorburn RJ, Lipscomb AP, Stewart AL, et al. Timing and antecedents of periventricular haemorrhage and of cerebral atrophy in very preterm infants. Early Hum Dev 1982;7:221–238.
49. Hill A, Volpe JJ. Seizures, hypoxic-ischemic brain injury, and intraventricular hemorrhage in the newborn. Ann Neurol 1981;10:109–121.
50. Lou HC. On the pathogenesis of germinal layer hemorrhage in the neonate. APMIS Suppl 1993;40:97–102.
51. Funato M, Tamai H, Noma K, et al. Clinical events in association with timing of intraventricular hemorrhage in preterm infants. J Pediatr 1992;121:614–619.
52. Kosmetatos N, Dinter C, Williams ML, et al. Intracranial hemorrhage in the premature. Its predictive features and outcome. Am J Dis Child 1980;134:855–859.
53. Ment LR, Stewart WB, Duncan CC, et al. Beagle puppy model of perinatal cerebral infarction. Acute changes in cerebral blood flow and metabolism during hemorrhagic hypotension. J Neurosurg 1985;63:441–447.
54. Gunkel JH, Banks PL. Surfactant therapy and intracranial hemorrhage: review of the literature and results of new analyses. Pediatrics 1993;92:775–786.

55. Ferrari B, Tonni G, Luzietti R, et al. Neonatal complications and risk of intraventricular-periventricular hemorrhage. Clin Exp Obstet Gynecol 1992;19:253–258.

56. Horbar JD, Pasnick M, McAuliffe TL, et al. Obstetric events and risk of periventricular hemorrhage in premature infants. Am J Dis Child 1983;137:678–681.

57. Guzzetta F, Shackelford GD, Volpe S, et al. Periventricular intraparenchymal echodensities in the premature newborn. Critical determinant of neurologic outcome. Pediatrics 1985;78:995–1006.

58. Jakobi P, Weissman A, Zimmer EZ, et al. Survival and long-term morbidity in preterm infants with and without a clinical diagnosis of periventricular, intraventricular hemorrhage. Eur J Obstet Gynecol Rep Biol 1992;46:73–77.

59. Perlman JM, Lynch B, Volpe JJ. Late hydrocephalus after arrest and resolution of neonatal post-hemorrhagic hydrocephalus. Dev Med Child Neurol 1990;32:725–729.

60. Slabaugh RD, Smith JA, Lemons J, et al. Neonatal intracranial hemorrhage and complicating hydrocephalus. J Clin Ultrasound 1984;12:261–266.

61. Ment LR, Duncan CC, Scott DT, et al. Posthemorrhagic hydrocephalus. Low incidence in very low birth weight neonates with intraventricular hemorrhage. J Neurosurg 1984;60:343–347.

62. Blankenberg FG, Norbash AM, Lane B, et al. Neonatal intracranial ischemia and hemorrhage: diagnosis with US, CT, and MR imaging. Radiology 1996;199:253–259.

63. Guit GL, van de Bor M, den Ouden L, et al. Prediction of neurodevelopmental outcome in the preterm infant. MR-staged myelination compared with cranial US. Radiology 1990;175:107–109.

64. Naulty CM, Gaiter JL, Chang CS, et al. Developmental outcome of infants with grade III intraventricular hemorrhage. South Med J 1983;76:158–162.

65. Williamson WD, Desmond MM, Wilson GS, et al. Survival of low-birth-weight infants with neonatal intraventricular hemorrhage. Outcome in the preschool years. Am J Dis Child 1983;137:1181–1184.

66. Rajani K, Goetzman BW, Kelso GF, et al. Prognosis of intracranial hemorrhage in neonates. Surg Neurol 1980;13:433–435.

67. Papile LA, Munsick-Bruno G, Schaefer A. Relationship of cerebral intraventricular hemorrhage and early childhood neurologic handicaps. J Pediatr 1983;103:273–277.

68. Donn SM, Roloff DW, Goldstein GW. Phenobarbitone and neonatal intraventricular haemorrhage [letter]. Lancet 1982;1:1240–1241.

69. Vohr BR, Garcia-Coll C, Mayfield S, et al. Neurologic and developmental status related to the evolution of visual-motor abnormalities from birth to 2 years of age in preterm infants with intraventricular hemorrhage. J Pediatr 1989;115:296–302.

70. Lin JP, Goh W, Brown JK, et al. Heterogeneity of neurological syndromes in survivors of grade 3 and 4 periventricular haemorrhage. Childs Nerv Syst 1993;9:205–214.

71. Bozynski ME, Nelson MN, Rosati-Skertich C, et al. Two year longitudinal followup of premature infants weighing less than or equal to 1,200 grams at birth: sequelae of intracranial hemorrhage. J Dev Behav Pediatr 1984;5:346–352.

72. Bozynski ME, Nelson MN, Genaze D, et al. Intracranial hemorrhage and neurodevelopmental outcome at one year in infants weighing 1200 grams or less. Prognostic significance of ventriculomegaly at term gestational age. Am J Perinatol 1984;1:325–330.

73. Krishnamoorthy KS, Kuban KC, Leviton A, et al. Periventricular-intraventricular hemorrhage, sonographic localization, phenobarbital, and motor abnormalities in low birth weight infants. Pediatrics 1990;85:1027–1033.

74. Holt PJ. Posthemorrhagic hydrocephalus. J Child Neurol 1989;4:S23–S31.

75. Olsen P, Paakko E, Vainionpaa L, et al. Magnetic resonance imaging of periventricular leukomalacia and its clinical significance in children. Ann Neurol 1997; 41:754–761.
76. Gibson JY, Massingale TW, Graves GR, et al. Relationship of cranial midline shift to outcome of very-low-birth-weight infants with periventricular hemorrhagic infarction. J Neuroimaging 1994;4:212–217.
77. Ross G, Boatright S, Auld PA, et al. Specific cognitive abilities in 2-year-old children with subependymal and mild intraventricular hemorrhage. Brain Cogn 1996;32:1–13.
78. Selzer SC, Lindgren SD, Blackman JA. Long-term neuropsychological outcome of high risk infants with intracranial hemorrhage. J Pediatr Psychol 1992;17: 407–422.
79. Lowe J, Papile L. Neurodevelopmental performance of very-low-birth-weight infants with mild periventricular, intraventricular hemorrhage. Outcome at 5 to 6 years of age. Am J Dis Child 1990;144:1242–1245.
80. Miller VS. Pharmacologic management of neonatal cerebral ischemia and hemorrhage: old and new directions. J Child Neurol 1993;8:7–18.
81. Ment LR, Oh W, Ehrenkranz RA, et al. Antenatal steroids, delivery mode, and intraventricular hemorrhage in preterm infants. Am J Obstet Gynecol 1995; 172:795–800.
82. Leviton A, Kuban KC, Pagano M, et al. Antenatal corticosteroids appear to reduce the risk of postnatal germinal matrix hemorrhage in intubated low birth weight newborns. Pediatrics 1993;91:1083–1088.
83. Leviton A, Pagano M, Kuban KC, et al. The epidemiology of germinal matrix hemorrhage during the first half-day of life. Dev Med Child Neurol 1991;33:138–145.
84. National Institutes of Health. Consensus Statement: Effect of Corticosteroids for Fetal Maturation on Perinatal Outcomes. Bethesda, MD: National Institutes of Health, 1994.
85. Ment LR, Oh W, Ehrenkranz RA, et al. Low-dose indomethacin and prevention of intraventricular hemorrhage: a multicenter randomized trial. Pediatrics 1994; 93:543–550.
86. Ment LR, Oh W, Ehrenkranz RA, et al. Low-dose indomethacin therapy and extension of intraventricular hemorrhage: a multicenter randomized trial. J Pediatr 1994;124:951–955.
87. Ment LR, Vohr B, Oh W, et al. Neurodevelopmental outcome at 36 months' corrected age of preterm infants in the Multicenter Indomethacin Intraventricular Hemorrhage Prevention Trial. Pediatrics 1996;98:714–718.
88. Shankaran S, Cepeda E, Muran G, et al. Antenatal phenobarbital therapy and neonatal outcome: I. Effect on intracranial hemorrhage. Pediatrics 1996;97: 644–648.
89. Barnes ER, Thompson DF. Antenatal phenobarbital to prevent or minimize intraventricular hemorrhage in the low-birthweight neonate. Ann Pharmacother 1993;27:49–52.
90. Kaempf JW, Porreco R, Molina R, et al. Antenatal phenobarbital for the prevention of periventricular and intraventricular hemorrhage: a double-blind, randomized, placebo-controlled, multihospital trial. J Pediatr 1990;117:933–938.
91. The EC Ethamsylate Trial Group. The EC randomised controlled trial of prophylactic ethamsylate for very preterm neonates: early mortality and morbidity. Arch Dis Child Fetal Neonatal Ed 1994;70:F201–F205.
92. Chen JY. Ethamsylate in the prevention of periventricular-intraventricular hemorrhage in premature infants. J Formos Med Assoc 1993;92:889–893.
93. Cooke RW, Morgan ME. Prophylactic ethamsylate for periventricular haemorrhage. Arch Dis Child 1984;59:82–83.

94. Chiswick M, Gladman G, Sinha S, et al. Vitamin E supplementation and periventricular hemorrhage in the newborn. Am J Clin Nutr 1991;53:370S–372S.
95. Law MR, Wijewardene K, Wald NJ. Is routine vitamin E administration justified in very low-birthweight infants? Dev Med Child Neurol 1990;32:442–450.
96. Fish WH, Cohen M, Franzek D, et al. Effect of intramuscular vitamin E on mortality and intracranial hemorrhage in neonates of 1000 grams or less. Pediatrics 1990;85:578–584.
97. Thorp JA, Parriott J, Ferrette-Smith D, et al. Antepartum vitamin K and phenobarbital for preventing intraventricular hemorrhage in the premature newborn: a randomized, double-blind, placebo-controlled trial. Obstet Gynecol 1994;83:70–76.
98. Morales WJ, Angel JL, O'Brien WF, et al. The use of antenatal vitamin K in the prevention of early neonatal intraventricular hemorrhage. Am J Obstet Gynecol 1988;159:774–779.
99. Castillo M, Fordham LA. MR of neurologically symptomatic newborns after vacuum extraction delivery. AJNR Am J Neuroradiol 1995;16:816–818.
100. Govaert P, Vanhaesebrouck P, de Praeter C. Traumatic neonatal intracranial bleeding and stroke. Arch Dis Child 1992;67:840–845.
101. Huang CC, Shen EY. Tentorial subdural hemorrhage in term newborns. Ultrasonographic diagnosis and clinical correlates. Pediatr Neurol 1991;7:171–177.
102. de Sousa C, Clark T, Bradshaw A. Antenatally diagnosed subdural haemorrhage in congenital factor X deficiency. Arch Dis Child 1988;63:1168–1170.
103. Hanigan WC, Powell FC, Miller TC, et al. Symptomatic intracranial hemorrhage in full-term infants. Childs Nerv Syst 1995;11:698–707.
104. Hayashi T, Hashimoto T, Fukuda S, et al. Neonatal subdural hematoma secondary to birth injury. Childs Nerv Syst 1987;3:23–29.
105. Perrin RG, Rutka JT, Drake JM, et al. Management and outcomes of posterior fossa subdural hematomas in neonates. Neurosurgery 1997;40:1190–1200.
106. Govaert P, Van De Velde E, Vanhaesebrouck P, et al. CT diagnosis of neonatal subarachnoid hemorrhage. Pediatr Radiol 1990;20:139–142.
107. Babcock DS, Bove KE, Han BK. Intracranial hemorrhage in premature infants. Sonographic-pathologic correlation. AJNR Am J Neuroradiol 1982;3:309–317.
108. Palmer TW, Donn SM. Symptomatic subarachnoid hemorrhage in the term newborn. J Perinatol 1991;11:112–116.
109. Tanaka Y, Sakamoto K, Kobayashi S, et al. Biphasic ventricular dilatation following posterior fossa subdural hematoma in the full-term neonate. J Neurosurg 1988;68:211–216.
110. Williamson WD, Percy AK, Fishman MA, et al. Cerebellar hemorrhage in the term neonate: developmental and neurologic outcome. Pediatr Neurol 1985;1:356–360.
111. Negishi H, Lee Y, Itoh K, et al. Nonsurgical management of epidural hematoma in neonates. Pediatr Neurol 1989;5:253–256.
112. Barmada MA, Moossy J, Shuman RM. Cerebral infarcts with arterial occlusion in neonates. Ann Neurol 1979;6:495–502.
113. Fujimoto S, Yokochi K, Togari H, et al. Neonatal cerebral infarction: symptoms, CT findings and prognosis. Brain Dev 1992;14:48–52.
114. Tabbutt S, Griswold WR, Ogino MT, et al. Multiple thromboses in a premature infant associated with maternal phospholipid antibody syndrome. J Perinatol 1994;14:66–70.
115. Silver RK, MacGregor SN, Pasternak JF, et al. Fetal stroke associated with elevated maternal anticardiolipin antibodies. Obstet Gynecol 1992;80:497–499.
116. Perlman JM, Rollins NK, Evans D. Neonatal stroke: clinical characteristics and cerebral blood flow velocity measurements. Pediatr Neurol 1994;11:281–284.
117. Sran SK, Baumann RJ. Outcome of neonatal strokes. Am J Dis Child 1988;142:1086–1088.

118. Hernanz-Schulman M, Cohen W, Genieser NB. Sonography of cerebral infarction in infancy. Am J Roentgenol 1988;150:897–902.
119. Cowan FM, Pennock JM, Hanrahan JD, et al. Early detection of cerebral infarction and hypoxic ischemic encephalopathy in neonates using diffusion-weighted magnetic resonance imaging. Neuropediatrics 1994;25:172–175.
120. Groenendaal F, van der Grond J, Witkamp TD, et al. Proton magnetic resonance spectroscopic imaging in neonatal stroke. Neuropediatrics 1995;26:243–248.
121. Babcock DS. Sonography of the brain in infants: role in evaluating neurologic abnormalities. AJR Am J Roentgenol 1995;165:417–423.
122. Filipek PA, Krishnamoorthy KS, Davis KR, et al. Focal cerebral infarction in the newborn: a distinct entity. Pediatr Neurol 1987;3:141–147.
123. Trauner DA, Chase C, Walker P, et al. Neurologic profiles of infants and children after perinatal stroke. Pediatr Neurol 1993;9:383–386.
124. Wulfeck BB, Trauner DA, Tallal PA. Neurologic, cognitive, and linguistic features of infants after early stroke. Pediatr Neurol 1991;7:266–269.
125. Delgado MR, Riela AR, Mills J, et al. Discontinuation of antiepileptic drug treatment after two seizure-free years in children with cerebral palsy. Pediatrics 1996; 97:192–197.
126. Hanigan WC, Powell FC, Palagallo G, et al. Lobar hemorrhages in full-term neonates. Childs Nerv Syst 1995;11:276–280.
127. Adams C, Hochhauser L, Logan WJ. Primary thalamic and caudate hemorrhage in term neonates presenting with seizures. Pediatr Neurol 1988;4:175–177.
128. Roland EH, Flodmark O, Hill A. Thalamic hemorrhage with intraventricular hemorrhage in the full-term newborn. Pediatrics 1990;85:737–742.
129. de Vries LS, Smet M, Goemans N, et al. Unilateral thalamic haemorrhage in the pre-term and full-term newborn. Neuropediatrics 1992;23:153–156.
130. Govaert P, Achten E, Vanhaesebrouck P, et al. Deep cerebral venous thrombosis in thalamo-ventricular hemorrhage of the term newborn. Pediatr Radiol 1992; 22:123–127.
131. Rivkin MJ, Anderson ML, Kaye EM. Neonatal idiopathic cerebral venous thrombosis: an unrecognized cause of transient seizures or lethargy. Ann Neurol 1992;32:51–56.
132. Takashima S, Iida K, Deguchi K. Periventricular leukomalacia, glial development and myelination. Early Hum Dev 1995;43:177–184.
133. Wilson DA, Steiner RE. Periventricular leukomalacia: evaluation with MR imaging. Radiology 1986;160:507–511.
134. Skullerud K, Westre B. Frequency and prognostic significance of germinal matrix hemorrhage, periventricular leukomalacia, and pontosubicular necrosis in preterm neonates. Acta Neuropathol 1986;70:257–261.
135. Takashima S, Mito T, Houdou S, Audo Y. Relationship between periventricular hemorrhage, leukomalacia and brainstem lesions in prematurely born infants. Brain Dev 1989;11:121–124.
136. Tzogalis D, Fawer CL, Wong Y, et al. Risk factors associated with the development of peri-intraventricular haemorrhage and periventricular leukomalacia. Helv Paediatr Acta 1989;43:363–376.
137. Glauser TA, Rorke LB, Weinberg PM, et al. Acquired neuropathologic lesions associated with the hypoplastic left heart syndrome. Pediatrics 1990;85:991–1000.
138. Sinha SK, Davies JM, Sims DG, et al. Relation between periventricular haemorrhage and ischaemic brain lesions diagnosed by ultrasound in very pre-term infants. Lancet 1985;2:1154–1156.
139. Zupan V, Gonzalez P, Lacaze-Masmonteil T, et al. Periventricular leukomalacia: risk factors revisited. Dev Med Child Neurol 1996;38:1061–1067.
140. Perlman JM, Risser R, Broyles RS. Bilateral cystic periventricular leukomalacia in the premature infant: associated risk factors. Pediatrics 1996;97:822–827.

141. Rogers B, Msall M, Owens T, et al. Cystic periventricular leukomalacia and type of cerebral palsy in preterm infants. J Pediatr 1994;125:S1–S8.
142. Fawer CL, Diebold P, Calame A. Periventricular leucomalacia and neurodevelopmental outcome in preterm infants. Arch Dis Child 1987;62:30–36.
143. Volpe JJ. Value of MR in definition of the neuropathology of cerebral palsy in vivo. AJNR Am J Neuroradiol 1992;13:79–83.
144. Truwit CL, Barkovich AJ, Koch TK, et al. Cerebral palsy. MR findings in 40 patients. AJNR Am J Neuroradiol 1992;13:67–78.
145. Miller VS, Roach ES. Embolization and radiosurgical treatment of cerebral arteriovenous malformations. Int Pediatr 1992;7:173–180.
146. Lasjaunias P, Garcia MR, Rodesch G, et al. Vein of Galen malformation. Endovascular management of 43 cases. Childs Nerv Syst 1991;7:360–367.
147. Lylyk P, Vineula F, Dion JE, et al. Therapeutic alternatives for vein of Galen vascular malformations. J Neurosurg 1993;78:438–445.

10

The Electroencephalogram, Seizures, and Epileptic Syndromes in the Cerebral Palsies

Barry R. Tharp

The association of seizures and cerebral palsy was mentioned by Little in his classic paper on children with static deformities (cerebral palsy [CP]), in which he attributed the findings to "lesions of nervous centre."[1] He also inferred that the seizures "probably aggravate the disorder" by their impact on the lungs and heart. Seizures occur in 25–50% of individuals with CP and are seen more commonly in those persons in whom the pathologic process involves the cerebral cortical gray matter as opposed to the white matter. Aicardi[2] estimated that 34–60% of spastic hemiplegics have epilepsy, whereas the incidence is 50–90% in individuals with quadriplegia, 16–27% in diplegics, and 23–26% in dyskinetic CP patients. Seizures may first appear in the neonatal period and may be a symptom of an acute or chronic in utero hypoxic-ischemic encephalopathy, meningitis, stroke or a cerebral malformation, or a defect in neuronal maturation. Seizures may be limited to this period, recur in infancy or later in the first or second decades, or make their initial appearance later in life. In the more severe encephalopathies, seizures will begin at birth or in the first year of life and be life-long.

PATHOPHYSIOLOGIC OVERVIEW

Seizures are the result primarily of abnormal neuronal activity at the cortical or subcortical (thalamic) level. Epileptogenesis may be caused by groups of abnormally hypersynchronized neurons, abnormal transmitter production or postsynaptic sensitivity, abnormal neuronal membrane function, or abnormal dendritic activity with excessive presynaptic input to otherwise normal neurons. Generalized convulsive seizures (generalized tonic-clonic, tonic, and clonic), simple and complex partial seizures (without and with an alteration of consciousness, respectively), and drop attacks are the most commonly encountered seizure types in the child with CP and are caused by abnormal neuronal function primarily at the level of the neocortex or hippocampus, whereas nonconvulsive generalized seizures (i.e., absences [or petit mal]), which are not associated with CP, presumably are generated by abnormalities in the T-type calcium channels in thalamic neurons, perhaps with a concomitantly hyperexcitable neocortex. The generators of so-called atypical absence seizures (often seen in the Lennox-Gastaut syndrome and CP) are unknown but may involve the interaction of foci in the frontal lobes or other neocortical sites. The cerebellum and brain stem may modulate cerebral activity and, therefore, are indirect participants in cortically generated seizures (either inhibiting excessive neuronal discharge or assisting in the propagation of the seizure). The generally held belief is that seizures virtually never originate in these subcortical structures, but one report described cerebellar seizures in a child with a cerebellar ganglioma.[3]

GENETIC INFLUENCES

The focal or regional onset of seizures in the neocortex has, in the past, been attributed to structural pathology in these cells. The description of a benign focal (rolandic) epilepsy almost four decades ago expanded our concept of focal epilepsy to include an inherited epileptic disturbance in a population of microscopically normal neurons that disappears by the teen years or earlier.[4,5] A congenital biochemical or membrane defect now is considered the basis for the regional hyperexcitability of this and subsequently described partial epilepsies. Studies of several families with a dominantly inherited form of frontal lobe epilepsy have, for the first time, elucidated a specific membrane defect presumed to be responsible for focal seizures.[6] This epileptic syndrome is characterized by primarily nocturnal partial seizures and has been localized to chromosome 20q13.2. The neuronal nicotinic acetylcholine receptor α_4 subunit maps to the same region, and the gene is widely expressed in the brain, including all layers of the frontal cortex of animals.[7] Possibly, thalamocortical input to defective receptors leads to excessive neuronal discharge and seizures.

Genes that encode specific neurochemicals have also been described in several of the idiopathic generalized epilepsies.[8] These genetic disorders are familial, but only a small leap of imagination is required to incriminate similar cellular and membrane alterations after cortical insults such as ischemia, hypoxemia, or endotoxin damage, which are believed to be responsible for the neuronal injury that leads to the static encephalopathy of some CP patients.

Studies of large populations have confirmed that genetic influences are also at play in the epileptic disorders associated with the CPs. It is well known that probands with idiopathic epilepsy (syndromes with presumed genetic origin) and cryptogenic epilepsy (syndromes presumed to be nongenetic but for which insufficient evidence exists to allow assignment of an etiology) have an increased incidence of family members with seizures as compared with the normal population.[9–11] Risks of epilepsy are lower in the relatives of probands with symptomatic epilepsy (epilepsies with a known nongenetic etiology [e.g., meningitis or trauma]). Ottman and colleagues[10] studied the family incidence of epilepsy of 1,957 adults with epilepsy, very few of whom had an idiopathic epilepsy syndrome.

The risk of epilepsy was no higher in the relatives of those with *postnatal* insults (symptomatic seizures; 1.5%) than in the general population but was significantly increased in those with idiopathic or cryptogenic seizures (2.4-fold as compared with those with postnatal symptomatic epilepsy) as well as in a second group with a "neurodeficit from birth," which included children with CP (3.1-fold increased incidence as compared with the symptomatic group). The increased incidence in the CP group included relatives with idiopathic or cryptogenic seizures (SMR [standardized morbidity rate] of 3.8) as well as those whose seizures were believed to be secondary to a "neurodeficit from birth" (SMR of 10).[10]

These studies suggest that there may be a "shared genetic susceptibility to epilepsy and cerebral palsy,"[10] as had already been suggested in an analysis of the data from the National Perinatal Collaborative Project.[12] This latter study showed that the presence of one or more adverse neurologic outcomes, including CP, nonfebrile seizures, low IQ, and small head size, was twice as common in the offspring of women with seizures before or during their pregnancy. The consumption of antiepileptic medications did not play a role in the outcomes. Though CP was observed more frequently in the offspring of the women with seizures, the increase was not statistically significant except in the subtype mixed CP (spastic paresis with dyskinesia or ataxia).

LOCATION OF PATHOLOGIC PROCESS AND RISK OF SEIZURES

The location and extent of cortical injury or maldevelopment determines the risk for the future development of seizures. The neocortex—particularly the frontal, central, and temporal regions—and the limbic system—particularly the amygdalohippocampal complex—have the lowest threshold for seizure expression. When pathologic processes primarily involve subcortical nuclear groups and posterior fossa structures, seizures usually are absent (e.g., choreoathetotic and ataxic forms of CP). Primary white matter disease also is uncommonly associated with seizures until it is far advanced or encroaches on the neighboring cortex. In a magnetic resonance imaging (MRI) study of 30 children with spastic diplegia and MRI evidence of periventricular leukomalacia, only four (13%) had epilepsy.[13] These simple pathophysiologic facts allow one to make a reasonable prediction of the risk of seizures in infants with CP. The more severe and extensive the involvement of the neocortex or limbic system, the more likely is it that seizures will occur.

Nevo and associates[14] reported a retrospective analysis of 1,946 children referred to a developmental clinic in Tel Aviv. The cumulative risk of seizures by 5 years of age depended at least partially on the presumed extent of the pathologic process and the cause of the neurologic impairment. Risk in children with "pure" mental retardation (MR), CP without MR, and MR plus CP was 8%, 47%, and 68%, respectively, compared with 1% in those without CP or MR.

A large population-based study from the Mayo Clinic showed a similar correlation between seizure incidence and the severity of the CP.[15] The risk of developing seizures ranged from 12% in those with CP without MR to 52% in those with severe CP, many of whom had associated disabilities such as MR. Twenty-three percent of children with mild to moderate CP had seizures. Children with severe CP who were intellectually normal or mildly to moderately retarded usually did not suffer seizures. This latter group most likely had primary white matter pathology secondary to periventricular leukomalacia.

The extent and location of neocortical involvement determines the clinical manifestations of the CP and seizures and the extent of cognitive impairment. The imaging study complements the physical examination: The more abnormal the neocortical pathology on the scan, the more likely the occurrence of seizures. In a retrospective study of children with hemiparetic CP, Cohen and Duffner[16] found that 58% developed seizures. Those whose computed tomography (CT) scans were most abnormal were more likely to have seizures (86%), particularly if the electroencephalogram (EEG) contained paroxysmal discharges, than were those with normal or mildly abnormal CT scans (25%). The incidence of seizures was only 11% in children with a normal EEG and a normal or mildly abnormal CT scan.

Sussova and associates[17] studied 51 children with hemiparetic CP and found that 80% had "epileptic" abnormalities on the EEG but fewer than half had clinical signs of epilepsy. Clinical seizures were much more common in individuals with left-hemisphere involvement. These investigators also reported that all their subjects who had neonatal seizures developed such seizures later in life. (Others have found a lower incidence of seizure recurrence.)[17]

The incidence of seizures, therefore, is relatively low in dyskinetic CP, which primarily reflects involvement of subcortical gray matter. This form of CP had been closely linked to birth asphyxia, but some reports, including one about adults, has cast doubt on this association and suggested that this condition may be clinically and etiologically heterogeneous, occasionally very slowly progressive, and sometimes inherited.[18] In Fletcher and Marsden's series[18] of 24 patients referred with this diagnosis, an alternative diagnosis (i.e., Pelizaeus-Merzbacher disease, cerebellar degeneration with dystonia, or a probable mitochondrial disorder) was identified in three patients.

This latter study did not discuss EEG and evoked potential results, but other investigators have described in the slowly progressive syndromes specific neurophysiologic abnormalities that, if found in a patient with an atypical form of CP, should prompt further investigation. For example, in Pelizaeus-Merzbacher disease, the centrally mediated waves of the brain stem auditory evoked response often are absent and less striking changes in other evoked potentials are seen.[19] In several of the mitochondrial disorders, particularly the syndromes with myoclonic epilepsy and ragged-red fibers, the EEG contains generalized bursts of frontally dominant slow waves that, in later stages, include spikes.[20] High-amplitude quasi-periodic slow waves with admixed polyspikes over the posterior scalp areas are common in Alpers' disease.[21] These abnormalities are not necessarily diagnostic but, when recorded in a patient with assumed CP, particularly if the course is atypical or possibly progressive, should initiate a search for another etiology.

SEIZURES, CEREBRAL PALSY, AND PROGRESSIVE ENCEPHALOPATHY

Early onset of seizures in children with CP has been postulated to have a deleterious effect on subsequent development. Vargha-Khadem and colleagues[22] examined memory and neuropsychologic function in 82 hemiplegic children 11–12 years of age whose IQs fell within the normal range. They found that early damage to either brain hemisphere, even if extensive, resulted in relatively mild deficits if the child had not had seizures in the first 5 years of life, exclusive of febrile seizures. In contrast, lesions that were accompanied by early seizures resulted in a high incidence and degree of deficit that was unrelated to the side of the injury. This study suggests that the seizures per se caused neuronal damage and worsening of the child's cognitive function. An alternative explanation is that the pathologic lesions in the seizing children were located in areas of the brain more closely related to memory development (e.g., the limbic system) or that the damage actually was more extensive in the children with seizures but was not discernible on the CT. The CT and a measure of limb weakness were used by Vargha-Khadem and colleagues[22] to grade the extent of the brain lesion. These are not particularly accurate tools for assessing the extent of neocortical involvement. A dilated ventricle may be the result of primary white matter damage and might be associated with a severe hemiplegia, yet the cortex may be spared and the risk of seizures low. In contrast, mild cortical atrophy with relatively normal ventricular size may be associated with a mild hemiparesis and severe seizures.

Children with intractable seizures can manifest progressive cognitive deterioration, but this is the exception rather than the rule. The Landau-Kleffner syndrome is a rare example of progressive loss of language, presumably due to persistent epileptiform activity in a critical area of an immature and developing cortex. Little evidence exists to support the notion that seizure per se, even if intractable to antiepileptic medication, will lead to more seizures in the majority of children.[23]

The EEG may be helpful in recognizing a subtly progressive degenerative or metabolic disorder. If the background rhythms in serial EEGs deteriorate, usually in the form of decreased frequency of the dominant rhythms and loss of normal activity such as sleep patterns, one should suspect that the patient's encephalopathy is not static. The emphasis here is on the term *background rhythms,* because EEG *epileptiform* patterns (spikes, sharp waves, and bursts of spike and slow-wave activity) may change over time (days to years) in the child with idiopathic epilepsy or a static encephalopathy. These changes may include the location of focal discharges: A temporal spike might "disappear" and spikes "appear" in the parietal region in sequential tracings; generalized discharges might appear in a record that earlier had contained only focal spikes and vice versa; and epileptiform activity might "appear" where none had occurred in earlier tracings. These changes usually reflect the randomness of the EEG and may occur even in EEGs obtained hours apart. One should not determine that a child's neurologic condition has worsened solely on the basis of an EEG that shows epileptiform activity where none had existed previously or an increase in the abundance of spikes or the appearance of seemingly new foci. Fluctuation of epileptiform activity in serial records obtained over long intervals also may simply reflect normal maturational processes. The normality or abnormality of the background, however, usually does not change significantly over time in most children: That is, if the background is normal in earlier recordings, it usually remains normal in subsequent tracings.

The practitioner should bear in mind that abnormalities in the background may unexpectedly appear in children with static encephalopathies when the EEG is obtained immediately after a seizure (postictal slowing), when high levels of anticonvulsant medications are present (e.g., diffuse slowing is common with phenytoin intoxication and even with therapeutic levels of carbamazepine), when there is a metabolic perturbation such as high fever or electrolyte disturbance and, occasionally, because the tracings being compared have been recorded while the child is in a different state (e.g., alert or drowsy). The latter situation usually is characterized by an initial EEG obtained while the child sleeps after sedation and a later EEG obtained in an older child while the child is wakeful, the first showing a normal background and the other an abnormal background. The waking background probably would have been abnormal in the earlier tracings if the child had been able to cooperate for an awake recording. Remember that the child's state, medication consumption, and recent seizure history must be considered when serial EEGs are being compared.

MENTAL RETARDATION AND EPILEPSY

Seizures occur more frequently in children with MR.[24,25] Steffenburg and colleagues[25] found an incidence of "active epilepsy" of 2 per 1,000 in 98 retarded children in a population study involving more than 48,000 children (0.7 per 1,000 in the mildly retarded and 1.3 per 1,000 in the severely retarded). They found that a major contributor to the high incidence of seizures, particularly in the severely retarded population, was CP. In other studies of MR and epilepsy, the correlation with CP was strongest in those individuals in whom seizure onset occurred at an early age. The etiology of the seizures, other than the intellectual impairment, in those mentally retarded patients with an onset at a later age is often unknown.[26]

Goulden and associates[27] prospectively followed 221 children with MR to 22 years of age. They found a high correlation between CP and seizures. The cumulative risk of epilepsy at 5, 10, and 22 years was 28%, 31%, and 38%, respectively. Importantly, these researchers also found that the spontaneous remission rate of seizures was high: 56% in the group with MR without associated disabilities and 47% in those with MR and CP.

SEIZURE TYPES IN CEREBRAL PALSY

The types of seizures that accompany CP represent the entire gamut except for typical absences. Partial seizures with and without secondarily generalized clonic, tonic, and tonic-clonic seizures are most common, whereas atypical absences (episodes of staring with loss of awareness accompanied by slow spike and slow wave activity on the EEG), myoclonic seizures, drop attacks, and infantile spasms occur less frequently. Several common epileptic syndromes are also occasionally associated with CP, including the Lennox-Gastaut syndrome and infantile spasms. Usually, these syndromes—particularly the Lennox-Gastaut syndrome—are not associated with significant motor handicap. It is noteworthy that in most studies of CP and epilepsy, the cause of the encephalopathy is not known and the results of imaging studies, if done, are not reported. Migration disorders and other malformation processes may exist but might remain unrecognized if imaging is limited to CT, which may miss subtle anatomic abnormalities and show what appears to be nonspecific atrophic lesions.

In a retrospective study of 174 children with long histories of poorly controlled epilepsy, Aksu[28] compared 57 with CP and 117 with normal neurologic status (controls). All the children had CT scans. Most of the CP group had "secondary"* generalized seizures, including generalized tonic-clonic seizures (47%) of focal and multifocal origin, infantile spasms (28%), and the Lennox-Gastaut syndrome (18%). A few had partial seizures and "primary" generalized seizures. CT scans were abnormal in 77% of the CP children and in only 15% of the controls. The CT scans in the former group showed primarily focal or generalized atrophic lesions and a few examples of subdural hematoma, congenital abnormalities, hydrocephalus, and cerebellar atrophy. Mild generalized atrophy was the major abnormality in all but one of the control subjects. A family history of epilepsy existed in 16.4% of the CP children and 7.8% of the controls. Abnormal CT scans were more common in the CP children with seizure onset at an early age. As one might expect, the CP children experienced seizure onset at an earlier age, had seizures that were more difficult to control, and were more often on polytherapy. Complete seizure control was achieved in 52% of the controls as compared to only 14% of the CP children. Discontinuance of antiepileptic drugs after a 2-year seizure-free period was more successful in the control group.

OUTGROWING SEIZURES

Children will often "outgrow" their seizures by the second decade, regardless of etiology. Developmental changes in excitatory and inhibitory neurotransmitter systems may explain the age-related differences in the incidence of seizures.[29]

The tendency for seizures to regress and disappear in the first two decades occurs in children with severe encephalopathies and MR as well as in those with idiopathic and familial seizures, albeit at a lower rate. Huttenlocher and Hapke[30] analyzed 145 children younger than 13 years who had intractable seizures for at least 5 years (more than one seizure per month for at least 2

Secondary seizures are those due to a recognized brain lesion, as compared to *primary* seizures, which infers a genetic or idiopathic origin. *Secondarily generalized* refers to generalized convulsive or nonconvulsive seizures that are the spread of a partial seizure.

years, despite antiepileptic medication), some of whom had MR (IQ >30) and epileptiform EEG abnormalities. The group with normal IQs achieved seizure control at a rate of 4% per year, and approximately 25% followed for at least 18 years continued to have more than one seizure per year. Children with MR lost their seizures at a rate of 1.5% per year, and 70% continued to have at least one seizure per year after 18 years of follow-up. Remission rate in the total population was 35%.

MORTALITY, CEREBRAL PALSY, AND SEIZURES

Another indicator that epilepsy is associated with more severe forms of CP is the shortened life span of individuals with CP, epilepsy, and MR. A population-based survey from British Columbia looked at the life expectancy of individuals with CP.[31] The investigators found that patients with certain forms of CP (i.e., quadriplegia and diplegia) had shorter life expectancies than did individuals with hemiplegia, monoplegia, ataxia, and other forms. They also reported that individuals with epilepsy had a mortality somewhat more than twice that of the nonepileptic CP population. The conditions most strongly associated with reduced survival, in decreasing importance, were severe MR, CP other than hemiplegia and monoplegia, and epilepsy. Each variable was an independent predictor of survival. The mortality associated with MR and CP is particularly increased in individuals younger than 20 years but persists in older age groups to a lesser degree.[31,32]

EPILEPTIC SYNDROMES AND CEREBRAL PALSY

Individuals with CP may occasionally have seizures, clinical signs and symptoms, and EEG abnormalities that allow their condition to be classified as one of the epileptic syndromes.[9]

West Syndrome (Infantile Spasms)

The Commission on Classification and Terminology of the International League Against Epilepsy[9] states that West syndrome "consists of a characteristic triad: infantile spasms, arrest of psychomotor development, and hypsarrhythmia, although one element may be missing. Spasms may be flexor, extensor, lightening, or nods, but most commonly they are mixed. Onset peaks between 4 and 7 months and always occurs before the age of 1 year." The spasms typically occur in clusters, often immediately after awakening. Other seizures may precede and, in more than 50% of cases, follow the resolution of the spasms. Affected children are divided into two groups: The largest (80–90%) is *symptomatic*, with evidence of brain damage or a more specific etiology. In the smaller *cryptogenic* group, the etiology is not known and affected individuals are neurologically and developmentally normal before the onset of spasms. The latter group has a better long-term prognosis, particularly cognitive development, than does the symptomatic group, into which the CP patients fall. Included within the cryptogenic classification is a small group of persons with *idiopathic West syndrome* (IWS),[33] which is defined as normal development before the onset of symmetric spasms without other kinds of seizures, normal examination, normal imaging studies, lack of focal interictal or ictal EEG abnormalities, and persistence of hypsarrhythmia between consecutive spasms of a cluster (rather than a disappearance of the pattern during a run of spasms).[34] This latter point is somewhat controversial and needs confirmation with further studies.

The West syndrome has multiple causes, including many of those that are responsible for CP (e.g., hypoxic-ischemic encephalopathy, bacterial and viral meningoencephalitis, chromosomal syndromes, neurocutaneous disorders [particularly tuberous sclerosis], and various migration and developmental syndromes).[35–37] By definition, a specific etiologic diagnosis cannot be determined in the cryptogenic group. One positron emission tomography (PET) study, however, showed an extremely high incidence of focal and multifocal abnormalities in a large group of infants classified as cryptogenic on the basis of normal MRI and CT scans.[38] Chugani and Conti[38] reported that 92 of 95 infants with refractory cryptogenic infantile spasms (often with other seizure types) could be reclassified as symptomatic after PET scanning. They assumed that the abnormalities on PET represented areas of cerebral dysgenesis, on the basis of pathologic studies of tissue removed at surgery from another small group of children with intractable seizures, infantile spasms, and similar PET abnormalities[39] and the more than 40% incidence of malformations found at autopsy in infantile spasm patients.[40] The focal PET abnormalities in the surgical series represented cortical hamartomas or dysplasia, occasionally resembling that seen in tuberous sclerosis, and cystic-gliotic encephalomalacia, the latter attributed to an early-life ischemic or anoxic injury.

Riikonen[41] has noted that the incidence of infantile spasms has not changed significantly in the last 40 years, despite improvements in neonatal care and large drops in infant mortality. He found an incidence of 0.41 per 1,000 live births in all infants born in a Swedish county between 1960 and 1976 and 0.43 per 1,000 between 1977 and 1991, which suggests that the etiology of the spasms was of prenatal origin, as it is in the majority of individuals with CP.

Infantile spasms usually are symmetric extensor or flexor events with symmetric EEG abnormalities. The ictal EEG pattern is typically an abrupt symmetric drop in voltage of the interictal hypsarrhythmic pattern, often with superimposed fast activity, the so-called electrodecremental response, and a preceding or admixed high-voltage central slow wave. Asymmetric (>50% interhemispheric amplitude difference) and asynchronous (one hemisphere preceding the other by at least 100 milliseconds) EEG events are not uncommon and, in several studies, occurred in approximately 20% of patients.[42–44] Children with asymmetric spasms usually had significant and often focal pathologic findings on imaging studies and CP; in addition, many had focal seizures and other EEG abnormalities corresponding to the pathologic findings, which included a porencephalic cyst, residua of an infarction or hypoxic-ischemic encephalopathy, or a dysplastic lesion.[42,43,45]

Gaily and colleagues,[43] impressed by the association of agenesis of the corpus callosum in their patients with asynchronous spasms, suggested that delayed spread of seizures between the hemispheres was responsible for the asymmetric EEG and clinical spasms. They also remarked on the association of unilateral central region pathologic findings in children with frequent asymmetric and asynchronous spasms. These individuals often had a hemiparesis and showed stronger spasms on the hemiparetic side and the most prominent ictal discharges over the opposite, more abnormal, hemisphere. Focal pathology posterior to the central region or in the temporal lobes was never associated with asymmetric or asynchronous EEG ictal patterns. The researchers speculated that unilateral pathology in the primary sensorimotor cortex could trigger spasms as well as partial motor seizures. Noteworthy is the fact that the children in this study from the University of California, Los Angeles, probably represent a biased population, as they were referred for surgical treatment of their refractory infantile spasms partially on the basis of focal abnormalities on imaging studies, partial seizures, or asymmetric findings on neurologic examination.

Children with asymmetric spasms may respond favorably to adrenocorticotropic hormone (ACTH). Significant focal pathologic processes may often be associated with symmetric spasms but often manifest as asymmetric ictal EEG discharges or focal interictal background abnormalities.[46] Video EEG monitoring may be necessary, however, to demonstrate the asymmetric nature of spasms. Also, in many reports of infantile spasms, the ictal events are simply termed *generalized*. Though the long-term neurologic and cognitive outcome of individuals with asymmetric and asynchronous spasms usually is poor, exceptions do occur.[45]

Riikonen[47] presented data on 20- to 35-year follow-up of 214 infants with infantile spasms. Mortality was 31%, usually at a young age. Nonetheless, 33% were seizure-free at follow-up, particularly individuals of normal intelligence. Twenty-five patients were of normal intelligence, and 11 were only slightly impaired. Some of these latter individuals had motor handicaps consistent with CP, emphasizing the fact that CP and infantile spasms are not always associated with a poor long-term prognosis. All the adults with a favorable outcome experienced short lags between the onset of spasms and the initiation of ACTH therapy and had an excellent response to therapy.

In other studies,[36,48] more than 85% of children with infantile spasms, particularly those in the symptomatic group, are mentally retarded at follow-up examination. In addition, in our experience and that of others, motor dysfunction, which would meet the criteria for CP, occurs in more than 50%.

Lennox-Gastaut Syndrome

The Lennox-Gastaut syndrome (LGS) is uncommon, comprising less than 3% of childhood epilepsies. Its onset is in the preschool years, and it is characterized by tonic-axial seizures (tonic seizures significantly involving the truncal musculature), atonic seizures (drop attacks), and atypical absences. Other types of seizures, including myoclonic, generalized tonic-clonic, and partial, may occur. The EEG is characterized by an abnormal background, often with multi-focal epileptiform discharges, interrupted by bursts of symmetric and asymmetric, primarily frontal, slow (<3 cycles per second [cps]) spike and slow wave discharges (Lennox's "petit mal variant"). During sleep, bursts of fast activity at 10 cps (recruiting rhythm) may be associated with subtle tonic seizures. The syndrome is often, but not always, accompanied by MR, which may progress over the first one to two decades.

Unfortunately, the definition of LGS varies: Some researchers include children with slow-spike and slow-wave discharges on EEG only, regardless of seizure type or clinical concomitants, whereas others insist that a child have tonic seizures before he or she is classified as having this syndrome. These differences probably explain the wide variation in incidence figures.

Though neurologic abnormalities, including CP, occur in individuals with LGS, most patients have normal neurologic examinations or mild nonspecific motor dysfunction. Imaging studies often show mild, diffuse, and nonspecific atrophic changes. Tuberous sclerosis, the residual changes of perinatal and pre-natal infection, and trauma are uncommonly seen. Extremely rarely, major mal-formations, including Aicardi's syndrome and lissencephaly, are associated with LGS.[49] Infantile spasms (West syndrome) precede LGS in fewer than one-third of the cases.[50] In many of these individuals, the duration of the spasms gradually lengthens and blends imperceptibly into typical tonic seizures, occasionally characterized by sudden loss of tone (drop attack). The ictal EEG may still manifest the electrodecremental pattern that characterizes the typical spasms of infancy. In a study of "epileptic falls" in 15 children with LGS, Ikeno and associates[51] described seven with seizures characterized by flexor spasms that clinically and electrographically resembled infantile spasms who had previously experienced the West syndrome.

Chromosomal Syndromes

Although most children with a static encephalopathy escape a specific etiologic diagnosis, some are found to a have a chromosomal syndrome. Many children in this latter group have seizures and abnormal EEGs that are nonspecific and do not suggest a specific cause. Many reports[52,53] cite "diagnostic" EEG patterns in specific chromosomal syndromes, but none of the authors has looked at a large control population of retarded and motor-handicapped age-matched individuals in a blinded fashion. Certain types of EEG abnormalities may occur more commonly in certain syndromes, but whether a specific etiologic diagnosis can be made on the basis of the EEG alone is not clear.

Epileptiform activity characterized by centrally located spike and wave discharges resembling those seen in individuals with benign rolandic epilepsy have been reported in several chromosomal syndromes, including deletion of the long

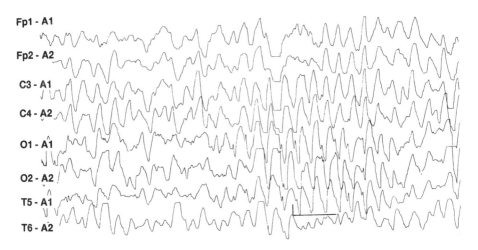

Figure 10.1 Three-year-old boy with Angelman syndrome due to a deletion of chromosome 15. Electroencephalographic background is markedly slow with runs of rhythmic, 3- to 4-cps activity admixed with spikes in the occipitotemporal regions bilaterally. Slower delta activity is present over the frontal regions. Calibration: 50 μV, 1 sec.

arm of chromosome 1, trisomy 9p, and Angelman syndrome.[52,53] Children with these disorders manifest significant motor delay, often with hypotonia, MR, and seizures, and frequently they are referred to CP clinics.

Angelman syndrome is characterized by relatively easily recognized neurologic, morphologic, ophthalmologic, and dermatologic features. One cause is a deletion of the proximal portion of the long arm of the maternally derived chromosome 15 (15q11–13). Other less common abnormalities of chromosome 15 include paternal uniparental disomy, translocations, and imprinting mutations.[54,55] Boyd and associates[56] described EEG abnormalities that were "sufficiently characteristic to help identify patients at an early age." The EEG patterns consisted of (1) high-voltage persistent rhythmic theta, (2) runs of high voltage (usually anterior delta) often admixed with spikes, and (3) spikes mixed with high-voltage (3–4 cps) components posteriorly and facilitated or seen only with eye closure (Figure 10.1).[56] The epileptiform activity is often striking and, at times, may be associated with jerky motor behavior that cannot be distinguished from myoclonus.[57] In patients affected by the latter condition, often quasi-continuous rhythmic myoclonus involving the face and upper extremities is seen, accompanied by rhythmic 5- to 10-Hz EEG activity. Occasionally, girls with Angelman syndrome may resemble those with Rett syndrome. The strikingly different EEG patterns in these two disorders are helpful in arriving at the proper diagnosis, particularly if the routine chromosomal analysis is normal.

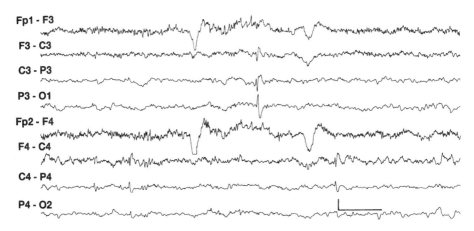

Fp1 - F3

F3 - C3

C3 - P3

P3 - O1

Fp2 - F4

F4 - C4

C4 - P4

P4 - O2

Figure 10.2 Three-year-old girl with Rett syndrome, stage 3. Electroencephalogram shows independent bilateral central and parietal spikes on a low-voltage background. Other portions of the tracing showed a poorly formed alpha rhythm and relatively normal sleep patterns. Calibration: 50 µV, 1 sec.

Rett Syndrome

The neurodevelopmental disorder known as *Rett syndrome* begins in the first or second year of life and occurs only in girls. The cause is unknown, and involved individuals often receive a diagnosis of CP because the clinical progression may be very slow and, therefore, missed. The characteristic clinical pattern includes hand and gait apraxia and hand stereotypies, dementia, unusual respiratory patterns while awake, and very slowly progressive motor impairment, including spasticity and dystonia. The correct diagnosis is made when one recognizes the relatively normal development in the first year of life, the slow decline in head circumference usually beginning at 4–6 months of age, and the slow deterioration of motor and cognitive development thereafter.

The EEG may aid in making the diagnosis of Rett syndrome (or, for that matter, other progressive neurometabolic or neurodegenerative disorders) when serial recordings show progressive deterioration of the background rhythms (Figure 10.2).[58]

In Rett syndrome, the EEG is normal in the earlier stages of developmental arrest but, as the child grows, the background rhythms deteriorate, with increased slowing and decrease or loss of normal age-appropriate activity and appearance of epileptiform activity. Some authors[58,59] have described a characteristic EEG progression with normal recordings in the first stage. Epileptiform activity and slowing of the background rhythms appear in stage 2, the former consisting of spikes and sharp waves in the central and temporal regions, which are increased in frequency during sleep and resemble the interictal discharges of benign partial epilepsy with centrotemporal spikes.[58,59] Hagne and colleagues[60] emphasized several EEG features that they found to occur commonly in Rett syndrome, including pseudoperiodic delta and theta bursts resembling those seen in subacute sclerosing panencephalitis, monorhythmic, 4- to 5-cps background slowing, and continuous, rhythmic, bilaterally synchronous and generalized 1-Hz spikes. The latter two patterns typically occur in the third and fourth stages of the syndrome. (For a detailed discussion of the stages of Rett syndrome, see Hagberg and Witt-Engerström.[61])

MALFORMATIONS OF CORTICAL DEVELOPMENT

Malformations of cortical development are increasingly recognized as a cause of severe static encephalopathy and epilepsy, particularly since the introduction of MRI.[62,63] Up to 25% of children referred to epilepsy centers with intractable partial epilepsy have been found to have focal cortical dysplastic lesions.[64] In most cases, the EEG abnormalities are rather nonspecific and may be surprisingly mild or absent, particularly in those individuals with MR only or in those with focal seizures and normal intelligence. Children with significant motor impairment and seizures, however, usually have abnormal EEGs, but these do not necessarily suggest the specific diagnosis. A review of all the disorders caused by aberrations in the various steps of proliferation, migration, and organization of the cerebral cortex is beyond the scope of this chapter. Here we concentrate on the entities most familiar to the clinician and often associated with severe epilepsy (Table 10.1).

Despite the apparent chaotic arrangement and abnormal morphology of neurons in areas of dysplastic and heterotopic cortex, epileptiform activity has been recorded from this tissue, in vitro and in vivo, that resembles activity seen in more "typical" epileptogenic regions. The intrinsic epileptogenicity of this tissue has been demonstrated by the application of a convulsant drug, 4-aminopyridine, to slices of dysplastic cortex removed at seizure surgery and the subsequent production of spontaneous seizure discharges.[65] Corticography during epilepsy surgery has also demonstrated seizures, interictal spikes, and bursting discharges from dysplastic cortex,[66] from heterotopic cortex in band heterotopia (the double-cortex syndrome),[67] and from subcortical heterotopic nodules.[68]

Hemimegalencephaly

Hemimegalencephaly, or unilateral megalencephaly, is an uncommon disorder characterized by enlargement of all or part of a cerebral hemisphere, sometimes with contralateral somatic hypertrophy. The mechanism responsible for this malformation is unknown, but defects in cell migration and neuronal and glial proliferation have been proposed. It may occur in some neurocutaneous syndromes, including the epidermal nevus syndrome.[69] Affected children

Table 10.1 Malformations of Cortical Development Associated with Epilepsy and Cerebral Palsy

Disorders of neuronal and glial proliferation
Hemimegalencephaly
Focal cortical dysplasia
Disorders of abnormal neuronal migration
Lissencephaly
Subcortical band heterotopia
Subependymal heterotopia
Abnormal cortical organization
Schizencephaly
Bilateral perisylvian syndrome

usually are retarded, manifest a contralateral hemiparesis, and suffer from refractory partial seizures or infantile spasms or both. Rare individuals with normal intelligence and easily controlled seizures have been reported.[70]

The EEG typically shows background abnormalities over the involved hemisphere, ranging from a mild increase in beta activity[70] to multifocal or diffuse hemispheric slowing with absence of all normal activity in wakefulness and sleep. Usually, abundant focal and multifocal spikes and sharp waves occur, occasionally having a pseudoperiodic appearance, and one sees asymmetric suppression-burst patterns and an unusual, diffusely distributed, high-voltage, alpha-like activity that is maximal in the involved hemisphere.[71] Hypsarrhythmia is seen in patients with spasms and may be asymmetric or, occasionally, unilateral.[72] Focal epileptiform abnormalities often accompany the abnormal background. Paladin and colleagues[71] suggested that the presence of an alpha-like pattern is associated with a better long-term prognosis, including better motor development and less severe seizures.

Focal Cortical Dysplasia

Cortical dysplasia is being recognized more frequently as a cause of seizures, particularly in patients with epilepsy that is difficult to control. In many seizure surgery centers, it has become one of the most common lesions removed from patients with intractable partial seizures.[73] In many such patients, the dysplastic tissue is not seen on standard MRI but is found at the time of operation or is suspected on the basis of hypometabolism on PET scans. The dysplastic areas are characterized by a lack of cortical lamination, abnormal giant neurons, and occasionally, large, bizarre eosinophilic balloon cells, sometimes resembling the changes seen more diffusely in tuberous sclerosis.[39] Dendrites and axons also are abnormal.

Most patients with focal cortical dysplasia present with seizures and minor to absent pyramidal findings, particularly those with dysplastic cortex in the perirolandic region. Visual-field defects, occasionally accompanied by a mild hemiparesis, have been described in individuals with occipital lobe malformations.[74] Many individuals are mildly retarded or have borderline intelligence, but a significant number, particularly those in whom the temporal lobes are involved, are of normal intelligence.[73]

The EEGs of patients with focal cortical dysplasia usually contain focal slowing or epileptiform activity that generally corresponds roughly with the site of the dysplastic lesion on MRI. The background activity is usually normal. The epileptiform activity may emerge on serial recording over years in some patients, whereas in others the abnormalities remain stable over many years.[75] The epileptogenic zone, particularly as seen on direct recordings from the neocortex at surgery, often extends well beyond the visible or MRI-delineated dysplastic area.

Lissencephaly

The most severe of the migration disorders associated with prolonged survival is the agyria-pachygyria (lissencephaly) complex.[76–79] Classic (type 1) lissencephaly occasionally is linked to chromosome 17 (Miller-Dieker syndrome). It also may be inherited as an X-linked recessive disorder and can occur in the same family in which individuals with subcortical band heterotopias are seen. Type 2 lissencephaly (cobblestone) is seen in children with congenital muscular dystrophies, muscle-brain-eye disease, and the Walker-Warburg syndrome.

Two types of abnormal EEG backgrounds have been described in lissencephaly. Infantile spasms with a characteristic hypsarrhythmic EEG pattern is commonly seen in young children. Others show high-voltage background rhythms, typically in the alpha and beta bands (Figure 10.3). Usually, this activity is quite continuous and is distributed diffusely over both hemispheres or is maximal in the frontal and central regions. High-voltage slower rhythms may be admixed with the faster activity or may dominate the background. The combination of these various patterns may lead to a background that resembles hypsarrhythmia. The faster background activity is perhaps more common in type 1 lissencephaly.

Sebire and colleagues[80] reported 43 children with extensive convolutional abnormalities who had developmental delay, hypotonia, and in 70%, seizures. In all patients, radiologic studies confirmed the absence or a paucity of cortical sulci and the absence or a reduction of interdigitation between gray and white matter. These researchers excluded patients with focal gyral abnormalities, Walker-Warburg syndrome, Fukuyama muscular dystrophy, cytomegalovirus embryofetopathy, and Zellweger syndrome. They separated their patients into two groups on the basis of the imaging features: Group A (30 children) showed bilateral and symmetric thickening of the neocortex, enlarged lateral ventricles, and sylvian fissures that are wider and more vertical than normal, whereas group B (13 children) showed heterogeneous imaging abnormalities differing from those in group A in at least one of the four major features: absence of the aforementioned sylvian fissure abnormalities, thin neocortex, normal-sized lat-

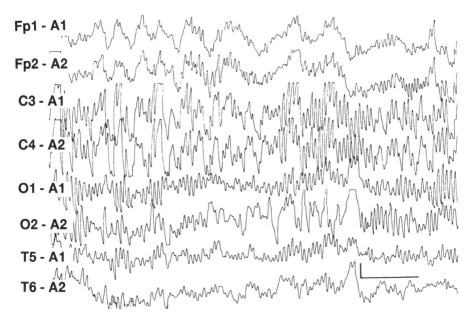

Figure 10.3 One-and-a-half-year-old boy with type 1 lissencephaly. Electroencephalogram shows virtually continuous high-amplitude (13- to 15-cps) rhythmic activity over both hemispheres, which is of maximal voltage in the central regions. Very slow delta activity is present anteriorly, whereas somewhat faster delta activity is present in the right occipital region. Calibration: 50 μV, 1 sec.

eral ventricles, and asymmetry of the brain defects. Five of these children also had brain stem defects.

Group B patients were more clinically impaired than were those in group A.[80] Twice as many in the former group never acquired the ability to sit and were microcephalic, and more had ocular motor impairment. Seizures were equally common in both groups. The types of seizures were similar as well and included infantile spasms, generalized seizures, and partial seizures. The seizures were more likely to be refractory in group B (100%, as compared to 55% in group A).

The authors described two distinct EEG features: high-amplitude (50- to 400-μV) rapid rhythms (9–22 Hz) and high-amplitude slow waves (delta and theta). The delta-theta rhythms were "generalized, asynchronous, continuous or discontinuous, and consisted of bursts of sharp theta waves (300–600 μV) intermingled with delta (400–600 μV)."[80] This latter pattern resembled hypsarrhythmia but lacked true epileptiform discharges. All children with rapid rhythms and 12 of the 13 with diffuse slow activity belonged to group A. The EEGs of group B patients showed focal and multifocal spikes and irregular spike and wave complexes on a slow background. The rapid rhythm pattern can also be seen in patients with other types of structural brain abnormality, including severe post–hypoxic encephalopathy.[81]

Band Heterotopia

Band heterotopia (double-cortex syndrome) is a relatively common migration disorder often associated with epilepsy and is characterized by variable cognitive impairment ranging from mild to severe retardation and often accompanied by a delay in the acquisition of motor milestones, hypotonia, poor coordination, and absent to mild pyramidal symptoms. The heterotopia typically consists of bilateral and symmetric bands or islands of neurons located in the centrum semiovale. The bands spare the striate and cingulate gyri and the medial temporal lobes. The overlying cortex, which usually is histologically normal, may be thinner than normal or pachygyric. Families have been reported in which subcortical band heterotopia occurs in the female family members and lissencephaly in the males.[82]

The EEG may be normal in less affected children or may manifest diffuse, usually nonfocal background abnormalities, particularly in those with the most severe cortical abnormalities (pachygyria, thicker heterotopic bands, and significant ventricular enlargement). Epileptiform activity may take the form of focal and multifocal spikes, generalized slow-spike and slow-wave activity (often associated with seizures typical of LGS), generalized polyspike and slow-wave discharges and, occasionally, 3- to 5-Hz spike and wave complexes. The focal spikes can arise from any brain region but, in some series, are most common in the frontal and temporal regions. A patient whose infantile spasms responded to corticosteroids has also been reported[83]; the EEG showed generalized 3- to 5-Hz spike and wave discharges. Most patients with partial and generalized seizures responded to conventional antiepileptic drugs, including those with LGS.[83,84]

Schizencephaly

The schizencephalies are a heterogeneous group of congenital disorders characterized by clefts lined by gray matter spanning the cerebral hemispheres from the pial surface to the lateral ventricle. The clefts either are opened to the subarachnoid space and associated with hydrocephalus (type 1) or are covered by a "pial-ependymal seam," with the two lips abutting through the majority of the cleft (type 2). The clefts often occur bilaterally and in all cortical regions but are most frequent in the parietal (72%), frontal (55%), and temporal lobes (22%).[85] They are considered to be developmental defects occurring at 3–5 months of gestation. The clefts may be associated with other malformations, including absence of the septum pellucidum and the corpus callosum, focal cortical dysplasia, hypoplasia of the optic nerves and, rarely, lissencephaly or extracranial abnormalities.[86–88] Some authors believe that the clefts are encephaloclastic lesions from intrauterine cerebral infarctions and that the term *schizencephaly* should be avoided.[89] Probably, the cleft, which is the result of a genetic or ischemic process and has onset at the end of the first or beginning of the second trimester, can originate from both of these causes.

Clinical abnormalities are varied, ranging from normal development to isolated partial seizures to more severe cognitive impairment and CP, particularly hemiparetic and quadriparetic CP. In a review of 47 cases, children with closed-lip schizencephaly were most likely to have a hemiparesis (72%), whereas the open-lipped group were more likely to have severely abnormal neurodevelopmental outcomes and hydrocephalus.[85] Forty-seven percent of the children had a spastic quadriparesis, including all 12 with bilateral open-lipped schizencephaly. Seizures occurred equally in all groups (unilateral, bilateral, closed or open lipped), with an overall incidence of 57%, and were not correlated with neurodevelopmental outcome. Seizures usually are partial, and secondary generalization may or may not occur; infantile spasms, generalized tonic-clonic, tonic, and atonic seizures occur less frequently. The EEG usually contains focal background abnormalities and epileptiform activity that correspond with the site of the cleft(s). The overall background rhythms may be normal.[85,86]

In several patients, mesial temporal sclerosis has been reported in addition to the clefts.[87] Extensive presurgical EEG monitoring is necessary in these patients to define the precise site of seizure onset prior to resective surgery. Resection of the temporal lobe rather than removal of tissue directly associated with the cleft may be accompanied by resolution of the seizures.[90]

Subependymal Heterotopia

Subependymal heterotopia is rare and usually occurs sporadically or can be inherited in an X-linked fashion.[91,92] The periventricular heterotopia may be unilateral or bilateral, and the MRI picture may be confused with tuberous sclerosis, particularly if the patient presents with seizures and MR. Though some patients have pyramidal signs including hemiparesis, the phenotype usually is mild, and many patients are normal or have seizures with normal neurologic examinations. The clinical picture is more severe in involved male individuals, though there is an overall female preponderance.

Patients experience a variety of seizure types. Partial seizures occur more often than others, though generalized seizures (both convulsive and nonconvulsive, including atypical absences) may occur. Seizures start after the age of 10 in approximately 80% of individuals. Many patients, even those with intractable seizures, are of normal intelligence, and few have motor syndromes.[91,92]

In light of the heterogeneous nature of the seizures, the EEG abnormalities not surprisingly are also variable, many showing normal background activity. The epileptiform activity consists of focal and multifocal spikes and sharp waves (in both the unilateral and bilateral forms of the syndrome) and generalized discharges (including, in some individuals, bilateral heterotopia and 3- to 4-Hz spike and wave activity indistinguishable from a primary generalized epilepsy).

A subgroup of patients with periventricular heterotopia have intractable complex partial seizures, and many will also show hippocampal atrophy on

MRI volumetric studies. Despite thorough preoperative neurophysiologic investigation that appeared to confirm the unilateral temporal lobe onset of ictal activity, these patients have done very poorly after surgical therapy, with most experiencing no reduction of seizures.[91] Surgical intervention therefore should probably be undertaken cautiously (with resection of the hippocampus and amygdaloid and as much of the heterotopic tissue as possible) or should not be performed at all in individuals with temporal lobe seizures and MRI evidence of contiguous or extratemporal dysgenesis or heterotopias.

Developmental Bilateral Perisylvian Dysplasia

Foix, Chavany, and Marie[93] described an acquired syndrome characterized by faciopharyngoglossomasticatory diplegia. Their cases and subsequent ones have usually been caused by bilateral strokes or encephalitis.[94] More recently, a similar syndrome often associated with seizures and MR has been reported and attributed to a restricted neuronal migration disorder with bilateral opercular polymicrogyria. Kuzniecky and associates[95] described this clinical spectrum in 31 patients, including mild to moderate MR in 75%, pyramidal signs (among them moderate quadriparesis) in 60%, and severe dysarthria and oromotor dysfunction (pseudobulbar paresis) in all patients. Seizures occurred in 87% (atonic and tonic drop attacks in 73%, brief atonic and atypical absence episodes in 62%, generalized tonic-clonic seizures in 35%, and brief tonic or atonic seizures or atypical absences in 80%). Partial seizures with or without secondary generalization occurred in 26%. Four individuals had an unusual seizure consisting of bilateral clonic contractions of the lips with spread to the face or perioral region.

The EEG background was normal in one-half of the patients. Interictal recordings most commonly demonstrated bilateral synchronous spike and sharp- and slow-wave, or polyspike and slow-wave discharges (2.5–3.0 Hz in 39% and slower in 27%). More than one-third had independent or bilateral multifocal epileptiform abnormalities involving the centrotemporoparietal regions without generalized discharges. The most common ictal abnormalities were "generalized low-voltage attenuation recruiting pattern," diffuse high-voltage fast activity, and a generalized 4- to 12-Hz polyspike and slow-wave discharge.

The clinical presentation, neurologic examination, MR, and generalized interictal EEG activity suggest a diffuse disturbance of cerebral function. CT scans may be unimpressive, and only MRI scans, often with special sequences that enhance the gray-white junction, will lead to the correct diagnosis. Many of the patients with intractable seizures, particularly those with drop attacks, will benefit from a corpus callosotomy.

CONCLUSION

Many neurologic syndromes and disorders may be associated with motor impairment and what appears to be a static encephalopathy. Among these are the progressive or relatively stable neurometabolic disorders, chromosomal syndromes, cerebral dysplastic disorders, and some hereditary neuromuscular syndromes. In this chapter, we have concentrated on the conditions that appear commonly in a CP clinic with the referral diagnosis of CP and that ultimately are found to have a recognizable etiology. A special focus was those disorders associated with epilepsy and in which the EEG may provide helpful and, rarely, diagnostic information. The EEG is a valuable tool for initially screening the patient with CP and seizures, the patient in whom a progressive disorder is suspected, and the patient who is having abnormal episodic behavior, including unusual activity during sleep, that cannot definitely be identified as seizure activity.[96]

REFERENCES

1. Wilkins R, Brody I. Neurological classics XV. Little's disease. Arch Neurol 1969; 20:217–224.
2. Aicardi J. Epilepsy in brain-injured children. Dev Med Child Neurol 1990;32: 191–202.
3. Harvey A, Jayakar P, Duchowny M, et al. Hemifacial seizures and cerebellar ganglioma: an epilepsy syndrome of infancy with seizures of cerebellar origin. Ann Neurol 1996;40:91–98.
4. Bray P, Wiser W. Evidence for a genetic etiology of temporal-central abnormalities in focal epilepsy. N Engl J Med 1964;271:926–933.
5. Nayrac P, Beaussart M. Les pointes ondes prerolandiques, expression EEG trés particulière. Etude électroclinique de 21 cas. Rev Neurol 1958;99:203–205.
6. Scheffer I, Bhatia K, Lopes-Cendes I, et al. Autosomal dominant nocturnal frontal lobe epilepsy. Brain 1995;118:61–73.
7. Steinlein O, Mulley J, Propping P, et al. A missense mutation in the neuronal nicotinic acetylcholine receptor α_4 subunit is associated with dominant nocturnal frontal lobe epilepsy. Nat Genet 1995;11:201–203.
8. Duchowny M, Harvey A. Pediatric epilepsy syndromes: an update and critical review. Epilepsia 1996;37:S26–S40.
9. Commission on Classification and Terminology of the International League Against Epilepsy. Proposal for revised classification of epilepsies and epileptic syndromes. Epilepsia 1989;30:429–445.
10. Ottman R, Annegers J, Risch N, et al. Relations of genetic and environmental factors in the etiology of epilepsy. Ann Neurol 1996;39:442–449.
11. Ottman R, Lee J, Risch N, et al. Clinical indicators of genetic susceptibility to epilepsy. Epilepsia 1996;37:353–361.
12. Nelson K, Ellenberg J. Maternal seizure disorder, outcome of pregnancy, and neurologic abnormalities in the children. Neurology 1982;32:1247–1254.
13. Fedrizzi E, Inverno M, Bruzzone M, et al. MRI features of cerebral lesions and cognitive functions in preterm spastic diplegic children. Pediatr Neurol 1996;15:207–212.
14. Nevo Y, Shinnar S, Samuel E, et al. Unprovoked seizures and developmental disabilities: clinical characteristics of children referred to a child development center. Pediatr Neurol 1995;13:235–241.
15. Kudrjavcev T, Shoenberg B, Kurland L, et al. Cerebral palsy: survival rates, associated handicaps and distribution by clinical subtype (Rochester, MN, 1950–1976). Neurology 1985;35:900–903.
16. Cohen M, Duffner P. Prognostic indicators in hemiparetic cerebral palsy. Ann Neurol 1981;9:353–357.

17. Süssová J, Seidl Z, Faber J. Hemiparetic forms of cerebral palsy in relation to epilepsy and mental retardation. Dev Med Child Neurol 1990;32:792–795.
18. Fletcher N, Marsden C. Dyskinetic cerebral palsy: a clinical and genetic study. Dev Med Child Neurol 1996;38:873–880.
19. Wang P, Young C, Liu H, et al. Neurophysiological studies and MRI in Pelizaeus-Merzbacher disease: comparison of classic and connatal forms. Pediatr Neurol 1995;12:47–53.
20. So N, Berkovic S, Andermann F, et al. Myoclonus epilepsy and ragged-red fibres (MERRF). Brain 1989;112:1261–1276.
21. Boyd S, Harden A, Egger J, Pampliglione G. Progressive neuronal degeneration of childhood with liver disease ("Alpers' disease"): characteristic neurophysiological features. Neuropediatrics 1986;17:75–80.
22. Vargha-Khadem F, Isaacs E, van der Werf S, et al. Development of intelligence and memory in children with hemiplegic cerebral palsy. The deleterious consequences of early seizures. Brain 1992;115:315–329.
23. Berg A, Shinnar S. Do seizures beget seizures? An assessment of the clinical evidence in humans. J Clin Neurophysiol 1997;14:102-110.
24. Forsgren L, Edvinsson S, Blomquist H, et al. Epilepsy in a population of mentally retarded children and adults. Epilepsy Res 1990;6:234–248.
25. Steffenburg U, Hagberg G, Viggedal G, Kyllerman M. Active epilepsy in mentally retarded children: I. Prevalence and additional neuro-impairments. Acta Pediatr 1995;84:1147–1152.
26. Brodtkorb E. The diversity of epilepsy in adults with severe developmental disabilities: age at seizure onset and other prognostic factors. Seizure 1994;3:277–285.
27. Goulden K, Shinnar S, Koller H, et al. Epilepsy in children with mental retardation: a cohort study. Epilepsia 1991;32:690–697.
28. Aksu F. Nature and prognosis of seizures in patients with cerebral palsy. Dev Med Child Neurol 1990;32:661–668.
29. Johnson M. Developmental aspects of epileptogenesis. Epilepsia 1996;37:S2–S9.
30. Huttenlocher PR, Hapke R. A follow-up study of intractable seizures in childhood. Ann Neurol 1990;28:699–705.
31. Crichton J, Mackinnon M, White C. The life-expectancy of persons with cerebral palsy. Dev Med Child Neurol 1995;37:567–576.
32. Forsgren L, Edvinsson S, Nystrom L, Blomquist H. Influence of epilepsy on mortality in mental retardation: an epidemiologic study. Epilepsia 1996;37:956–963.
33. Commission on Pediatric Epilepsy of the International League Against Epilepsy. Workshop on infantile spasms. Epilepsia 1992;33:195.
34. Dulac O, Plouin P, Jambaque I. Predicting favorable outcome in idiopathic West syndrome. Epilepsia 1993;34:747–756.
35. Tjiam A, Stefanko S, Schenk V, Vlieger M. Infantile spasms associated with hemihypsarrhythmia and hemimegalencephaly. Dev Med Child Neurol 1978;20:779–798.
36. Lombroso C. A prospective study of infantile spasms: clinical and therapeutic considerations. Epilepsia 1983;24:135–158.
37. Kuzniecky R, Andermann F, Guerrini R. Infantile spasms: an early epileptic manifestation in some patients with the congenital bilateral perisylvian syndrome. J Child Neurol 1994;9:420–423.
38. Chugani H, Conti J. Etiologic classification of infantile spasms in 140 cases: role of positron emission tomography. J Child Neurol 1996;11:44–48.
39. Vinters H, DeRosa M, Farrell M. Neuropathological study of resected cerebral tissue from patients with infantile spasms. Epilepsia 1993;34:772–779.
40. Jellinger K. Neuropathological aspects of infantile spasms. Brain Dev 1987;9:349–357.
41. Riikonen R. Decreasing perinatal mortality: unchanged infantile spasm morbidity. Dev Med Child Neurol 1995;37:232–238.

42. Drury I, Beydoun A, Garofalo EA, Henry TR. Asymmetric hypsarrhythmia: clinical, electroencephalographic and radiological findings. Epilepsia 1995;36:41–47.
43. Gaily E, Shewmon D, Chugani H, Curran J. Asymmetric and asynchronous infantile spasms. Epilepsia 1995;36:873–882.
44. Haga Y, Watanabe K, Negoro T, et al. Asymmetric spasms in West syndrome. J Epilepsy 1995;8:61–67.
45. Watanabe K, Haga T, Negoro T, et al. Focal spasms in clusters, focal delayed myelination, and hypsarrhythmia: an unusual variant of West syndrome. Pediatr Neurol 1994;11:47–49.
46. Alvarez L, Shinnar S, Moshe S. Infantile spasms due to unilateral cerebral infarcts. Pediatrics 1987;79:1024–1026.
47. Riikonen R. Long-term outcome of West syndrome: a study of adults with a history of infantile spasms. Epilepsia 1996;37:367–372.
48. Jeavons P, Bower B, Dimitrakoudi M. Long-term prognosis of 150 cases of "West syndrome." Epilepsia 1973;14:153–164.
49. Dulac O, N'guyen T. The Lennox-Gastaut syndrome. Epilepsia 1993;34:S7–S17.
50. Weinmann H. Lennox-Gastaut Syndrome and its Relationship to Infantile Spasms (West's Syndrome). In E Niedermeyer, R Degen (eds), The Lennox-Gastaut Syndrome. New York: Liss, 1988;301–316.
51. Ikeno T, Shigematsu H, Miyakoshi M, et al. An analytic study of epileptic falls. Epilepsia 1985;26:612–621.
52. Stern J. The epilepsy of trisomy 9p. Neurology 1996;47:821–824.
53. Vaughn B, Greenwood R, Aylsworth A, Tennison M. Similarities of EEG and seizures in del(1q) and benign rolandic epilepsy. Pediatr Neurol 1996;15:261–264.
54. Nicholls R, Shashidhar P, Gottlieb W, Cantu E. Paternal uniparental disomy of chromosome 15 in a child with Angelman syndrome. Ann Neurol 1992;32:512–518.
55. Smeets D, Hamel B, Nelen M, et al. Prader-Willi syndrome and Angelman syndrome in cousins from a family with a translocation between chromosomes 6 and 15. N Engl J Med 1992;326:807–811.
56. Boyd S, Harden A, Patton M. The EEG in early diagnosis of the Angelman (happy puppet) syndrome. Eur Pediatr 1988;147:508–513.
57. Guerrini R, DeLorey T, Bonanni P, et al. Cortical myoclonus in Angelman syndrome. Ann Neurol 1996;40:39–48.
58. Glaze D, Frost J, Zoghbi H, Percy A. Rett's syndrome. Correlation of electroencephalographic characteristics with clinical staging. Arch Neurol 1987;44:1053–1056.
59. Robb S, Harden A, Boyd S. Rett syndrome: an EEG study in 52 girls. Neuropediatrics 1989;20:192–195.
60. Hagne I, Witt-Engerström I, Hagberg B. EEG development in Rett syndrome. A study of 30 cases. Electroencephalogr Clin Neurophysiol 1989;72:1–6.
61. Hagberg B, Witt-Engerström I. Rett syndrome: a suggested staging system for describing impairment profile with increasing age towards adolescence. Am J Med Genet 1986;24:47–59.
62. Barkovich A, Kuzniecky R. Neuroimaging of focal malformations of cortical development. J Clin Neurophysiol 1996;13:481–494.
63. Kuzniecky R, Barkovich A. Pathogenesis and pathology of focal malformations of cortical development and epilepsy. J Clin Neurophysiol 1996;13:468–480.
64. Kuzniecky R, Murro A, King D, et al. Magnetic resonance imaging in childhood intractable partial epilepsy: pathologic correlations. Neurology 1993;43:681–687.
65. Mattia D, Olivier A, Avoli M. Seizure-like discharges recorded in human dysplastic neocortex maintained in vitro. Neurology 1995;45:1391–1395.
66. Palmini A, Gambardella A, Andermann F, et al. Intrinsic epileptogenicity of human dyplastic cortex as suggested by corticography and surgical results. Ann Neurol 1995;37:476–487.

67. Morrell F, Whisler W, Hoeppner T, et al. Electrophysiology of heterotopic gray matter in the "double cortex" syndrome. Epilepsia 1992;33(suppl 3):76.
68. Francione S, Kahane S, Tassi L, et al. Stereo-EEG of interictal and ictal electrical activity of histologically proved heterotopic gray matter associated with partial epilepsy. Electroencephalogr Clin Neurophysiol 1994;90:284–290.
69. Pavone L, Curatolo P, Rizzo R, et al. Epidermal nevus syndrome: a neurologic variant with hemimegalencephaly, gyral malformation, mental retardation, seizures, and facial hemihypertrophy. Neurology 1991;41:266–271.
70. Fusco L, Ferracuti S, Fariello G, et al. Hemimegalencephaly and normal intelligence. J Neurol Neurosurg Psychiatry 1992;55:720–722.
71. Paladin F, Chiron C, Dulac O, et al. Electroencephalographic aspects of hemimegalencephaly. Dev Med Child Neurol 1989;31:377–383.
72. Tjiam A, Stefanko S, Schenk V, Vlieger M. Infantile spasms associated with hemi-hypsarrhythmia and hemimegalencephaly. Dev Med Child Neurol 1978;20:779–798.
73. Wyllie E, Baumgartner C, Prayson R, et al. The clinical spectrum of focal cortical dysplasia and epilepsy. J Epilepsy 1994;7:303–312.
74. Kuzniecky R, Gilliam F, Morawetz R, et al. Occipital lobe developmental malformations and epilepsy: clinical spectrum, treatment, and outcome. Epilepsia 1997;38:175–181.
75. Raymond A, Fish D, Boyd S, et al. Cortical dysgenesis: serial EEG findings in children and adults. Electroencephalogr Clin Neurophysiol 1995;94:389–397.
76. Barkovich A, Koch T, Carrol C. The spectrum of lissencephaly: report of ten patients analyzed by magnetic resonance imaging. Ann Neurol 1991;30:139–146.
77. Barkovich A, Kjos B. Nonlissencephalic cortical dysplasias: correlation of imaging findings with clinical deficits. Am J Neuroradiol 1992;13:95–103.
78. Barkovich A, Kuzniecky R, Dobyns W, et al. A classification scheme for malformations of cortical development. Neuropediatrics 1996;27:59–63.
79. Gastaut H, Pinsard N, Raybaud Ch, et al. Lissencephaly (agyria-pachygyria): clinical findings and serial EEG studies. Dev Med Child Neurol 1987;29:167–180.
80. Sebire G, Goutieres F, Tardieu M, et al. Extensive macrogyri or no visible gyri: distinct clinical, electroencephalographic, and genetic features according to different imaging patterns. Neurology 1995;45:1105–1111.
81. Quirk J, Kendall B, Kingsley D, et al. EEG features of cortical dysplasia in children. Neuropadiatrie 1993;24:193–199.
82. Dobyns W, Andermann E, Andermann F, et al. X-linked malformations of neuronal migration. Neurology 1996;47:331–339.
83. Palmini A, Andermann F, Aicardi J, et al. Diffuse cortical dysplasia, or the 'double cortex' syndrome. Neurology 1991;41:1656–1662.
84. Burkovich A, Guerrini R, Battaglia G, et al. Band heterotopia: correlation of outcome with magnetic resonance imaging parameters. Ann Neurol 1994;36:609–617.
85. Packard A, Miller V, Delgado M. Schizencephaly: correlations of clinical and radiologic features. Neurology 1997;48:1427–1434.
86. Kuban K, Teele R, Wallman J. Septo-optic dysplasia–schizencephaly: radiographic and clinical features. Pediatr Radiol 1989;19:145–150.
87. Granata T, Battaglia G, D'Incerti L, et al. Schizencephaly: neuroradiologic and epileptologic findings. Epilepsia 1996;37:1185–1193.
88. Silengo MC, Lerone M, Pelizza A, et al. A new syndrome with cerebro-oculo-skeletal-renal involvement. Pediatr Radiol 1990;20:612–614.
89. Sarnat HB. Disorders of Neuroblast Migration. In Cerebral Dysgenesis: Embryology and Clinical Expression. New York: Oxford University Press, 1992; 250–252.
90. Silbergeld D, Miller J. Resective surgery for medically intractable epilepsy associated with schizencephaly. J Neurosurg 1994;80:820–825.

91. Li L, Dubeau F, Andermann F, et al. Periventricular nodular heterotopia and intractable temporal lobe epilepsy: poor outcome after temporal lobe resection. Ann Neurol 1997;41:662–668.
92. Raymond A, Fish D, Stevens J, et al. Subependymal heterotopia: a distinct neuronal migration disorder associated with epilepsy. J Neurol Neurosurg Psychiatry 1994;57:1195–1202.
93. Foix C, Chavany J, Marie J. Diplegie facio-linguo-masticatrice d'origine cortico-sous-cortical sans parlysie des membres. Rev Neurol 1926;33;214–219.
94. Grattan-Smith P, Hopkins I, Shield L, Boldt D. Acute pseudobulbar palsy due to bilateral focal cortical damage: the open opercular syndrome of Foix-Chavany-Marie. J Child Neurol 1989;4:131–136.
95. Kuzniecky R, Andermann F, Guerrini R, CBPS Multicenter Collaborative Study. The epileptic spectrum in the congenital bilateral perisylvian syndrome. Neurology 1994;44;379–385.
96. Kotagal S, Gibbons VP, Stith JA. Sleep abnormalities in patients with severe cerebral palsy. Dev Med Child Neurol 1994;36:304–311.

11

The Bladder and Genitourinary Tract in the Cerebral Palsies

Timothy B. Boone

Most children with cerebral palsy and normal cognition gain adequate urinary control during childhood. However, up to 30% of children with cerebral palsy suffer from lower urinary tract dysfunction.[1] The exact incidence is unknown, as few studies have focused on incontinence, the principal bladder dysfunction prompting referral to a specialist for diagnosis and treatment. In this chapter, we describe the neurologic basis of micturition, review the literature pertinent to bladder dysfunction in cerebral palsy, and review some treatment protocols for achieving urinary control.

MICTURITION: NEUROANATOMY AND PHYSIOLOGY

Urinary storage and expulsion is governed by a complex array of pathways in both the somatic and autonomic nervous systems, the latter composed of sympathetic and parasympathetic fibers. Urinary continence in childhood occurs with maturation of the cortical pathways regulating the micturition center in the brain stem. An understanding of the neuroanatomy and neurophysiology of the lower urinary tract will allow the practicing clinician to pinpoint the site of voiding dysfunction, weigh the risk to renal function, and plan effective therapy.

The human bladder is a hollow, smooth-muscled organ lined with watertight urothelium. The smooth-muscle bundles coalesce, creating a single unit without defined muscle layers. The bladder's smooth muscle, or detrusor, is innervated by the parasympathetic and sympathetic nervous symptoms. A third, noncholinergic, nonadrenergic system has been proposed, although the clinical importance of this purinergic system has yet to be defined. The bladder is characterized by its ability to accommodate a large volume of urine at low pressure. Ureteral transport of urine is unidirectional, and the vesicoureteral junction prevents urinary reflux back toward the kidneys, thereby reducing the risk of infection, pyelonephritis, and renal scarring. During the storage phase of micturition, continence is achieved by specialized zones in the urethra. Smooth-muscle fibers circle the bladder neck, forming the proximal or internal urethral

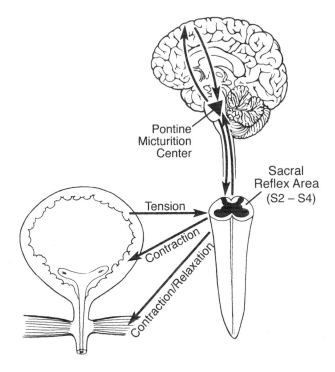

Figure 11.1 Pathways for micturition.

sphincter. This sphincteric unit is densely innervated by adrenergic fibers from the sympathetic nervous system. Just distal to the bladder neck is a second continence zone, the external urethral sphincter. This external urethral sphincter consists of an inner smooth-muscle layer encircled by specialized striated muscle. The striated portion of the external urethral sphincter is innervated by the somatic nervous system and is under voluntary control. During bladder filling, both continence zones increase their resistance, and no spontaneous contractions of the bladder should occur.

Parasympathetic neurons in the sacral spinal cord (S2–S4) provide the autonomic motor fibers to the bladder. Sympathetic fibers originate from T12 to L2, and their primary target for innervation is the bladder neck or proximal urethral sphincter. Figure 11.1 illustrates the pathways for micturition. Afferent and efferent tracts run the length of the spinal cord from the pontine reticular formation to the sacral nuclei subserving micturition. The pontine micturition center in the brain stem coordinates the bladder and urethral sphincters, assuring coordinated bladder contraction with simultaneous relaxation of the sphincters. Neurologic lesions or injury to the pathways between the pons and sacral cord can lead to a state of detrusor-sphincter dyssynergia whereby the bladder contracts against a closed sphincter mechanism, thereby creating elevated bladder

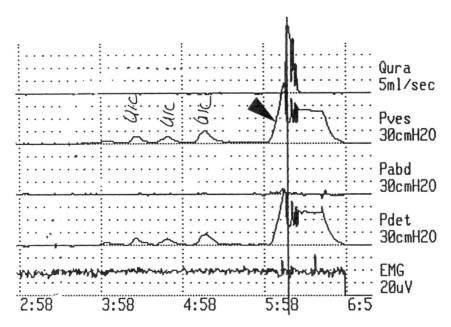

Figure 11.2 Evidence of detrusor hyperreflexia in a child with cerebral palsy who was unable to inhibit the onset of bladder contractions voluntarily. Onset of such contractions caused urinary incontinence. (Qura = flow rate; Pves = bladder pressure; Pabd = abdominal pressure; Pdet = subtracted bladder pressure; EMG = pelvic floor electromyography. The handwritten notation [UIC] indicates instances of uninhibited contraction.)

pressure with significant risk to renal function. Cortical pathways modulate the pontine micturition center to control the voiding reflex. Because coordination of the bladder and sphincters is localized to the pons, all suprapontine injuries or lesions lead to synergistic voiding, although reflex voiding may trigger without voluntary control. In general, the majority of suprapontine sites projecting to the micturition center are inhibitory.

In summary, as the bladder fills, afferent impulses are transmitted to the spinal cord along mixed, sympathetic, and parasympathetic nerves. These pathways converge on the pontine micturition center, where the voiding reflex is constantly inhibited by higher input until it is appropriate to void. When cortical loss of inhibition occurs, a synergistic void can take place, completely emptying the bladder. However, the reflex is spontaneous (without voluntary control). The resultant detrusor hyperreflexia causes clinical symptoms of frequency, urgency, and urge incontinence. Laboratory evaluation with urodynamic studies may reveal these sudden precipitous bladder contractions. Figure 11.2 is an illustration of detrusor hyperreflexia in a child with cerebral palsy. The child was unable to inhibit the onset of bladder contractions voluntarily, and the onset of such contractions caused urinary incontinence.

CEREBRAL PALSY
AND BLADDER DYSFUNCTION

The literature regarding neurogenic bladder dysfunction in cerebral palsy is sparse. This is largely due to the fact that most children with cerebral palsy achieve total urinary control. Table 11.1 is a compilation of six studies involving 205 patients with cerebral palsy. Most of the studies focused on children with voiding problems, so the overall incidence of neurogenic bladder dysfunction in cerebral palsy is unknown. Across the series, the incidence of incontinence ranged from 26% to 100%, urinary urgency or frequency from 5% to 56%, hesitancy from 3.5% to 52%, and urinary retention from 2% to 7%. Urodynamic studies were performed on 133 of 205 children with cerebral palsy. Detrusor hyperreflexia was the most common cystometric finding, occurring in 17–87% of the children.

The exact incidence of urinary incontinence has never been determined, but McNeal and associates[1] suggest that 36% of children with cerebral palsy have voiding symptoms suggestive of neurogenic bladder dysfunction. These investigators screened 50 children with cerebral palsy for bladder dysfunction, including stress incontinence, dribbling, persistent enuresis, or urinary urgency. Eighteen children had symptoms severe enough to warrant urologic evaluation. Thirteen children underwent urodynamic evaluation, which revealed hyperreflexive bladder contractions in 31%. Uninhibited bladder contractions from hyperreflexia occurred more commonly in children with the greatest impairment, according to Vining's classification system.[2] McNeal and colleagues[1] noted a significant incidence of bladder dysfunction in their children with cerebral palsy. Effective therapy required accurate evaluation of the urologic symptoms, using urodynamic equipment.

Drigo and associates[3] emphasized the correlation between incontinence and recurrent urinary tract infection (UTI) in 20 children with severe cerebral palsy. Voiding cystourethrography revealed vesicoureteral reflux in 35% of the children. Urodynamic studies showed detrusor hyperreflexia in all the children and evidence of detrusor-sphincter dyssynergia in 20%. A state of generalized hypertonicity in which the pelvic floor was involved contributed to impaired emptying of the bladder and postvoiding residual urine. The authors attributed the combination of vesicoureteral reflux and the residual urine to recurrent UTIs.[3]

Mayo[4] studied 23 children with cerebral palsy who were referred because of lower urinary tract symptoms. Difficulty voiding was the primary presenting symptom of voiding dysfunction. Unlike all other published series, Mayo emphasized that hesitancy (problems initiating a urinary stream) is a very common problem in symptomatic children with cerebral palsy. Moreover, he attributed the problem with initiating micturition to nonrelaxation of the pelvic floor, as opposed to classic detrusor-sphincter dyssynergia. Mayo[4] noted urgency with hyperreflexia when the bladder was full in half the patients who experienced difficulty initiating a urinary stream. A neurologic insult between the pontine micturition center and the sacral spinal cord is required to induce detrusor-sphincter

Table 11.1 Bladder Dysfunction in Cerebral Palsy

Study	Date	Patients (no.)	Male-Female Ratio	Mean Age	Inconti-nence	Reflux	Urgency and Frequency	Hesitancy	Reten-tion	DH	DESD
McNeal et al.[1]	1983	45	24/26	13.4	26	N/A	18	N/A	N/A	31 (n = 13)	0
Decter et al.[5]	1987	57	28/29	8.0	86	N/A	5	3.5	2	71 (n = 49)	14
Drigo et al.[3]	1988	20	13/7	5.5	100	35	N/A	N/A	N/A	80 (n = 9)	20
Mayo[4]	1992	23	12/11	<20	48	N/A	48	52	0	35 (n = 23)	0
Reid & Borzyskowski[6]	1993	27	9/18	9.9	74	11%	U: 37 F: 56	11%	7	87 (n = 27)	25
Sweetser et al.[7]	1995	33	N/A	N/A	67	N/A	U: 18 F: 6	N/A	N/A	17 (n = 12)	8

Urodynamics (%) spans the columns: Incontinence, Reflux, Urgency and Frequency, Hesitancy, Retention, DH, DESD.

U = urgency; F = frequency; N/A = not applicable; DH = detrusor hyperreflexia; DESD= detrusor external-sphincter dyssynergia.

dyssynergia. Other investigators[3,5-7] have reported dyssynergia as a urodynamic finding in children with cerebral palsy and voiding dysfunction. How this can occur is open to speculation, given the need for a concurrent anoxic injury to the spinal cord at the time of initial neurologic insult. Mayo's theory of nonrelaxation of the sphincter with pelvic floor hypertonus that causes difficulty with urination is a more possible cause.

Decter and colleagues[5] in 1987 evaluated dysfunctional voiding in 57 patients with cerebral palsy. Urinary incontinence was the presenting complaint in 49 of 57 patients (86%). An upper motor neuron lesion with associated detrusor hyperreflexia was diagnosed using urodynamic studies in 86% of the children. Eleven percent of the children had electromyographic evidence of incomplete lower motor neuron involvement of the external urethral sphincter. A complete lower motor neuron injury to the sphincter was never demonstrated. The presence of detrusor hyperreflexia and associated uninhibited bladder contractions made control of urination and continence very difficult to achieve in these children. More importantly, although only 10 children had evidence of a UTI, 83% of this subgroup had structural damage from abnormal micturition with infection. Radiologic evaluation is mandatory in children with cerebral palsy, dysfunctional voiding symptoms, and a UTI.

Daytime urinary incontinence was the primary presenting symptom in a series of 27 children referred to Reid and Borzyskowski.[6] Urinary frequency (56%) and urgency (37%) were common symptoms, followed by difficulty initiating micturition in 11% of the patients. Video-urodynamic studies were abnormal in 85% of the children. In these children, detrusor hyperreflexia and reduced bladder capacity were the most common findings. Five of the children had detrusor-sphincter dyssynergia. Reid and Borzyskowski[6] suggest that a concurrent hypoxic injury to the spinal cord pathways between the sacral cord and pons may induce dyssynergic voiding. Only one child in their series had vesicoureteral reflux, and this child had evidence of detrusor-sphincter dyssynergia with loss of renal function.

Video-urodynamic studies were used to evaluate bladder function in 12 children before selective sacral dorsal rhizotomy to control spasticity in cerebral palsy.[7] Sweetser and associates found incontinence to be the major symptom in 67% of the patients and encountered no problems relating to difficulty in initiating micturition. Dyssynergia was identified in one child, although he was able to empty his bladder well despite high voiding pressures. Almost half of the children with spasticity showed improvement in bladder control after sacral dorsal rhizotomy, and no child was noted to sustain permanent damage to the urinary tract.

Overall, the limited studies of lower urinary tract function in children with cerebral palsy reveal a consistent pattern of detrusor hyperreflexia when incontinence is the urologic problem. Most children who demonstrate cognition sufficient to toilet train will gain bladder control. Those who do not should be evaluated by urodynamic studies, which might reveal the specific bladder dysfunction. The neurologic basis for detrusor-sphincter dyssynergia in cerebral palsy remains an enigma based on the pathophysiology of cerebral palsy. Future

Table 11.2 Modes of Treatment Used in 69 Children with Cerebral Palsy

Anticholinergics	54
Adrenergics	1
Antibiotics	2
Intermittent catheterization (ICP)	10
ICP + anticholinergics	4
Frequent voiding schedule	8
Behavior modification	6
Surgery	3
No treatment	7

Sources: Adapted from RM Decter, SB Bauer, S Khosbin, et al. Urodynamic assessment of children with cerebral palsy. J Urol 1987;138:1110–1112; and RM Decter, SB Bauer, S Khosbin, et al. Urodynamic assessment of children with cerebral palsy. J Urol 1987;138:1110–1112.

studies should address this problem, although treatment can still be directed appropriately, as described in the next section. All children with voiding symptoms and infection should be studied with a urodynamic workup, a voiding cystourethrography, and upper tract imaging.

TREATMENT

The cornerstone of treatment for voiding dysfunction in cerebral palsy is accurate analysis of the child's intelligence and support structure. Because most children will gain normal urinary control and many of the severely affected will not be amenable to therapy (other than diapering or chronic indwelling catheters), treatment primarily is directed at children with symptomatic or structural urinary tract problems who can follow a regimen of medications and intermittent catheterization. First, all children must be screened for UTI. Infection may be the sole cause for recurrent incontinence with frequency and urgency. Simple communication with caregivers or better access to bathroom facilities may go a long way toward effectively remedying urinary incontinence.[8] Children with sterile urine and voiding symptoms should undergo urodynamic testing to guide therapy.

Like many other children with neuropathic bladders, ileal conduit urinary diversion for children with voiding problems and cerebral palsy was for many years the gold standard for managing incontinence and protecting renal function.[9,10] Long-term follow-up, however, revealed disastrous results, with a significant proportion of the patients losing renal function to chronic infection and stone disease.[11] Newer treatment regimens are centered on preventing infection, achieving or improving continence, and limiting surgical intervention. Only two studies have taken urodynamic data from children with cerebral palsy and then applied the findings to treatment protocols: Tables 11.2 and 11.3 are a compilation of treatment data from Decter and colleagues[5] and Reid and Borzyskowski.[6]

Detrusor hyperreflexia is the most common urodynamic finding in all children with voiding symptoms and cerebral palsy. Anticholinergic and antispas-

Table 11.3 Findings with Nonsurgical Treatment at Follow-Up in 37 Children

Dry	8
Much improved	21
Slightly improved	4
Unchanged	4

Sources: Adapted from CJD Reid, M Borzyskowski. Lower urinary tract dysfunction in cerebral palsy. Arch Dis Child 1993;68:739–742; and RM Decter, SB Bauer, S Khosbin, et al. Urodynamic assessment of children with cerebral palsy. J Urol 1987;138:1110–1112.

modic medications can be used to control uninhibited contractions and the symptoms of urgency and urge incontinence. Oxybutynin, propantheline, and hyoscyamine are examples of common pharmaceutical agents used to treat detrusor hyperreflexia. Residual urine volumes should be monitored in children taking anticholinergic medications, as the reduction in bladder contractility may lead to poor emptying of the bladder. Intermittent catheterization is an important adjunctive therapy for children who retain urine before or after the institution of bladder-relaxant medication. In many cases, the parents or caregivers will have to be instructed in the technique of clean, intermittent catheterization. Chronic indwelling catheters should be avoided whenever possible, because the infection rate over time is 100%. Other long-term risks with chronic indwelling tube drainage include pyelonephritis, bladder stones, urethral erosion, and squamous cell carcinoma of the bladder. When chronic indwelling tube drainage is needed, a suprapubic tube is preferable to a urethral catheter. Suprapubic tubes are easier to manage and change on a 4- to 6-week regimen.

Diapering may be the only management option in severely debilitated children. As long as harmful bladder pressures are not occurring during storage of urine and emptying is complete, then diapering can be a safe alternative to tube drainage. Skin breakdown is the only other major concern, and the child must be carefully monitored for signs of sore formation.

In summary, treatment of voiding symptoms in children with cerebral palsy should be guided by the urodynamic evaluation of their bladder function. All infections of the urinary tract mandate a search for voiding dysfunction and coexisting vesicoureteral reflux.

REFERENCES

1. McNeal DM, Hawtrey CE, Wolraich ML, Mapel JR. Symptomatic neurogenic bladder in a cerebral-palsied population. Dev Med Child Neurol 1983;47:612–616.
2. Vining F, Accardo P, Rubenstein J, et al. Cerebral palsy—a pediatric developmentalist's overview. Am J Dis Child 1976;130:643–649.
3. Drigo P, Seren F, Artibani W, et al. Neurogenic vesicourethral dysfunction in children with cerebral palsy. Ital J Neurol Sci 1988;9:151–154.
4. Mayo ME. Lower urinary tract dysfunction in cerebral palsy. J Urol 1992;147:419–420.

5. Decter RM, Bauer SB, Khosbin S, et al. Urodynamic assessment of children with cerebral palsy. J Urol 1987;138:1110–1112.

6. Reid CJD, Borzyskowski M. Lower urinary tract dysfunction in cerebral palsy. Arch Dis Child 1993;68:739–742.

7. Sweetser PM, Badell A, Schneider S, Badlani GH. Effects of sacral dorsal rhizotomy on bladder function in patients with spastic cerebral palsy. Neurourol Urodyn 1995;14:57–64.

8. Bellinger MF. Myelomeningocele and Neurogenic Bladder. In JY Gillenwater, JT Grayhack, SS Howards, JW Duckett (eds), Adult Pediatric Urology, vol 2 (2nd ed). St. Louis: Mosby, 1991;2063.

9. Cass AS, Geist RW. Results of conservative and surgical management of the neurogenic bladder in 160 children. J Urol 1972;107:865–868.

10. Waldbaum RS, Muecke EC. Management of the congenital neurogenic bladder in children. J Urol 1972;108:165–166.

11. Hill JT, Ransley PG. The colon conduit: a better method of urinary diversion? Br J Urol 1983;55:629–631.

12

Feeding the Child with Cerebral Palsy

Carlos H. Lifschitz, Kerrie K. Browning, Ingrid Linge, Ann R. McMeans, and Catherine Loren Turk

Children with cerebral palsy often have associated feeding and swallowing difficulties.[1] Common problems affecting feeding include tongue thrusting, prolonged or exaggerated bite reflex, abnormally increased or decreased gag reflex, tactile hypersensitivity, and drooling.[2] Coughing, chronic wheezing, or bronchitis can be secondary to aspiration during swallowing or gastroesophageal reflux. An oromotor evaluation and clinical feeding assessment can provide valuable information regarding the oral phase of swallowing, but it may fail to identify disorders in the pharyngeal and esophageal phases of swallowing, such as aspiration, which may be detected with a videofluoroscopic study.

To help a family overcome the problems that arise in feeding a child with cerebral palsy, a team approach should be implemented. This team should include all relevant health care professionals and the patient's family. The professional members of the feeding team should include a gastroenterologist, occupational therapist, speech therapist, dietitian, nurse, and psychologist. The evaluation should encompass the patient's ability to suck, masticate, swallow, control head and trunk, maintain nutritional status, and sustain an adequate level of consciousness (neurologic status). The family's desires and expectations in regard to the child's feeding capabilities should also be considered.

CLINICAL EVALUATION

The first step in evaluating the feeding of a child with cerebral palsy is the gathering of information regarding any known problem, the family's or primary physician's concerns, and any previous evaluations or tests performed. Caregivers should be asked whether the patient suffers from recurrent episodes

This chapter was originally published by the U.S. Department of Agriculture, Agriculture Research Services (USDA/ARS), Children's Nutrition Research Center, Department of Pediatrics, Baylor College of Medicine, and Texas Children's Hospital. Funding has been provided in part by the USDA/ARS Cooperative Agreement No. 58-6258-6100. The contents of this work do not necessarily reflect the views or policies of the U.S. Department of Agriculture, nor does mention of trade names, commercial products, or organizations imply endorsement by the U.S. government. The authors thank James Carter, M.A., for critical review and Leslie Loddeke for editorial assistance.

of wheezing, coughing (particularly during or immediately after meals), or chronic bronchitis, which may be the result of aspiration. A history of recurrent otitis media or hoarseness might also indicate alterations in the swallowing mechanism. Other important questions must address the potential existence of behaviors such as excessive crying, irritability, refusal to eat, interruption of feeding before the meal is completed, or waking in the middle of the night. Caregivers may report behavioral changes in children with severely compromised neurologic status that may be too subtle to be detected by health care providers who are not familiar with the child.

Whenever feeding problems are identified, an evaluation by specialized professionals is required. An occupational therapist or speech therapist with expertise in the area of feeding should perform an assessment of the child's development and environment, followed by a clinical feeding evaluation, which should include an examination of the oral musculature, posture control, and respiration. The location in which the evaluation takes place must be quiet, comfortable, spacious, and devoid of interference from telephones, beepers, and an excessive number of observers or passersby. Depending on the facility, the clinical feeding evaluation may be completed in collaboration with other members of the feeding team, some of whom may be present in the evaluation room or observing through a one-way mirror or a television monitor.

Knowledge of the child's development is important for the information it provides about the child's cognitive, psychosocial, and physical status—information that is essential in deciding how to interact with the child, plan the program, and set goals. An assessment of the child's cognition and psychosocial status usually is gained through an interview, clinical observations, and a review of the medical history. History of vomiting or regurgitation during or after feeding is important to assess fully the scope of the patient's problems. When considering the child's physical development, an examination of muscle tone is usually necessary. Changes in the child's muscle tone usually relate to the types of feeding problems present. Therefore, management of muscle tone is essential, because tonal abnormalities greatly affect feeding ability.

Characteristics of a child with hypertonicity may include a retracted lower jaw, tongue thrusting, extended neck and trunk, and retracted arms with legs in extension. An increase in muscle tone inhibits normal feeding patterns because the child is unable to use a chin-tuck position, in which the neck is slightly flexed. The tongue, jaw, lips, and oral musculature need a point of stability from which to function; this stability normally is provided by the chin-tuck position. Children with hypotonicity demonstrate different types of problems, such as weak oral musculature. The child may be unable to maintain an adequate anterior lip seal, so that liquid or food escapes from the mouth. The child with low muscle tone often develops abnormal patterns to create a point of stability, such as fixing the tongue against the hard palate. This position prevents the child from spontaneously opening the mouth to receive either the nipple or a spoon and contributes to problems associated with the development of adequate suction when expressing milk from the nipple or with clearing the spoon.

A child with cerebral palsy may have fluctuating muscle tone, which contributes to difficulty maintaining or assuming a stable, seated posture, another important consideration when evaluating the child's feeding potential. The inability to maintain proximal stability affects the efficiency of the oral structures and their relationships in feeding.

In addition to determining the child's abilities and difficulties in feeding, a dietitian should perform an assessment of nutritional status and, if it proves deficient, an estimation of the child's energy needs. Accurate determination of the energy needs of a child with cerebral palsy is difficult because of the lack of consensus regarding an adequate and practical assessment method. Estimation of energy needs can be made from long-term growth history, dietary history, basal energy expenditure, or various other calculations.[3-6] Anthropometric measurements are sometimes of limited value in nutrition assessment because of varying growth patterns in children with cerebral palsy as compared to children without cerebral palsy.[7]

Many children with cerebral palsy tend to be underweight and short relative to standard references for growth. Most reference data on children's growth use as their basis the general pediatric population, not children with cerebral palsy. The National Child Health Statistics standard reference scale can be useful for following long-term growth and for making assessments in cerebral palsy patients but should not be used to evaluate growth, as it too is based on the normal pediatric population.[8] Obtaining height measurements in children with cerebral palsy is also difficult.[9] When contractures prevent standard measurement with a stadiometer, alternate measurements can be performed for linear growth assessment, such as upper arm length,[4] lower leg length,[5] or segmental body measurements.[3] These measurements are most valuable for long-term follow-up. Skinfold thickness may overestimate body fat because fat folds have been shown to increase over paralyzed limbs.[10]

If the parent or other caregiver is a good historian, and weight records are available, a history of weight gain or loss can be used for the energy needs assessment, without length measurements. If a trend in weight loss or gain is seen, energy intake can be adjusted. Clinical judgment of ideal body weight based on weight for age (usually between the tenth and fiftieth percentile for age on the National Child Health Statistics scale[7]) can also be used to begin the assessment of energy needs, especially in patients with no weight history or records. A complete nutritional history also is helpful in the assessment of energy needs.

Several practical methods exist for estimating energy needs in children with cerebral palsy and, with proper follow-up, a child's energy needs can be adjusted as necessary. One method, recommended by Cully and Middleton,[6] uses kilocalories per centimeter of height. For children 5–11 years of age, a calorie intake of 13.9 kcal/cm is recommended for mild to moderate motor dysfunction, and 11.1 kcal/cm is recommended in cases of severe motor dysfunction.[6] This requires a segmental length or a supine length, if possible, and is limited by the age of the child. Guidelines by Pemberton and colleagues[11] recommend 10 kcal/cm for cerebral palsy with decreased levels of activity, 15 kcal/cm for cerebral palsy with normal or increased levels of activity, and up to 6,000 kcal/day for adolescents with athetoid cerebral palsy. Another means of assessment of energy needs is the Krick method[3]:

$$\text{Basal energy expenditure (estimated for pediatric patients)} \times$$
$$\text{tone factor} \times \text{activity factor} + \text{growth factor}$$

Assessment of energy needs and losses in children with cerebral palsy vary; one method of assessment may be preferable to another, depending on the patient and information available.

An assessment of the interactions between the child and caregivers will indicate the emotional support being provided for the child. Feelings of guilt, manipulation of the caregiver by the child, or unusual demands by other family members on a tacitly designated caregiver may create situations that require the intervention of a psychotherapist. Information on the availability of resources in the home and immediate community is helpful in planning the necessary intervention strategies. The assistance of a social worker may be required.

RADIOLOGIC EVALUATION OF SWALLOW FUNCTION

The information gathered from the parents, in conjunction with the rest of the medical history and results of the clinical evaluation, will determine whether a videofluoroscopic swallow function test must be performed. The purpose of the videofluoroscopic contrasted swallow function study, commonly referred to as a *modified barium swallow study, swallow function study,* or *oropharyngeal motility study,*[12] is to objectively evaluate the oral preparatory, oral transit, and pharyngeal phases of the swallow. Steps of the normal swallow mechanism are described in Table 12.1. Many patients show no clinical signs of swallowing difficulty, such as coughing and choking, but have recurrent pneumonia, upper respiratory infection, or chronic congestion. Such children may have "silent" aspiration (no protective cough reflex), which might be identified on a swallow function study.

Limited information regarding the esophageal phase of the swallow is obtained during a swallow function study. For more complete and accurate information about the esophageal phase, an upper gastrointestinal series should be performed and interpreted by a radiologist.

The swallow function study typically is performed by a radiologist and a speech therapist trained in the evaluation of dysphagia. Studies usually are performed according to the protocol described by Logeman.[13] This protocol calls for the use of a systematic checklist by which to evaluate the oral and pharyngeal phases of swallowing. The child is placed in an upright, seated position. Modifications in positioning often are made, such as placing support behind the head and neck (to minimize hyperextension) or at the feet (to obtain optimal posi-

Table 12.1 Stages of Swallowing in Infants

Oral preparatory phase
>This phase involves the manipulation of food in the mouth to form a bolus. With bottle presentation, minimal time may be necessary. With thicker consistencies, however, the amount of time needed to prepare the bolus increases.

Oral phase
>This phase should take 1 second.
>During this phase, the bolus is propelled to the pharynx. The soft palate begins to elevate to close off the nasopharynx.

Pharyngeal phase
>This phase also takes only 1 second in normal infants.
>The material may descend to the level of the valleculae before eliciting a swallow reflex; however, no delay at this level should be seen. The swallow reflex is triggered, such that the posterior tongue moves to approximate the posterior pharyngeal wall.
>As with the adult swallow, the following occur simultaneously:
>>laryngeal elevation
>>velopharyngeal closure
>>downward tipping of epiglottis
>>true and false vocal fold closure
>>initiation of pharyngeal peristalsis
>>relaxation of the cricopharyngeal sphincter to allow material to flow into the esophagus

Esophageal phase
>Peristaltic movement through the entire esophagus occurs in 6–10 seconds.

Note: The radiologist or physician interprets the esophageal phase.
Source: Adapted from JA Logeman. Appendix B: Videofluorographic Worksheet. In Manual for the Videofluorographic Study of Swallowing. Austin, TX: PRO-ED, 1993;157–162.

tioning for feeding). Information collected at the time of the clinical evaluation may be useful for better positioning of the child during the radiologic evaluation. Infants are positioned by side-lying at a semireclined angle to best mimic a normal feeding position. Lateral radiographic views of the swallowing mechanism are obtained. Anteroposterior views may be assessed if asymmetries are suspected.

Various food and liquid consistencies are given, depending on the age and ability of the child. Information regarding the consistencies that the child finds easy or difficult to swallow should be obtained during the clinical feeding evaluation and used during the swallow study. Foods and liquids are mixed with liquid barium or barium paste. Approximately three swallows of each consistency are administered.

To limit radiation exposure, the swallow study should not last more than 2 minutes. Images of the swallows are videotaped, reviewed, and analyzed by the speech therapist and the radiologist. The results, taken in concert with those of the clinical feeding evaluation, are used to identify problems and to formulate an appropriate plan of care for the child. Results and recommendations then are reported to other health care professionals involved in the care of the child.

Table 12.2   Criteria for Swallow Function Study Referral

Choking with feeds
Coughing with feeds
Apnea with feeds
Bradycardia or tachycardia during feeds
Audible respiration
Wet, gurgling vocal quality
Refusal to eat
Excessive drooling, inability to handle secretions
Recurrent upper respiratory infections, pneumonia, congestion, asthma
Poor weight gain
Nasal regurgitation
Frequent emesis
Failure to thrive
Feeding longer than 30 minutes

Swallow study results have led to alterations in a child's diet, elimination of certain dietary consistencies secondary to aspiration, and position changes for optimal feeding. The information, in conjunction with that gained from clinical feeding evaluation, can help facilitate overall health. Monitoring of a child's swallowing ability should be conducted at periodic intervals using videofluoroscopic studies as well as clinical observation, to facilitate changes in dietary textures or to determine whether oral feedings can be either initiated or continued safely. Modern electronic equipment is available to integrate results from radiologic, manometric, and swallow sounds into one recording. Clinical signs of swallowing dysfunction, requiring referral for a swallow function study, often include behaviors such as those described in Table 12.2.

Published research regarding videofluoroscopic assessment of dysphagia in children with cerebral palsy is scarce, most likely because of the heterogeneity of problems that affect children in whom cerebral palsy is diagnosed. A few studies have been published on specific swallowing problems documented radiographically in children with cerebral palsy.[14–16] According to Griggs and associates,[16] 70% of children with cerebral palsy aspirated during a swallow function study, 60% of whom had silent aspiration. These statistics argue for performance of a videofluoroscopic swallow function study in any child with cerebral palsy whose medical history is suspect.

Rogers and colleagues[14] completed a retrospective review of clinical evaluations and swallow function studies performed in 90 children with cerebral palsy. These investigators found that all had abnormal oral and pharyngeal phases of swallowing, 97% of the children demonstrated a delayed initiation of the swallow reflex, and 58% had pharyngeal residue after the swallow. Of the 38% who aspirated during or after the swallow, 97% displayed silent aspiration. The consistency most commonly aspirated was that of liquids.

Mirrett's group,[15] using contrasted radiologic swallow studies, evaluated 22 children with severe spasticity. They found that 95.4% of the children had oral phase abnormalities, 90.1% demonstrated delayed initiation of the swallow reflex, 77.3% had pharyngeal residue after the swallowing event, and 77.3% demonstrated aspiration, which in 68.2% was silent. In addition, 68% had documented gastroesophageal reflux. Another interesting finding was that reduced pharyngeal clearance was the only statistically significant predictor of aspiration.

OTHER MEDICAL EVALUATION

A bronchoscopy may be indicated whenever aspiration cannot be demonstrated by a swallow function study in a patient who presents symptoms compatible with aspiration. The search for lipid-laden macrophages in bronchial washings[17] or chronic bronchial inflammation diagnosed by bronchoscopy may support the diagnosis of aspiration. Performance of direct visualization of the epiglottis by nasolaryngoscopy while the patient swallows a colored liquid usually is difficult in children with cerebral palsy because of their inability to comply with a visual examination. This test, however, may be helpful in detecting aspiration of small amounts of liquid.

Recurrent otitis media or hoarseness may also be secondary to the misdirection of liquids while swallowing. In this case, consultation with an otorhinolaryngologist may help in establishing the diagnosis. Patients who are reported to have experienced a change in behavior, such as onset of excessive crying, irritability, refusal to eat, interruption of feedings before the meal is completed, or waking in the middle of the night, may have esophagitis secondary to gastroesophageal reflux. Empiric treatment with an antacid, an H_2 blocker, and anti–gastroesopheal reflux medication such as cisapride or a similarly acting drug can be attempted as a noninvasive way to support the diagnosis of esophagitis. If treatment fails, referral to a gastroenterologist for possible endoscopy is warranted. Studies that may be indicated include upper endoscopy, 24-hour esophageal pH monitoring, esophageal manometry, and determination of upper esophageal sphincter pressure and function.

INTERVENTION

Several types of intervention might be necessary for a patient with cerebral palsy who is affected with feeding problems. Such interventions are related to posture, tone, suck, gastroesophageal reflux, nutritional status, psychosocial status, and other medical problems.

Nonmedical Intervention

The feeding specialist's plan of intervention may include manipulation of posture and positioning to elicit more normal tonal patterns, provision of oral exercises to improve oral motor skills, prescription of adaptive aids as compensatory measures, and education of others regarding developmentally appropriate eating behaviors and patterns. Throughout the process, the feeding specialist works with the child and family as part of the team. Occupational therapists employ techniques such as neurodevelopmental therapy, positioning, sensory integration, and joint mobilization to normalize muscle tone as much as possible.

Recommendations should take into account evaluation of the child's eating environment. An optimal environment includes appropriate physical and emotional support for the child. The physical environment, such as appropriate seating and eating surfaces, is equally important when working toward normal muscle tone. Guidelines for positioning a child for feeding include the following: (1) upright position with alignment of the head and neck neutral to the trunk; (2) no rotation in the trunk; (3) symmetric shoulders; (4) arms at the child's sides with elbows flexed; (5) thighs fully supported by the seated surface and knees flexed; and (6) feet in contact with a solid surface. The child may need external support to achieve this position. Positioning aids such as a wheelchair seating system, rolled cushions, or custom seats may be used. In some cases, deviations from these guidelines are necessary to achieve a more optimal feeding position. These circumstances will depend on the child's structural anatomy; for example, the child with a fixed scoliosis might require special seating to accommodate the trunk. Sometimes adaptations to the physical environment and specialized equipment such as built-up eating utensils or a plate guard may be all that are necessary to allow the child independence in gaining eating skills.

Feeding a child with cerebral palsy can become a difficult and time-consuming process, and it may overwhelm parents. The child may provide few cues as to hunger or fulfillment and, consequently, may not be provided with an appropriate amount of food.[18] The feeding specialist can teach cues of satiety, information on more efficient methods of feeding, and optional positioning of the child. Specific intervention with the caregiver may be necessary and could include relaxation techniques, time management, or arranging respite for the caregiver.

Medical and Surgical Intervention

Patients with suspected or proved gastroesophageal reflux may undergo a therapeutic trial with a combination of drugs (antacids; mucosal surface protectors such as sucralfate, prokinetics, or medications to increase the tone of the lower esophageal sphincter; and H_2 or acid pump inhibitors). When medical therapy to treat gastroesophageal reflux fails, a fundoplication is warranted. Parents should be told that recurrent pneumonia, bronchitis, or reactive airway disease due to aspiration of secretions will not necessarily be resolved by fundoplication but, at best, will be improved by diminishing the gastroesophageal reflux component.

In patients with poor nutritional status whose energy needs are unlikely to be met by mouth, a gastrostomy should be recommended. Because many parents are reluctant to accept a gastrostomy, the benefits must be clearly explained to the family while their wishes are continually borne in mind. Even in those children with cerebral palsy who are fed successfully by mouth at the expense of the almost full-time dedication of the caregiver (usually the mother), a gastrostomy may shorten the feeding time. This will allow more time for caregivers to attend to their other children in the family and to themselves and will diminish the stress imposed by the difficult task of successfully feeding the patient.

Dietary Intervention

Energy needs and losses in a child with cerebral palsy can vary depending on the severity and type of disability.[19,20] Children with severe hypertonia and athetoid movements can expend energy far in excess of perceived needs and current intake.[21] In children with spastic cerebral palsy, energy needs can be far lower than the recommended dietary allowances, leading to a risk for obesity.[21] Poor feeding skills can increase energy needs and losses in any child with cerebral palsy.

After energy needs have been assessed in a patient, a feeding plan can be implemented. A patient may need only an addition of high-calorie foods to his or her diet or a change in food textures and consistencies (e.g., switching from a solid to a thick or thin puree) to increase energy intake.

Many children with cerebral palsy need supplemental or full feedings via nasogastric, gastrostomy, or jejunostomy tubes.[10,22] These feedings may have to be adjusted depending on formula tolerance and weight gain. Nasogastric feedings, which should be used for a limited time only, may be indicated in the newborn period; prolonged use may lead to aversive oral behaviors. Definition of the term *prolonged*, however, is difficult, though it could be considered to mean more than 8–10 weeks. Nasogastric feedings might be indicated to provide additional calories for "catch-up" in a patient who is recovering from another illness or surgery but who is expected to return to a basal level of intake, or who has a respiratory illness and is transiently unable to take enough volume by mouth. Nasogastric feedings could also be used to determine whether a patient can handle appropriate amounts of bolus feeds and, by extension, to determine whether a fundoplication will be necessary or whether a gastrostomy (percutaneous or surgical) will suffice.

The decision to perform a fundoplication is not always easy, but it is even more complex in a patient with cerebral palsy. Many of these patients swallow abundant air and, after the fundoplication, may be unable to burp the air out, become bloated, and remain uncomfortable. In addition, patients with cerebral palsy have a higher tendency than do neurologically normal patients to develop postprandial retching, a difficult problem that exasperates many parents. Follow-up to assess weight gain and growth in these children is a very important aspect of care.

Psychosocial Intervention

Disruption of the usual family dynamics caused by a child with a severe medical condition may result in a wide range of psychosocial and financial problems. In our experience, feeding problems are the source of parents' feelings of poor parenting and inadequacy. In many cases, feeding by mouth is the only skill that children with cerebral palsy will demonstrate, and parents will insist in feeding by mouth despite the lengthy, unrewarding feeding sessions and recurrent episodes of aspiration pneumonia. At times, management of this situation can become difficult, particularly if school personnel refuse to administer oral feedings to a child with cerebral palsy because of the risk of aspiration while the parents insist that at home the child handles oral feedings well.

Frustration and anger are not unusual in a family dealing with a child with a severe illness, particularly if the patient loses previously acquired skills such as eating. A psychotherapist may help in these situations. A social worker might assist by identifying and organizing the available community services to meet the individual needs of a patient.

In conclusion, it is important for children with cerebral palsy to have a feeding evaluation, because inadequate feeding skills, dysphagia, and excess feeding time can contribute significantly to poor weight gain and growth, parental exhaustion, and disruption of family life. Feeding evaluations are necessary to diagnose such conditions as gastroesophageal reflux, which can lead to inadequate weight gain and growth because of a child's refusal to eat. Parents need to be educated as to the nature of the problems, the potential solutions, and the likelihood of resolving the problems. In our experience, even minor improvements in feeding are received with gratitude by the caregivers of children with cerebral palsy.

REFERENCES

1. Arvedson JC. Management of Swallowing Problems. In JC Arvedson, L Brodsky (eds), Pediatric Swallowing and Feeding; Assessment and Management. San Diego: Singular Publishing Group, 1993;364–365.
2. Mueller H. Feeding. In NR Finnie (ed), Handling the Young Cerebral Palsied Child at Home. New York: Dutton, 1975;119–121.
3. Krick J, Murphy PE, Markham JFB, et al. A proposed formula for calculating energy needs of children with cerebral palsy. Dev Med Child Neurol 1992;34:481–487.
4. Belt B, Ekvall S, Cook C, et al. Linear growth measurement: a comparison of single arm-length and arm span. Dev Med Child Neurol 1986;28:319–324.
5. Spender QW, Cronk CE, Charney EB, et al. Assessment of linear growth of children with cerebral palsy: use of alternative measures for height or length. Dev Med Child Neurol 1989;31:206.
6. Cully WJ, Middleton TO. Caloric requirements of mentally retarded children with and without motor dysfunction. J Pediatr 1969;75:380.
7. Admunson JA, Sherbondy A, Van Dyke DC, et al. Early identification and treatment necessary to prevent malnutrition in children and adolescents with severe disabilities. J Am Diet Assoc 1994;94:880–883.
8. Krick J, Murphy-Miller P, Zeger S, et al. Pattern of growth in children with cerebral palsy. J Am Diet Assoc 1996;96:680–685.
9. Feucht S. Assessment of growth. Nutr Focus 1989;4:1–8.
10. Isaacs JS, Georgeson KE, Cloud HH, Woodall N. Weight gain and triceps skinfolds fat mass after gastrostomy placement in children with developmental disabilities. J Am Diet Assoc 1994;94:849–854.

11. Pemberton CM, Moxness KE, German MJ, et al. Developmental Disability. In Mayo Clinic Diet Manual (6th ed). Toronto: BC Decker, 1988;320.

12. American Speech, Language, and Hearing Association. Instrumental diagnostic procedures for swallowing. Draft for peer review. ASHA 1991;33:67–73.

13. Logeman JA. Appendix B: Videofluorographic Worksheet. In Manual for the Videofluorographic Study of Swallowing. Austin, TX: PRO-ED, 1993;157–162.

14. Rogers B, Arvedson J, Buck G, et al. Characteristics of dysphagia in children with cerebral palsy. Dysphagia 1994;9:69–73.

15. Mirrett PL, Riski JE, Glascot J, et al. Videofluoroscopic assessment of dysphagia in children with severe cerebral palsy. Dysphagia 1994;9:174–179.

16. Griggs CA, Jones PM, Lee RE. Videofluoroscopic investigation of feeding disorders in children with multiple handicaps. Dev Med Child Neurol 1989;31:303–308.

17. Nussbaum E, Maggi JC, Mathis R, Galant S. Association of lipid-laden alveolar macrophages and gastroesophageal reflux in children. J Pediatr 1987;110:190–194.

18. Krieger I. Nutrition and the Central Nervous System: Paediatric Disorders of Feeding, Nutrition, and Metabolism. New York: Wiley, 1982;156–157.

19. Azcue MP, Zello GA, Levy LD, Pencharz PB. Energy expenditure and body composition in children with spastic quadriplegic cerebral palsy. J Pediatr 1996;129:870–876.

20. Stallings VA, Zemel BS, Davies JC, et al. Energy expenditure of children and adolescents with severe disabilities: a cerebral palsy model. Am J Clin Nutr 1996;64:627–634.

21. Bandini L, Patterson B, Ekvall SW. Cerebral Palsy. In SW Ekvall (ed), Pediatric Nutrition in Chronic Disease and Developmental Disorders. New York: Oxford University Press, 1993;165–172.

22. Lifschitz CH. Enteral feeding in children. Ann Nestle 1988;46(2):73–81.

13

Neurorehabilitation for the Child with Cerebral Palsy

Barry S. Russman and Mark Romness

The term *cerebral palsy* refers to a motor dysfunction that exists secondary to a central nervous system abnormality.[1] The central nervous system abnormality is static. The diagnosis is established by a history of motor "delay" and confirmation that the patient is not losing function. The neurologic examination establishes that the deficit is secondary to a central nervous system abnormality and not due to a problem in the motor unit. Attempts should be made to establish an etiology. Such associated problems as learning disabilities and epilepsy should be identified. A rehabilitation program that is optimistic but at the same time realistic can now be developed. In fact, the use of the term *cerebral palsy* suggests that a rehabilitation program will be of benefit to the patient and family. The rehabilitation program is developed by a team of knowledgeable specialists including a pediatric neurologist, orthopedist, physical therapist, occupational therapist, speech therapist, clinical nurse specialist, a pediatric neurosurgeon, and a physiatrist.

Many caveats must be considered as the neurorehabilitation program is being developed. First, muscle tone will change over time. Dystonia or spasticity commonly develops in the hypotonic child during the early first decade of life. Further, athetosis or chorea may develop during the same period. These changes should not suggest a degenerative disease unless the patient loses function.

Second, if there is function loss, one must ensure that this loss is related to changing muscle tone or contracture development and not to a loss of skills secondary to a degenerative process. For example, progressive ataxia might suggest Louis-Barr syndrome, or Freidreich ataxia. Increasing spasticity with a loss of function might suggest progressive lateral sclerosis.

A third caveat holds that nonambulation might develop in patients who are only marginally ambulatory, presumably related to an increase in body mass.

Fourth, contractures will develop in patients with cerebral palsy because of abnormal tone and growth. This is an especially important issue in the spastic patient; contractures do not commonly develop in the patient with dystonia, as patients with the latter problem, especially when in the supine position, remain hypotonic.

The fifth and final caveat states that the neurorehabilitation program will change over time. During the first 2 years of life, emphasis is on an infant stimulation program that stresses more than just improving motor deficits. Educating the parents about cerebral palsy, showing how positioning can be an effective way of helping the child be mobile, encouraging parent-child interaction, and demonstrating muscle stretching are aspects of an infant stimulation program. Also during this period, cognitive impairments will be identified and appropriate referrals made.

At ages 2–5 years, rapid growth occurs in the patient, and muscle tone will develop or worsen, not only leading to the development of contracture but also resulting in a decrease in mobility. As one develops a program to control this muscle tone, the most important question to be answered is: Can I improve the patient's function and decrease the patient's disability by altering muscle tone? Not uncommonly, what actually is preventing the patient from performing certain functions is lack of motor control or lack of sensation and not abnormal muscle tone.[2]

Between 5 and 10 years of age, the child begins to approach his or her adult height. At this time, definitive orthopedic intervention can be considered; as already noted, contracture development occurs as a result of abnormal muscle tone in combination with growth.

As the child approaches the teen years, issues of sitting and hygiene care are important considerations, especially in the nonambulatory patient. Problems of pain secondary to spasticity or dystonia must be addressed. Finally, altering the patient's tone and position might allow the patient to function more readily.

TYPES OF INTERVENTION

Most treatment programs for patients with cerebral palsy are based on experience rather than on data-based research. Within the last 10 years, efforts to correct this glaring deficiency have been made. Outcome scales that can be used for research as well as for clinical care have been developed, validated, and shown to be reliable. Over time, use of these outcome scales should lead to the development of critical pathways for patient care on the basis of data.[3]

The traditional interventions used to treat cerebral palsy include physical therapy (PT), orthoses, and orthopedic surgery. Muscle tone management, by way of selective dorsal rhizotomy, botulinum toxin (BTX) injections, and intrathecal administration of baclofen, has dramatically altered the traditional approach to the management of cerebral palsy. Using the paradigm of Goldberg,[4] outcome of such interventions can be assessed as follows:

1. Has there been a technical success? For example, if botulinum toxin was injected into the gastrocnemius muscle, was there improvement in the range of motion of the ankle joint?
2. Was there an improvement in function? For example, did the patient fall less frequently, and was there an increase in endurance?
3. Was the patient, parent, or caregiver satisfied with the outcome?

4. Was the cost of the intervention reasonable? The answer to this question usually necessitates an answer to a second question: What is the cost of an alternative therapy program or the cost to the patient and family if no therapy was rendered?

Physical Therapy

The primary goals of a PT program are to minimize the impairment, reduce the disability, and optimize function.[5] A review of the very early intervention programs is provided by Weiss and Betts.[6] Early programs emphasized passive range-of-motion exercises and use of braces to prevent contractures and to inhibit abnormal muscle function, a program developed by Phelps. It was expected that once these objectives were met, the normal muscles would provide the necessary functions for the child to attain his or her milestones. In the 1940s, Deaver promoted a program that emphasized functional abilities rather than movement patterns. Extensive bracing was used to prevent abnormal motor movements from interfering with function. At nearly the same time, Fay developed the prototype of what became known as the *Doman-Delacato* or *patterning program*. Other therapeutic approaches in vogue at that time included provision of a sensory input (including stroking, icing, and heat) to promote a motor output, a program developed by Rood. In the late 1950s, the Bobaths[7] developed the neurodevelopmental treatment program. The methods employed in this program attempt to inhibit abnormal infantile reflexes such as the tonic neck and Moro reflex and to promote (i.e., facilitate) more normal movement patterns such as the righting reflex.

Published studies suggest that, for some patients, certain therapeutic programs may make a difference in the patient's outcome. In a 1962 retrospective review, Paine[8] noted that individuals receiving intensive PT had fewer contractures compared with those who did not follow a therapeutic program but that both treated and untreated patients required a similar number of surgical procedures. Wright and Nicholson[9] reported that treatment programs did not affect range of motion or influence the retention or loss of developmental reflexes. On the other hand, some possible benefit was found for those children who had quadriparesis in the first year of life. Scherzer and colleagues[10] found a strong trend toward improvement in motor status and social motivation after treatment among those children with cerebral palsy who had a normal IQ, as compared with findings in a control group.

Many studies of therapeutic programs, on the other hand, have reached negative conclusions regarding the beneficial effect of such programs on the eventual motor outcome of the patient.[11] However, in reviewing the benefits of any program, more than the motor outcome must be considered. The psychological impact of rearing a disabled child can be devastating. This subject has been the focus of several studies. Breslau and associates,[12] in a study addressing the issue of psychological stress in mothers whose children are disabled, concluded that the specific diagnosis did not cause as much stress as expected among mothers; however, the dependency of the disabled child on the mother in helping him or her accomplish activities of daily living was significantly correlated with maternal stress. A therapeutic program might be extremely helpful in these cases, not necessarily to stimulate development but rather to offer parents easier ways to work with their child.

Selective Dorsal Rhizotomy

Selective dorsal rhizotomy (SDR) involves the cutting of approximately 50% of the dorsal roots, thus decreasing the muscle tone in the lower extremities. The theory is that as a result of the decrease in the muscle tone, discomfort or pain will be alleviated and sitting posture or gait will improve. The ideal candidate is a child who has normal or near-normal strength in the lower extremities and who has not developed fixed contractures so that the alteration of tone will lead to the desired improvements in function.[13]

Several studies during the late 1990s have begun to validate this type of intervention. A randomized clinical trial comparing SDR to intensive PT found a definite decrease in muscle tone 1 year later in those patients who received the operation as compared to the PT group.[14] Further, the surgical group showed significant improvement in motor skills as measured by a gross motor function measure scale.[15] Whether there was a major clinical improvement in the patients was unclear from the article.

In a second study, 178 patients who underwent SDR were analyzed retrospectively; the consideration was determining the percentage of these patients who would need orthopedic intervention.[16] Thirty-eight percent of the 178 patients had at least one orthopedic intervention before or after SDR. If the rhizotomy was performed before age 4, only 22% required orthopedic intervention, whereas if the procedure was performed after that age, the percentage requiring intervention climbed to 45%. Unfortunately, as the authors discussed, historical control data for the rate of orthopedic surgery in children with spastic cerebral palsy is not readily available.[16] Nevertheless, they cite two studies, one that revealed that 61% of children have undergone orthopedic intervention by age 8 years and a second that reported that 20% of children who underwent orthopedic surgery and who were younger than 5 years required repeat operative intervention.[17,18] The authors concluded that early SDR possibly could prevent the need to undergo orthopedic intervention.

The short-term complications of SDR are infection and excessive weakness, which can adversely affect function. The long-term complications of SDR are just beginning to be appreciated. Spondylolisthesis and spondylolysis as well as severe lumbar lordosis have been reported.[19,20]

Botulinum Toxin

BTX is a medication that inhibits the release of acetylcholine from the presynaptic site at the muscle nerve junction. Injecting BTX into a specific muscle leads to a weakening of that muscle. A combination of muscle weakening and strengthening of the agonist muscle will minimize or prevent contracture development with bone growth. This type of intervention is used when a limited number of muscles are causing deformities—for example, if the gastrocnemius muscle is causing a toe-heel gait or hamstring contracture is responsible for a crouch gait. Recovery of the muscle tone occurs because of the sprouting of the nerve terminals, a process that peaks at approximately 60 days.[21] Uncontrolled studies have shown efficacy of BTX therapy when the agent is used appropriately.[22,23]

This type of intervention may also be used for upper-extremity deformity secondary to abnormal muscle tone and bone growth. A common presentation of upper-extremity deformity is of shoulder adduction and internal rotation, elbow flexion, forearm pronation, and wrist and finger flexion as well as thumb adduction and flexion. Using a randomized, double-blind approach, Corry and colleagues[24] studied 14 patients with upper-extremity deformities treated with BTX. The injections were most effective in correcting elbow flexion contracture and thumb adduction contracture. We have been impressed that injection of BTX into the elbow flexors, in addition to causing relaxation of the injected muscles, provides ease of underarm care because of a decrease in muscle tone of the shoulder adductors. Fine-motor function, not surprisingly, was not helped as BTX can alter only tone and not motor control.

Complications from BTX injections are almost nonexistent. The pain is minimal, usually lasting no more than 5 minutes. Efficacy is seen within 48–72 hours and may last 2–4 months. The number of months or years that treatment continues depends on the degree of abnormal muscle tone, the response of the patient, and the ability to achieve and then maintain the desired result.

Intrathecal Baclofen Infusion

Baclofen, a gamma-aminobutyric acid agonist, administered intrathecally via an implanted pump, has been helpful to patients whose increase in muscle tone is more generalized and is interfering with function. As baclofen does not cross the blood-brain barrier very effectively, large doses must be used to achieve success, as compared to administering baclofen intrathecally (ITB). Invariably, the patient on oral medication becomes lethargic.

Candidates for ITB can be divided into two groups. Group 1 consists of ambulatory patients whose gait is adversely affected by the muscle tone and who have some underlying muscle weakness.[25] Rhizotomy in these patients is contraindicated as the procedure invariably will result in muscle weakness, possibly causing an ambulatory patient to become nonambulatory. Group 2 consists of those patients whose generalized tone interferes with activities of daily living such as hygiene, transferring from a chair to a bed, or simply maintaining the body in a safe, upright position. One patient in our program is an example of spectacular success of ITB treatment. With minimal excitement, this patient would arch the back and extend the arms as he was being transported in his wheelchair and passing through doorways, inevitably resulting in bruising of his extremities. The use of ITB moderated the muscle tone enough so that this was no longer a problem.

The procedure of intrathecal baclofen administration initially was developed in the 1980s as a way of controlling severe muscle spasms in patients with spinal cord injury. Since the early 1990s, its use in the appropriately selected cerebral palsy patient has been shown to be efficacious. Furthermore, the pump and the catheters have been perfected so that breakage and malfunctioning of the equipment now is almost nonexistent.

Oral Medications

The use of oral medication in the treatment of abnormal tone has been disappointing. For spasticity, dantrolene, baclofen, and diazepam have been used. Tinizide, a new antispasmodic, has been shown to be useful in some patients with spinal cord injury and multiple sclerosis, but no studies are available concerning the use of this medication in treating cerebral palsy. Medications for the dyskinesias, including dystonia, athetosis, and hemiballismus, have been equally disappointing.[26]

Other Treament Modalities

Transcutaneous electrical stimulation, as advocated by Pape and associates,[27] consists of a low-level electric stimulus to the nonspastic antagonist muscles for prolonged periods while the patient sleeps. The theory is that this form of treatment will strengthen the stimulated muscles, which in turn will overcome the effect of the spastic muscles, thereby improving the patient's function. Unfortunately, research that supports the theoretical basis of this treatment is lacking. Most of the information regarding success of this type of intervention is anecdotal.

Two interesting ideas related to treatment of cerebral palsy have been raised in articles that pertain to PT programs. The first study addressed the issue of whether early intervention, before clinical evidence of cerebral palsy, might be of benefit.[28] Treatment was started on the basis of abnormal cranial ultrasonography. However, 30 months after the intervention was initiated, no difference between the patients who received early intervention and the control group were noted.

Another study has suggested that establishing goals for an intervention program and working with the patient and parents to achieve the functional outcome without emphasizing the methods might be more efficacious than using the traditional forms of therapy such as muscle stretching and a neurodevelopmental treatment program.[29] In fact, a short-term study using this approach did demonstrate efficacy. The authors concluded that the development of specific goals rather than merely providing therapy to increase movement should be considered in future studies.

APPLICATION OF INTERVENTIONS TO SPECIFIC PROBLEMS

PT is useful in all forms of cerebral palsy as both a treatment modality and as a way of monitoring the affected child's progress. Likewise, occupational and speech therapy are helpful when upper-extremity and speech function are impaired, respectively. The other modalities discussed earlier have been found to have specific areas of clinical relevance. The goal of all treatment modalities should be improved function and independence.

Diplegia

By definition, the lower extremities of the diplegic patient are more involved than are the upper extremities. These children typically walk later than does the normal child and have abnormal muscle tone in the lower extremities. Abnormal muscle tone may be noted in the upper extremities as well. However, much of the functional limitation in both the upper and lower extremities is related to a lack of motor control, which may give the patient the appearance of clumsiness and lack of dexterity.

The risk for contracture development is related to the amount of voluntary control, the amount of abnormal tone, and growth of the patient. Contractures may be static, as defined by limitations of range of motion on passive clinical examination, or contractures may be dynamic, wherein the limitation in range of motion is noted with activity such as walking. Contractures develop with growth, and patients are at highest risk for static contracture development during their rapid-growth years.

The role of PT in diplegia is to prevent contracture development through range-of-motion and strengthening exercises of opposing muscle groups. Isolated muscle control training in therapy also is useful for patients who do not exhibit good voluntary movement of selected muscle groups. Unfortunately, despite excellent compliance and diligence in such therapy, contractures may develop, presumably related to the degree of spasticity, although studies validating these observations are lacking.

Orthoses are useful during the early ambulatory stages to assist with stability, similar to the use of training wheels on a bicycle. Stability is obtained by preventing the equinus position of the foot and by providing structural support across the ankle. As the patient ages, orthoses may be used during the day to prevent dynamic equinus positioning and provide dorsiflexion assistance or may be used at night merely to prevent equinus contractures. An ankle-foot orthosis is the primary orthotic appliance used in cerebral palsy. Bracing above the knee rarely is indicated.

If the patient with diplegia has contractures that are limiting function or developing into true fixed contractures, then additional treatment modalities must be considered. The administration of BTX for dynamic gastrocnemius contractures has been found to be useful if the patient has an adequate range of ankle movement.[21,23] BTX can help prevent both the equinus positioning of the ankle and hyperextension of the knee in stance that is due to gastrocnemius overactivity. BTX may also be helpful for hamstring contractures if these are believed to be the main contributor to the crouch gait position. Further, BTX injections into the hip adductor muscles may limit "scissoring."

If fixed contractures are present, BTX has not been found to be effective unless combined with or following the use of stretching casts to correct the fixed contractures (according to personal experience). If the contractures cannot be improved with casting or BTX, then surgical intervention should be considered. All nonsurgical strategies should be tried if the patient is younger than approximately 6 years. Usually, nonoperative therapies are effective in children younger than 6 years, and the risk for recurrent contractures is higher for orthopedic procedures performed in patients in this age group.[30]

Before surgical intervention is attemped, a gait analysis is recommended.[31] This laboratory procedure affords the surgeon a more objective method of determining what types of operations would be of greatest benefit to the patient.

SDR should be considered for the patient with spastic diplegia who has lower-extremity spasticity but good underlying voluntary muscle strength. An important consideration is selection of the patient who has pure spasticity with no signs of rigidity and who does not use the spastic muscle activity for functional means. ITB has not been used extensively with spastic diplegia. However, it might be considered in the patient who has a mixed pattern of muscle tone or in a patient in whom it is not possible to define how much of his or her function is related to spastic muscle tone and how much is related to voluntary muscle strength. The advantage of baclofen is that the response may be titrated by adjusting the delivered dose.

Quadriplegia

All four extremities are more or less equally involved in quadriplegia. The abnormal muscle tone usually consists of a combination of spasticity and dystonia. In addition to the dystonia, other dyskinesias such as hemiballismus, chorea, athetosis, and tremor may be present. Most of these patients are nonambulatory or are ambulatory with functional limitations. The main long-term goal for patients with quadriplegia is communication. Ambulation is less important in these patients, although the ability to bear weight and to ambulate minimally does help function in the long term if it means less assistance is required from caregivers. Contractures develop with a quadriplegic's growth and must be monitored to prevent limitations in activities of daily living. Contractures also need to be addressed if they cause secondary problems such as hip dislocations or skin pressure areas.

Initially, intervention consists of an infant stimulation program, with the emphasis on positioning to compensate for the retained primitive reflexes as well as for muscle strengthening. Tone management becomes an issue commonly by age 3 or 4 years, as many of the patients are hypotonic before development of the abnormal tone. In addition to physical and occupational therapy, orthoses often are needed to prevent the development of fixed contractures. Daytime orthoses are designed to assist with activities, whereas the use of night-time orthoses is focused more on preventing development of contractures. Stretching casts may be used for more severe contractures in an attempt to prevent worsening of the contracture, which would necessitate surgical intervention. BTX may be useful if a specific muscle group is found to interfere with activities. As in the patient with diplegia, BTX is more effective if the contractures are dynamic in nature rather than static.

SDR usually is not appropriate for patients with quadriplegia, as it does not provide a substantial amount of tone reduction in the upper extremities. Rhizotomy may be considered if there is difficulty with perineal care because of severe adductor tone, or if severe contractures are leading to hip problems or lower-extremity positioning difficulties.

Medication delivered orally, in high enough doses to alter tone so that management can be enhanced, has been unsuccessful in our experience, because such side affects as lethargy are considerable. ITB has been very successful in the management of diffuse spastic and dystonic tone. Improved upper-extremity and lower-extremity function has been observed. In addition, caregivers find that daily activities are much easier as there is less resistance from the patient; a better sitting position and improved use of the upper extremities has been noted. Unfortunately, the current size of the pump used to administer ITB prevents use of this treatment method in the smaller patient (usually younger than 5 years) with severe muscle tone problems.

If the quadriplegic patient develops hip subluxation or dislocation despite tone management, then orthopedic surgery is necessary. Likewise, if the patient develops significant scoliosis secondary to the abnormal tone, spinal fusion may be indicated. This procedure leads to an improved sitting position, allowing use of the upper extremities for functional activities rather than for body support.

Hemiplegia

Patients with hemiplegia typically have significant upper-extremity involvement that limits two-handed activities. Owing to the limited function and abnormal tone of the affected limb, contractures tend to develop in the neglected extremity. An occupational therapist can help by teaching the patient to use the involved upper extremity in daily activities. Having received instruction in muscle control activities and range-of-motion exercises, the patient will find more use for the extremity.

Dynamic splints are often required for assistance in functional activities, and static resting splints are used to prevent the development of fixed contractures. These orthoses are often fabricated by the occupational therapist unless the increase in tone is such that the use of higher-strength plastics is required. These then are made by an orthotist.

If a specific muscle group is limiting function, then BTX may aid in controlling the tone in this one muscle group. BTX has been found to be useful for the biceps as well for wrist flexors and extensors. If the patient uses the upper extremity well yet has limitations in grasp due to poor wrist dorsiflexion, then a tendon transfer to assist in wrist flexion might be considered. Preoperative evaluation for this procedure requires careful assessment of finger and wrist mobility and control. Additional contractures may also have to be addressed surgically.

In the lower extremity, common problems are poor motor control about the knee, ankle, and foot. Patients so affected often develop contractures of the hamstrings and have dynamic contracture of the rectus femoris. Equinovarus deformity is common in the foot and ankle. Most often, the tone is more abnormal distally than proximally. Ankle-foot orthoses are useful to assist with dorsiflexion and to prevent equinovarus positioning of the foot. The ankle-foot orthosis also provides some control of the knee; as stated previously, bracing above the knee is rarely indicated in cerebral palsy. Casting may be necessary for fixed contracture about the foot and ankle, and BTX is useful for dynamic contractures. As in the patient with diplegia, surgical procedures should be considered if the deformities cannot be controlled by nonoperative means. The use of SDR and ITB has not been described in patients with hemiplegia.

One problem that is fairly unique to patients with hemiplegia is a leg length discrepancy, the involved leg being shorter. This condition is usually a combination of a true leg length discrepancy and a functional discrepancy due to the contractures in the extremity. The discrepancy should be treated only if the true leg length discrepancy is greater than 1 cm or if functional problems are associated with the discrepancy. That the involved leg is shorter is beneficial for clearance during gait, and so the goal should not be to equalize the leg lengths but to keep the involved extremity approximately 1 cm shorter than the other leg. Some of this discrepancy will be compensated by an orthosis. Rarely is surgical intervention necessary to equalize leg lengths; however, such therapy could be considered in the highly functional patient with a moderate discrepancy. Again, the goal would be to correct the involved leg length to just less than 1 cm shorter than the unaffected leg.

CONCLUSION

Neurorehabilitation programs for cerebral palsy should emphasize maximizing function within the recognized limits of the patient's deficits. Although this chapter has highlighted management of the patient's physical needs, communication and emotional issues must be addressed and incorporated into a comprehensive program. Maximizing the patient's physical abilities involves PT programs, appropriate use of orthoses, tone management, and surgical intervention. Our experience suggests that no one specialist has the broad perspective needed to meet all of a patient's needs. The team approach appears to be extremely effective.

REFERENCES

1. Nelson KB, Ellenberg JH. Epidemiology of cerebral palsy. Adv Neurol 1974;19: 421–435.
2. Landau WM. Spasticity: the fable of a neurological demon and the emperor's new therapy. Arch Neurol 1974;31:217–219.
3. Campbell SK. Quantifying the effects of interventions for movement disorders resulting from cerebral palsy. J Child Neurol 1996;11:S61–S70.
4. Goldberg MJ. Measuring outcomes in cerebral palsy. J Pediatr Orthop 1991; 11:682–685.
5. Barry MJ. Physical therapy interventions for patients with movement disorders due to cerebral palsy. J Child Neurol 1996;11:S51–S60.
6. Weiss H, Bettis HB. Methods of rehabilitation in children with neuromuscular disorders. Pediatr Clin North Am 1967;14:1009–1017.
7. Bobath B. The very early treatment of cerebral palsy. Dev Med Child Neurol 1996; 9:373–393.
8. Paine RS. On the treatment of cerebral palsy: the outcome of 177 patients, 74 totally untreated. Pediatrics 1962;29:605–616.
9. Wright T, Nicholson J. Physiotherapy for the spastic child: an evaluation. Dev Med Child Neurol 1973;15:146–163.
10. Scherzer AL, Mike V, Jolson J. Physical therapy as a determinant of change in the cerebral palsied infant. Pediatrics 1976;58:47–52.
11. Palmer FB, Shapiro BK, Wachtel RC. The effects of physical therapy on cerebral palsy. A controlled trial in infants with spastic diplegia. N Engl J Med 1988; 318:803–808.
12. Breslau N, Staruch KS, Mortimer EA. Psychological stress in mothers of disabled children. Am J Dis Child 1982;136:682–686.
13. Abbott R. Sensory rhizotomy for the treatment of childhood spasticity. J Child Neurol 1996;11:S36–S42.
14. Steinbock P, Reiner AM, Beauchamp R, et al. A randomized clinical trial to compare selective posterior rhizotomy plus physiotherapy with physiotherapy alone in children with spastic diplegic cerebral palsy. Dev Med Child Neurol 1997;39:178–184.
15. Russell D, Rosenbaum PL, Cadman D, et al. The gross motor function measure: a means to evaluate the effects of physical therapy. Dev Med Child Neurol 1989; 18:341–352.
16. Chicoine MR, Park TS, Vogler GP, Kaufman BA. Predictors of ability to walk after selective dorsal rhizotomy in children with cerebral palsy. Neurosurgery 1996;38: 711–714.
17. Norlin R, Tkaczuk H. One-session surgery for correction of lower extremity deformities in children with cerebral palsy. J Pediatr Orthop 1985;5:208–211.
18. Watt JM, Robertson CMT, Grace MGA. Early prognosis for ambulation of neonatal intensive care survivors with cerebral palsy. Dev Med Child Neurol 1989;31: 766–773.
19. Peter JC, Hoffman EB, Arens LJ. Spondylolysis and spondylolisthesis after five-level lumbosacral laminectomy for selective posterior rhizotomy in cerebral palsy. Childs Nerv Syst 1993;9:285–287.
20. Crawford K, Karol LA, Herring JA. Severe lumber lordosis after dorsal rhizotomy. J Pediatr Orthop 1996;16:336–339.
21. Cosgrove AP, Corry IS, Graham HK. Botulinum toxin in the management of the lower limb in cerebral palsy. Dev Med Child Neurol 1994;36:386–396.
22. Cosgrove AP, Graham HK. Botulinum toxin A prevents the development of contractures in the hereditary spastic mouse. Dev Med Child Neurol 1994;36:379–385.

23. Koman LA, Mooney JF III, Smith BP, et al. Management of spasticity in cerebral palsy with botulinum-A toxin: report of a preliminary, randomized, double-blind trial. J Pediatr Orthop 1994;14:299–303.

24. Corry IS, Cosgrove AP, Walsch EG, et al. Botulinum toxin A in the hemiplegic limb: a double-blind trial. Dev Med Child Neurol 1997;39:185–193.

25. Albright AL. Intrathecal baclofen in cerebral palsy movement disorders. J Child Neurol 1996;11:S29–S35.

26. Prazantelli MR. Oral pharmacology for the movement disorders of cerebral palsy. J Child Neurol 1996;11:S13–S22.

27. Pape KE, Kirsch SE, Galil A, et al. Neuromuscular approach to the motor deficits of cerebral palsy: a pilot study. J Pediatr Orthop 1993;13:628–633.

28. Weindling AM, Hallam P, Gregg J, et al. A randomized controlled trial of early physiotherapy for high-risk infants. Acta Paediatr 1996;85:1107–1111.

29. Bower E, McLellan DL, Arney J, Campbell MJ. A randomized controlled trail of different intensities of physiotherapy and different goal-setting procedures in 44 children with cerebral palsy. Dev Med Child Neurol 1996;38:226–237.

30. Bleck EE. Orthopedic Management in Cerebral Palsy. Oxford: MacKeith, 1987.

31. Gage JR. Gait Analysis in Cerebral Palsy. Oxford: MacKeith, 1991.

14

Role of Occupational Therapy, Physical Therapy, and Speech and Language Therapy in the Lives of Children with Cerebral Palsy

Linda Pax Lowes and Sharon M. Greis

Occupational therapists (OTs), physical therapists (PTs), and speech and language pathologists (SLPs) are integral members of an interactive health care team that can help optimize the potential of children with cerebral palsy. Collectively, therapists are concerned with the promotion of development, acquisition of functional skills, prevention or correction of deformity, and patient and family education. The early onset and chronic nature of cerebral palsy leads to a variety of interactions with the health care team at different stages in the child's life. Although most children with cerebral palsy will be involved with therapy at various intervals, the duration of service periods will vary with each child. The members of a child's health care team at any given time are determined by the needs of the child and can change over the course of the child's development. Throughout the changes, however, the child and family remain at the center of this interdisciplinary team.

REFERRAL TO THERAPY

Physicians generally are the first to provide information to a family after the diagnosis of cerebral palsy has been made and, therefore, they often have the opportunity to introduce a family to other members of the health care team. Cerebral palsy is known to be associated with developmental delay; therefore, an interdisciplinary evaluation that might include physical, occupational, and speech therapy is warranted as soon as possible after the diagnosis is made.[1] A child could also be referred directly to therapy if an expedient interdisciplinary evaluation is not possible. The most obvious reason for referral would be a motor or speech problem in a child or a family's difficulty in caring for a child. The therapist can provide parental instruction, direct treatment, or referral to a community agency, or can recommend adaptive equipment to facilitate care of a child. The therapist can be a resource for other agencies and individuals who can provide assistance, information, or support for a family.

An obvious delay is not the only reason for referral to a therapist. If a child is displaying atypical or unusual movement patterns, has reached a plateau in development, or is exhibiting behaviors such as inattentiveness or impulsivity not commensurate with chronologic age, referral is also indicated.[1] The therapist can provide information about a child's current level of development, activities to promote continued development, and interventions to prevent deformity. He or she can perform standardized developmental assessments to confirm whether a delay or atypical development is present or to alleviate concerns. This information can assist the family in making decisions about the needs of the child and also can serve as a baseline measurement of the child's abilities. If warranted, pediatric therapists are able to provide direct intervention through the use of play activities, to work with an infant toward maximizing abilities and preventing deformity. Referral to a therapist does not mean that a child will automatically be enrolled in a lengthy course of therapy. The therapist may provide information to the parents, develop a home program for the parents, or (in the United States) refer the child to a federally funded early-intervention program. The role of the therapist and the intensity of intervention will change as a child's needs change.

If the parent or physician believes that the child could benefit from therapy, the referral should be made as early as possible, as the current belief is that early intervention optimizes the beneficial effects of therapy.[2] Early referral allows the family to be instructed in practices that might prevent deformities, such as exercises to maintain range of motion or avoidance of practices that can contribute to decreased range of motion such as W sitting. Early referral also can permit the therapist and family to intervene to encourage the child in developing movements that promote function. For example, infants with cerebral palsy commonly prefer supine positioning because they find it difficult to lift the head in a prone position or to use the arms to push the body up. The parents, therefore, might avoid the prone position to keep the infant from complaining, unaware that for an infant with cerebral palsy, prone positioning is important to develop head control and upper-extremity strength as well as to decrease the natural hip flexion contracture with which full-term babies are born. Early referral to therapy can provide this information as well as techniques for positioning the infant in modified prone positions that the child can more easily tolerate but that also have the desired developmentally beneficial effects.

ROLE OF INDIVIDUAL DISCIPLINES

Although OTs, PTs, and SLPs work as part of an interdisciplinary team, each discipline has a specific area of expertise. Areas of specialized evaluation and treatment that might be addressed by therapists are identified in Table 14.1. Several areas, such as feeding, assistive technology, and adaptive equipment, appear under more than one therapeutic discipline as these often are optimally addressed by an

Table 14.1 Areas of Specialization for Occupational, Physical, and Speech-Language Therapists

Occupational Therapy	Physical Therapy	Speech-Language Pathology
Motor skills—concentration on fine-motor skills	Motor skills—concentration on gross-motor skills	Communication, language
Adaptive equipment		Augmentative communication equipment
Positioning and seating	Adaptive equipment	Sign language
Feeding	Positioning and seating	Feeding
Self-care, activities of daily living	Oromotor skills	Oromotor skills
Orthotics—generally upper extremity	Functional skills	Respiration
Sensory integration	Orthotics—generally lower extremity	Phonation
Augmentative communication	Sensory integration	Articulation
Range of motion	Pain management	Swallowing
Visuomotor perception	Gait analysis and training	Videofluoroscopy interpretation
	Balance	Sensory integration
	Fitness	
	Posture and biomechanical alignment	
	Range of motion	

interdisciplinary team. Different disciplines might approach each area from a different perspective or might share their approach to that area. Overlap occurs especially in some treatment areas in pediatric therapy (see Table 14.1).

Physical Therapists

In general, PTs work on the child's gross motor abilities such as rolling, crawling, standing, and walking. The PT has expertise in typical and atypical development and can perform standardized assessments to identify delay or aberration, to document progress, and to assist in planning. The PT also can evaluate posture and movement patterns and can develop treatment activities to promote efficient movements. In children with cerebral palsy, this is especially beneficial during gait.

The PT might be involved in computerized gait analysis or can use low-technology methods such as videography or footprint analysis to help to determine ways to optimize gait efficiency. This might include recommendations for exercises, orthotics, or ambulation aids.

In addition to motion analysis, cardiopulmonary efficiency and endurance and muscle strength can be evaluated and enhanced through individualized, age-appropriate, play-based exercise programs. Range-of-motion limitations can also limit the child's ability to move efficiently. Therapists are knowledgeable about techniques to increase range of motion, such as passive or active stretching and positioning or splinting equipment.

The PT can evaluate the child's sensory system to determine whether a primary sensory deficit is present or whether the child is having difficulty processing sensory information.

Function can be enhanced through the use of adaptive equipment to promote independence or through environmental modifications. PTs can assist the family with selection and fitting of adaptive equipment, including wheelchairs and other specialized seating systems, positioning aids such as a standing frame, and self-care aids such as bath chairs or lift devices. Ambulation aids such as walkers and lower-extremity orthotics can also benefit children with cerebral palsy. PTs can provide expertise in the appropriate selection of such aids and can fabricate many lower-extremity orthotics.

Environmental modifications might be necessary for older children with cerebral palsy who are more significantly physically challenged. PTs can assist with recommendations for transportation or architectural modifications in many environments such as the home, school, or playground. The recommended modifications can be as simple as installing grab bars in the bathroom or adding a ramp entrance, to more extensive changes such as assuring that space and height requirements are met so that individuals in a wheelchair can access and maneuver within the home.

Occupational Therapists

In an interdisciplinary team, some overlap or sharing of service delivery is possible because the different disciplines communicate with one another and have developed a collaborative relationship. Nonetheless, the primary focus of therapy will differ among disciplines. In general, OTs focus on fine-motor and perceptual skills, sensory processing, and self-care activities. The OT can also perform standardized developmental assessments and can evaluate movement patterns in an effort to develop strategies to promote efficiency. Hand skills necessary for school activities such as writing as well as those necessary for the child's performance of self-care activities such as dressing or feeding can be evaluated. The OT can then develop activities to address the physical limitations that are hindering a given function or can recommend adaptive equipment to simplify a task. The OT has extensive knowledge of adaptive equipment that can be used to simplify such self-care activities as feeding, grooming, and dressing. The OT can optimize the child's functional skills by selecting equipment that is most complementary to the child's abilities. Additionally, OTs can be a resource for wheelchair selection and fitting and have expertise in upper-extremity orthotic selection and fabrication. Upper-extremity orthotics can be used to position the hand optimally for function or can be used to increase or maintain range of motion.

The OT is also trained to evaluate the child's sensory system to determine whether a primary sensory deficit is present or whether a child has difficulty processing sensory information. *Sensory integration* refers to the ability to evaluate the relative importance of all sensory inputs acting on the body, on the basis of the child's current posture, previous movement experiences, and movement expectations.[3] A child with cerebral palsy may experience sensory integration dysfunction as a result of central nervous system damage, or sensory integration dysfunction might develop secondary to the limited sensory experiences that these children have as a result of their limited motor abilities.[2,3] This sensory integrative dysfunction can manifest in poor motor coordination. Sensory integrative therapy therefore is directed at facilitating the child's organization and processing of proprioceptive, tactile, and vestibular information to promote appropriate postural responses, awareness of the environment, and improved motor planning.[4]

Speech and Language Pathologists

The SLP is concerned primarily with diagnosis and treatment of oromotor function for feeding, speech production, language development, and communication. SLPs can work with a child on both verbal and augmentative communication to promote the optimal level of communication. Oromotor treatment can be directed toward vocalization through effective phonation, articulation and word formation, feeding, swallowing function, and control of drooling.

Forms of augmentative communication include sign language, simple communication boards that allow children to point to symbols to express desires, or computerized systems that allow more sophisticated nonverbal communication. The SLP also evaluates a nonverbal child's receptive language abilities and prerequisite motor skills, such as use of eye gaze and pointing ability, to determine the type of assistive technology that would be most appropriate. In most U.S. states, grant moneys are available for school-aged children who are candidates for a communication system. The use of assistive technology for communication in a nonverbal child also requires the input of an OT, to assess the child's motor skills for selection of the optimal computer interface device. A variety of interface devices are available and can be operated by hand motion, head movement, eye gaze, or breath control.

Assistive technology is an example of areas in which experts from all three disciplines—physical, occupational, and speech and language therapy—work together to enhance the child's functional use of a device. For optimal functional use of a device, the child requires proper wheelchair positioning, sufficient head and trunk control or support, the optimal interface tool to access the system, and the appropriate computerized equipment and language program for age-appropriate communication at home and at school.

Combined Therapies

Either OTs or SLPs generally perform the treatment of feeding and swallowing disorders. Each of these specialists is trained in the anatomy, pathology, and function of the oral mechanism and in the processes that affect feeding and swallowing. Feeding and swallowing disorders are a specialty area for which therapists might prepare themselves on the basis of interest and experience as well as local practice.

Poor growth and nutritional deficiency are associated with children with severe cerebral palsy.[5] Oromotor and swallowing dysfunction, as well as gastrointestinal problems, are the cause of difficult and lengthy mealtimes and result in inadequate caloric intake. These problems are handled most effectively by a multidisciplinary feeding team composed of parents, dietitians, medical specialists, psychologists, and social workers.[6,7] OTs and SLPs generally function as feeding therapists on these teams, providing intervention and performing videofluoroscopy of the swallow.

A PT might serve as part of the interdisciplinary team to select an appropriate supportive seating system so that the child has a stable base of support from which to hold his or her head steady and coordinate the chewing and swallowing mechanism. The PT might also work with the child on head and trunk control, to enable the child to chew his or her food more effectively. (As illustration of the importance of a stable base of support, imagine trying to perform a precision activity such as threading a needle. This task is accomplished much more easily if one is seated in a chair with elbows supported on a tabletop than if one is standing on one foot. The chair and tabletop provide a stable base of support from which the hands can be controlled. Standing on one foot provides less stability, and more effort is exerted to maintain balance, which distracts from the task of threading the needle.) A child with cerebral palsy can have poor head and trunk control and sitting balance. Putting the child in a stable supportive seating system enhances his or her ability to use the upper extremities to manipulate feeding utensils and to chew and swallow.

Even with a stable seating system, however, a child with cerebral palsy can experience difficulty with the fine-motor skill of self-feeding. The OT might be involved with feeding by working with a child's upper-extremity control. Finally, the SLP can be involved with the coordination of the chewing and swallowing of the food. A child who has had a delayed start at oral feeding owing to a complicated neonatal period or prolonged tube feeding might have developed a heightened sensitivity to oral stimulation.[8] Such a child may therefore reject food that is placed in the mouth. Therapists can develop a program to desensitize the child and promote oral feeding.

Feeding is just one example of how the multifactorial nature of cerebral palsy requires intervention from a team of health care professionals. Children who exhibit poor growth should be referred for a feeding evaluation, which will provide information to the physician and family for determining the cause of the problem, appropriate treatment strategies, and the possible need for supplemental feeding.

Despite the differences between therapy disciplines, the focus of therapy services over the course of the child's development is, foremost, the use of age-appropriate, play-based activities to enhance the child's development and functional skills, to remedy or prevent impairment, and to provide patient and family education. The specific area of intervention and the method for accomplishing it might vary as the child develops or might be specific to each discipline, but the overall goal remains constant.

THE DISABLING PROCESS

To understand the role of therapy, one must understand the disabling process associated with cerebral palsy. The National Center for Medical Rehabilitation and Research (NCMRR) has presented a five-level taxonomy of the disabling process that can be used to clarify levels of intervention.[9] The success of the individual is determined through a complex interaction of the five levels of the NCMRR taxonomy. Those levels are pathophysiology, impairment, functional limitations, disability, and societal limitation. The pathophysiology level deals with the cellular changes associated with cerebral palsy. For example, a child might present with ischemic changes to the brain white matter or basal ganglia. In the neonatal period, medical treatment often is directed at preventing or minimizing these pathophysiologic changes. Such changes in the brain are one way to describe or evaluate a child with cerebral palsy.

The second level in the NCMRR model, impairment, deals with manifestations of the pathophysiologic changes seen at the organ or tissue level. The child with ischemic brain damage might present with a variety of impairments, such as decreased range of motion, poor balance, or an articulation problem. Traditionally, the prevention or remediation of secondary impairments has been an important area of therapy evaluation and intervention. For example, a PT or OT might perform, or instruct the family in performing, range-of-motion exercises to increase or maintain optimal muscle length. Additionally, the therapist might educate the family about ways to minimize the risk of impairments, such as by avoiding contributory habits or postures such as W sitting to diminish the risk of contractures. The therapist also advises the family about when to seek additional medical attention for developing medical problems.[10] Evaluation of impairments can be used also to direct treatment. Although correlation between levels of impairment and functional abilities has been documented, simple remediation of impairments may be insufficient to maximize the child's abilities.[11,12]

Functional limitation is the next level in the taxonomy and can occur as a result of one or more impairments. Not all impairments result in a functional limitation, however. For example, a slight elbow contracture may not prevent the child from performing functional activities. As the impairment progresses, however, it may prevent self-dressing. The remediation of functional limitations is a critical area addressed by therapists who work with children with cerebral palsy, in efforts to maximize the child's abilities. Examples of functional limitations exhibited by a child with ischemic changes in the brain are the inability to walk fast enough to keep up with peers and the inability to dress independently. The functional limitation of inefficient walking could be caused by impairments such as poor force production or poor standing balance, whereas the inability to dress independently could be attributable to poor fine-motor control or to range-of-motion limitations. Oromotor functional limitations might include unintelligible speech or inefficient feeding.

If a functional limitation cannot be remedied or compensated for through the use of assistive devices, a disability results. Disabilities prevent children from fulfilling normal life roles, such as playing or attending school, and can affect the child's and the family's quality of life.[10] A functional limitation such as the inability to walk independently, if not remedied or compensated for, might lead to the child's inability to participate on a school sporting team. Likewise, the functional limitation of unintelligible speech might prevent the child with cerebral palsy from communicating with peers and therefore lead to limited socialization.

Societal limitations are the final level of the disabling taxonomy and include architectural barriers and discrimination based on prejudice or ignorance. If a child who uses a wheelchair for mobility cannot get to the classroom because it is located up a flight of stairs, a societal limitation is present. Another example of a societal limitation is a day-care policy that prohibits enrollment of a child who is not independent with toileting. Remedying societal limitations generally is out of the direct scope of therapy services but can be addressed through problem identification and community or political action.[10] The therapist can assist this process by evaluating the problem, serving as a resource for the community, and providing advocacy training to the family.

THERAPY EVALUATION AND TREATMENT MODELS

The domains of the NCMRR[9] disabling process model with which therapists are most likely to be involved are disability, functional limitation, and impairment. This framework is used to guide evaluation and treatment planning. To initiate an evaluation, the therapist directs the child or family member to explain why treatment is desired. This uncovers the disability that the child is experiencing. Children rarely identify an impairment, such as decreased range of motion, unless they are repeating something they have been told by another professional. Once the disabilities have been identified, the therapist assists the child and family in identifying strengths and weaknesses. The family's responses direct the focus of the evaluation. Such *family-centered intervention* empowers the child and family to direct therapy, thereby avoiding therapist biases. Finally, the family identifies its goals for therapy.

After the family determines the therapy goals, specialized evaluations may be performed to identify the functional limitations or impairments that might be preventing the child from functioning up to his or her maximum potential. The evaluation procedures also help to determine the feasibility of and requirements for attaining the family's goals. The results of the evaluation then are conveyed to family members to allow them to make decisions about the child's course of care. The therapist's role is to provide the results of the evaluation in an informative, unbiased, and nonjudgmental manner that will allow the family to make an educated decision.

If it is decided that the child should receive therapy services, decisions will have to be reached regarding possible focuses of intervention and settings in which the services will be provided.

Focuses of Intervention

Several types of intervention are used by therapists: promoting development, remedying impairments, and teaching compensations. The focus of therapy can be primarily one type of intervention or a combination of all three. For example, it is common for an SLP to teach a compensatory skill such as sign language while also working on verbal communication. This combination approach maximizes the child's overall communication repertoire while the child works toward verbal communication.[13]

Therapy that is directed at promoting development could include task-specific functional training as well as remediation of limiting impairment. For example, if the child's goal were independent ambulation, a PT might include range-of-motion and strengthening exercises as well as gait training in the treatment protocol. Promoting the child's development requires that the therapist analyze the functional activity and identify the essential components of the task. Therapy then can be directed at enabling the child to perform each of the necessary components or the task can be altered through the use of adaptive equipment. For example, the PT might also recommend a specific type of walker for the child to use.

Teaching compensations also might involve using adaptive equipment. If the family agrees that independent ambulation is not a practical form of mobility for the child, a compensation such as instruction in maneuvering a power wheelchair may be the focus of therapy. Teaching compensations does not negate the importance of impairment remediation, however. For example, increasing the child's range of motion might still be a focus to provide sufficient flexibility for optimal positioning in the wheelchair.

Intervention Settings

Service Delivery in a Medical Setting

Therapy services are provided in a variety of settings, depending on the age and physical condition of the child. The child with cerebral palsy will most likely first encounter a therapist in a hospital, rehabilitation center, or extended care facility. If the newborn is critically ill at birth and requires intervention in a neonatal intensive care unit (NICU), therapists should be consulted to evaluate the neonate. Therapists in the NICU can evaluate the neonate's response to the environment and minimize the traumatic effect of that environment, enabling the neonate to conserve energy and sleep more.[14] Adapting lighting, noise levels, intervention schedules, or positioning can reduce the physiologic stress to the infant, which in turn can decrease irritability and may improve oxygen saturation.[14]

Therapy intervention in the NICU also can aid in preventing secondary impairment and promoting function. For example, in addition to encouraging self-calming, proper positioning can prevent development of range-of-motion limitations and can maintain optimal muscle length for movement. As the neonate's medical condition allows, the therapist also can perform range-of-motion exercises, chest physical therapy, oromotor facilitation, and sensorimotor stimulation.[14] Sensorimotor stimulation is designed to encourage the child to maintain his or her behavioral state through self-calming activities (e.g., getting the hand to the mouth or swaddling) and to promote interaction such that parent-infant attachment is fostered. When the child becomes more medically stable, sensorimotor stimulation can also be used to promote motor development.[14]

Children with cerebral palsy who require medical intervention such as orthopedic surgery receive acute care and rehabilitation therapies in a hospital setting or outpatient clinic, to help restore function while the child heals and gains strength. Range-of-motion exercises, splinting, strengthening, ambulation training, and functional skill training are some of the interventions that may be provided. The child frequently receives several therapy sessions per day. Both postoperative therapy and neonatal therapy follow a medical model of service delivery and provide one-to-one intervention directed toward the specific medical needs of the child.

Developmental stimulation or functionally based therapy can also be provided through the medical model. The medical model of service delivery allows the parents and child input into the goals and intensity of the therapy services. This in contrast to educationally based therapy, in which the goals still are influenced by the parents and child but the goals must enhance the child's benefit from the academic curriculum. In the United States, this benefit of medical model therapy has been tempered by the increasing influence of third-party payers, because in the medical model, rehabilitation services generally are funded through private insurance, medical assistance programs, or private payment.

Service Delivery in an Educational Setting

Therapy services are available also to children with cerebral palsy who are not receiving medical or surgical care in a hospital. These services are provided in a more natural environment for the child, such as the home, preschool, community day-care facility, or school. In the United States, federal legislation and public laws now mandate that all children with special needs are entitled to free and appropriate public education. To enable students to access and benefit from public education, therapy services are frequently needed and therefore also are mandated as one of the related services that a school system must provide.

School Settings   On November 29, 1975, the Education for All Handicapped Children Act (PL 94-142)[15] was passed in the United States, which provided children between the ages of 5 and 21 years a free and appropriate public education. If an appropriate program is not available in a school district, then that school district must provide funding for an appropriate private school edu-

Table 14.2 Related Services Provided Through Federally Funded Education Programs for Children with Special Needs

Family training, counseling, and home visits
Special instruction
Speech pathology
Audiology
Occupational therapy
Physical therapy
Psychological services
Service coordination
Medical services for diagnosis or evaluation
Early identification, screening, and assessment services
Health services necessary to enable benefit from early intervention
Social work services
Assistive technology devices and services
Transportation services

cation. Children with cerebral palsy may enter regular education or special education classes with supportive therapy services. A psychological evaluation by the school district determines the eligibility for regular or special education. Occupational therapy, physical therapy, and speech therapy are all available to the child under the provision of related services, regardless of whether the child is placed in regular or special education. Additional related services are listed in Table 14.2. The levels of therapy services in the school district are determined on the basis of the educational relevance of the service, as opposed to having rehabilitative relevance. The therapy needs of a child must be directly related to that child's ability to benefit from school. For example, if a child with quadriplegia has a functional form of mobility, such as using a power wheelchair, and can move freely around the classroom, working on independent ambulation may not be educationally relevant, even though it may be medically beneficial to the child. If the parents and child would like to develop the child's ambulation skills, they may need to supplement the educationally based therapy with some additional therapy outside of the school. The child might continue to receive therapy in the school, but the goals would be related to the child's academic performance only. For example, the child might receive range-of-motion therapy to allow optimal seating in the wheelchair or transfer training to allow independent use of the restroom while at school.

Early Intervention Educational and therapeutic programming for children birth to 5 years of age who are exhibiting developmental delays is known as *early intervention* (EI). The Individuals with Disabilities Education Act (IDEA; PL 102-119),[16] which was reauthorized by the U.S. Congress in June 1997, provides funding to the states for programs to support and improve early intervention and special education for infants, toddlers, children, and youth with disabilities[17] (see

Table 14.2). Two separate programs are in place for children between the ages of birth and 5 years: the birth to 3-year program and the 3- to 5-year program. The distribution agency for the federal early-intervention funds generally is different for the two programs. The distribution agency for federal funds can vary between states but may be managed through a local mental health and mental retardation agency or through the department of education.

Reauthorization of IDEA emphasized serving infants and toddlers with disabilities in their natural environments, with a focus on the family. Individual states develop their own laws to implement IDEA, although the basic elements remain the same across states. Eligibility criteria for early intervention also vary among the states but can include a documented developmental delay, a diagnosis that predisposes the child to developmental delay, or informed clinical opinion. Many states use as their yardstick a 25% delay or a delay of one standard deviation below the mean in one or more of the developmental areas of physical development, cognitive development, communication, social or emotional development, or adaptive development (self-care).[18]

Cerebral palsy constitutes a diagnosis that predisposes a child to a developmental delay. Therefore, families should be informed about the availability of early intervention services and referred for an intake evaluation after the diagnosis has been made. A child who is suspected of having cerebral palsy may also be referred to early intervention before a formal diagnosis is made, using the informed clinical opinion provision. For example, findings of hypertonicity and atypical primitive reflexes in a premature infant might be used to refer a child. Health care professionals in the United States are encouraged to contact their state agencies to determine the eligibility requirements in their individual states.

The early intervention services that each child will receive depends on the individual needs of the child but might include special instruction, physical therapy, occupational therapy, and speech therapy (see Table 14.2).[19] In the birth to 3-year age group, these services frequently are provided in the home. Once again, the services that the infant will receive are based on the family's identified need and developmental area of greatest concern. For example, if a child of 2 years is unable to communicate verbally and cannot sit up, physical and speech therapy may be identified by the team as the most appropriate services. These services are identified in the development of an Individualized Family Service Plan (IFSP), which is the foundation of family-centered early intervention services.[19] The IFSP is a written agreement between the parents and the early intervention team that documents the child's current level of abilities, the family's needs and goals for the child, the service delivery plan and timeline to meet the needs and goals, and a means for evaluating the child's progress.[18]

The early intervention setting for children 3–5 years of age may be a center-based program (a preschool for children with special needs), or services such as therapy or special instruction can be provided at a community-based preschool or day-care facility or in the child's home. In the United States, federal law mandates that services be provided in the least restrictive environment available to the child,[16] which is defined as the environment that allows a child the most access to interactions with typically developing peers and opportunities similar to those of the child's peers while still meeting the unique needs of the child with cerebral palsy. Special services, such as therapy or special instruction, are provided to improve the child's level of function while playing and learning with typically developing peers in the least restrictive environment. The severity of a child's impairment would influence the type of setting that might be most appropriate for meeting developmental needs. For example, a child with age-appropriate cognition who is ambulatory with the aid of a walker might function more actively in a community day-care center than would a child with severe cognitive limitations and no form of independent mobility. The Americans with Disabilities Act of 1990 (ADA; PL 101-336),[20] however, mandates that most children with special needs have access to the preschool setting of their choice, regardless of severity of the disability.

The type and amount of service that a toddler receives, regardless of the setting, are identified on an Individual Education Plan (IEP). The IEP document is similar to an IFSP in that it is an agreement between the family and the early intervention team that lists the child's current level of performance, the family's goals for the child, the service delivery plan to meet those goals, and a plan for re-evaluation.

In the United States, services to children in the educational environment are funded through federal law. As funding expires, Congress must reauthorize moneys to continue these crucial services to children. Health care providers are encouraged to stay abreast of reauthorization timelines and political trends to ensure that funding in not decreased or eliminated. If health care professionals continue to contact their local politicians and continue to help families to advocate for themselves, children with cerebral palsy will continue to benefit from the worthwhile services provided in the educational setting.

REFERENCES

1. Hock-Long L. Guidelines for Referral. In LA Kutz, PW Dowrick, SE Levy, ML Batshaw (eds), Handbook of Developmental Disabilities: Resources for Interdisciplinary Care. Gaithersburg, MD: Aspen, 1996;27–28.
2. Foltz LC, DeGangi G, Lewis D. Physical Therapy, Occupational Therapy and Speech and Language Therapy. In E Geralis (ed), Children with Cerebral Palsy. Kensington, MD: Woodbine House, 1991;209–260.
3. Bradley NS. Motor Control: Developmental Aspects of Motor Control in Skill Acquisition. In SK Campbell (ed), Physical Therapy for Children. Philadelphia: Saunders, 1994;787–822.
4. Olney SJ, Wright MJ. Cerebral Palsy. In SK Campbell (ed), Physical Therapy for Children. Philadelphia: Saunders, 1994;489–524.
5. Patrick J, Boland M, Stoski D, Gordon M. Rapid correction of wasting in children with cerebral palsy. Dev Med Child Neurol 1986;28:734–739.
6. Arvedson J, Brodsky L (eds). Pediatric Swallowing and Feeding Assessment and Management. San Diego: Singular Publishing, 1993.
7. Wolf LS, Glass LP. Feeding and Swallowing Disorders in Infancy: Assessment and Management. Tucson, AZ: Therapy Skill Builders, 1992.
8. Palmer MM, Heyman MB. Assessment and treatment of sensory- versus motor-based feeding problems in very young children. Infants Young Children 1993;6:67–73.

9. National Institutes of Health. Research Plan for the National Center for Medical Rehabilitation Research (NIH Pub. No. 93-3509). Bethesda, MD: National Institutes of Health, 1993.

10. Palisano RJ, Campbell SK, Harris SR. Clinical Decision-Making in Pediatric Physical Therapy. In SK Campbell (ed), Physical Therapy for Children. Philadelphia: Saunders, 1994;183–204.

11. Butler PB, Thompson N, Major RE. Improvement in walking performance of children with cerebral palsy: preliminary results. Dev Med Child Neurol 1992;34:567–576.

12. Damiano DL, Kelly LE, Vaugh CL. Effects of quadriceps femoris muscle strengthening on crouch gait in children with spastic diplegia. Phys Ther 1995;75:658–667.

13. MacDonald JD, Gillette Y. Communicating with persons with severe handicaps: roles of parents and professionals. J Speech Hear Disord 1986;11:255–265.

14. Kahn-D'Angelo L. The Special Care Nursery. In SK Campbell (ed), Physical Therapy for Children. Philadelphia: Saunders, 1994;787–822.

15. Education of All Handicapped Children Act, Public Law 94-142, 89 Stat. 773-796, 1975.

16. Individuals with Disabilities Education Act, Public Law 102-119, 105 Stat. 587-608, 1991.

17. Aleman SR, Jones NL. Individuals with Disabilities Education Act reauthorization legislation: an overview. Congressional Research Service Report for US Congress, 1997;1–14.

18. Effgen SK. The Educational Environment. In SK Campbell (ed), Physical Therapy for Children. Philadelphia: Saunders, 1994;847–872.

19. Solomon R. Pediatricians and early intervention: everything you need to know but are too busy to ask. Infants Young Children 1986;7:38–51.

20. Americans with Disabilities Act, Public Law 101-336, 42nd Congress, Sec 12101, 1990.

Index

Note: Page numbers followed by f *indicate figures; page numbers followed by* t *indicate tables.*